Touch Me! I'm for Real

Jean Barrett Groves

PAGE PUBLISHING, INC.
New York, NY

First originally published by Page Publishing, Inc. 2019

ISBN 978-1-64462-937-6 (Paperback)
ISBN 978-1-64462-938-3 (Digital)

Printed in the United States of America

This book is dedicated to my dear husband and
sons. Thanks for your loving support.

Extend your hand,
Take mine,
See how I feel.
Hold me,
Taste me,
Touch my heart,
Know that I'm for real!

—Jean Barrett Groves

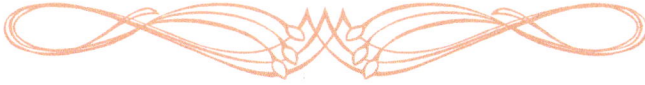

CONTENTS

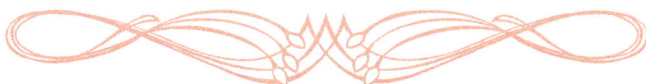

PROLOGUE

HAVE you ever asked yourself, "Who am I? Where did I come from? What gives my life worth?" Most people have. But questions like these are hard to answer when deep-seated issues mar the way we view ourselves.

My quest for positive identity began as a young girl born in poverty at a time when the doors of opportunity were barely screeching open. My parents came north in search of equality, after fleeing bias in the segregated South. Mom's goal was to buy a nice home in a neighborhood of her choice so we could grow up and "be somebody." They struggled to cross lines seemingly etched in granite that kept blacks locked in the urban ghettoes of the '50s. As we slowly inched our way out, she held tightly to her one valued possession—a rich heritage of faith left to her by my grandmother. But there was alcoholism in the family and marital problems that left scars on us as children. In those yearling years, I began looking for focus and direction but wound up at age twenty-one as a divorced welfare mother with a blighted future. Education and achievement, I was told, would allow me to rise above my station and bring respectability. So I pushed past hardships as a single parent and earned two degrees. Following graduation, I went into teaching, which added greatly to my esteem. Yet that sense of worth was tied mainly to my image as a college-educated black professional and performance as a working mother able to manage career and parenting responsibilities while going on with my studies. I was hard into competing, accumulating, and achieving. In so doing, I tried to be found worthy.

But my sense of personal value was immediately placed in jeopardy when I developed dual disabilities. Once I couldn't perform as I used to, away went the job title and income. My image cracked; I became obviously disabled and confined to a wheelchair. The things I'd placed my hopes in suddenly disappeared—things I used to define my *worth*. It was a painful climb back up to find acceptance, normalcy, and a new direction.

This book talks a lot about pain and how I translated it into purpose. Disability forced me to find new answers to those old questions. Finding oneself is often a lifelong process. Sometimes just when you think you know who you are, life slips in and gives you one of those one-two punches that knock you flat on your face for a while. This story tells how I got up after a fall. It talks about dealing with those challenges that seem so unfair, when dreams are shattered, work life is cut off, and you must face the horror of isolation and loneliness alone; about how to find hope amid the ruins of your life and rebuild; about the battle we all must inevitably fight to discover who we are, to sing the one song only we can sing, and finally to leave the stage, not with a standing ovation but with as much dignity as possible.

In today's society, image and performance seem to be everything, and there is little tolerance for failure. So many suffer feelings of inadequacy, since childhood (i.e., "I don't fit in," "I'm not good enough," or "I can't measure up) in relationships at home, at work, or in society. They harbor a sense of lack or brokenness, live in anger and vulnerability, and strive to hide their limitations. For some, these issues center around class or race. For others, being in a new season of life or at a crossroad has brought difficult challenges.

I hope to shed light on the lives of many who struggle to love and accept themselves because of feeling they somehow miss the mark. I drown out the negative tape that plays down on the inside, which always reminds me of my weaknesses, mess-ups, and imperfections by changing the things I look at, focus on, think about, listen to, and hang around also the people I allow to influence me. I now listen to the voice of my faith, and I'm working on deepening my knowledge base. Renewing one's thoughts brings a fresh attitude. I am no longer ashamed of who I am, how I look, where I am from, what I don't have, or what I can't do because I've discovered I am divinely designed just right for God's own purposes, and He alone holds my destiny. I believe any individual who has been made to feel less, for lack of things or inability to perform, can find worth in Christ.

This book offers a unique point of view. It doesn't discuss disability as a "condition" to try to escape from or reinforce a view of the disabled as superstars divinely compensated for our lack. Rather, it presents the visceral side of what it is like to live with it and shows that disability must be reconquered daily as you press on toward your dreams. It depicts the stages one passes through in the process of illness—from denial and anger, to acceptance, adjustment, acquisition of knowledge, and learning coping skills.

Touch Me! I'm for Real is also a story of pride written to inspire others. It presents my family, who descended from slaves. It is about denial of entry into society and the hang-ups we inevitably carry; about admiring unlikely people, not the rich and famous, but my poor black grandma, who lived in a shack; about looking back and being proud of from whence I've come. In the process of answering the question "Who am I?" it holds up a mirror for all to look deeply into themselves, open up, and disclose failures and vulnerabilities.

Despite vocal inability, writing has given me a voice and a greater sense of value. God touched me and helped me to put my thoughts on paper. I've turned my childhood love of stories into this spiritual journal to share with you. It is a dream come true, and I thank God for developing my text! I invite you to look past my tattered cover and read my life as a book. Enter my little sphere and see the world through my eyes. Let me give you my perceptions and truths. I hope it yields insight to someone who's walking where I've been. By unveiling my experience as a woman of color with physical limitations in a deeply personal way, I put you in touch with what it feels like to be me. Draw near for the sake of getting to know who I am. Let it penetrate your heart and bring understanding and sensitivity. One day when you reach one of life's inevitable transitions, you too will have to define who you are and what is meaningful and find how you can make a contribution that will change someone's world for the better. Don't discount yourself and focus on your lack or inadequacies. Don't be overcome by your inabilities and fears. Look past whatever negative thoughts have been governing your life. Give your needs to God and trust Him to turn things around. He has good things He wants to lead you into.

Atlanta, 2018
Jean Barrett Groves

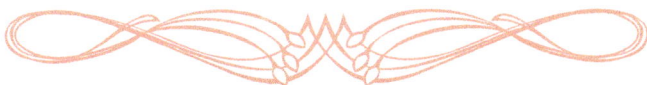

CHAPTER ONE
Beginnings

AN awe-inspiring atomic smasher exploded the year I was born, 1949.

But I was hardly one to make such a big to-do about (just a poor black girl born in the ghetto of New York City at a time when white society felt folks like us were good for nothing but cooking meals and cleaning stools, maybe a little singin' and dancin' on the side). Loretta Jean was my given name, second daughter of Andrew and Ernestine Farmer. My sister, Fay, arrived two years earlier, and my brother, Andre, three years later. Three would be the number of children born to my mother, unlike her mother who had seven.

Mom and Dad were Southerners who came with the wave of black immigrants from rural farm towns of the South to the northern cities during the war years in search of factory jobs and a better standard of living. Dad had been an army sergeant in World War II, serving in China, Burma, and India. He returned to the States in 1946 and married my mother on the advice of a fortune-teller, so he said. True or not, it was a story often retold—much to our delight—upon inquiring how they met. I suspect it may have been fanciful, conjured up to amuse, giving their relationship a mystical origin. As children, we loved to cuddle around, listening to wild tales of Dad's exploits overseas that led to the Indian woman in the tent who saw his bride in the trailing lines of his palm and told him her name. He returned, found her, and made her his bride. Of course, the details changed with each telling as he at times added and at other times took away to suit his fancy. We asked Mom to support his claim, but she would only swat the air and say "Get out of here!" with a knowing smile that went along with the game.

Dad's ability to laugh at life was his strength. A connoisseur of good times, he preferred the company of people, eating, dancing, and making merry so as not to succumb to life's problems. Mom, on the other hand, was hardworking and earnest like her name—Ernestine. The one who strived always to better our surroundings, she championed work and most of the responsibility for the household. While she struggled to accomplish set goals, Dad—content with whatever condition he found himself—survived no matter what, often with the help of a little drink. Certainly they were the descendants of a long line of survivors who had worked the cotton fields of the South, sunup and sundown, driven by strong faith that the Lord would see them through.

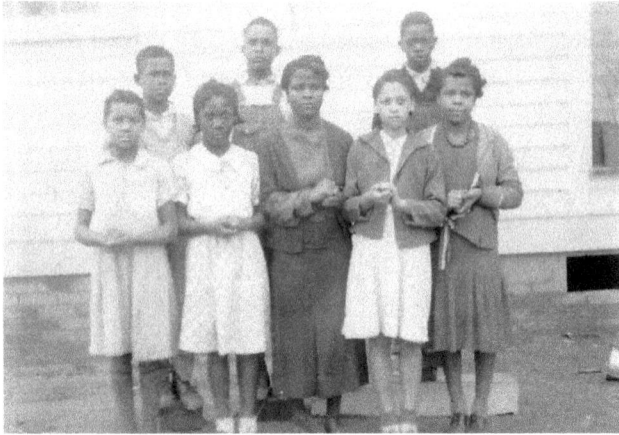

My mother, her classmates, and teacher back in The South in 1937.

My mom's parents, William and Fannie Rankin, were farm laborers and cotton pickers who sold vegetables on the roadsides of Greensboro, North Carolina, to support the family. Their eldest children picked and sold alongside forfeiting the opportunity to go to

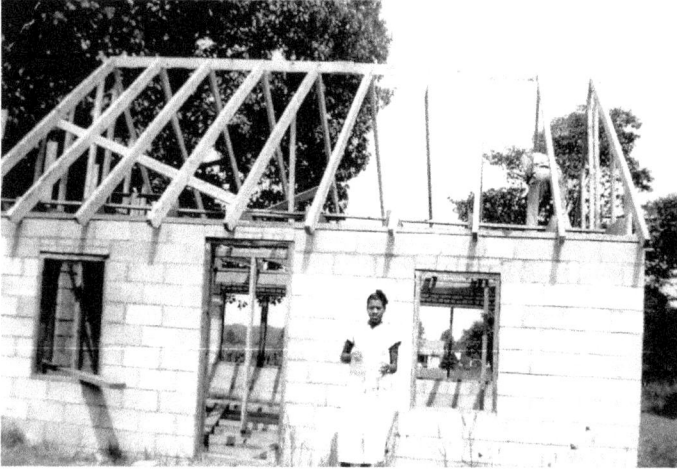

Mom and Dad's first home in the country built from scratch.

school. Mom, being near the youngest, was fortunate to attend and finish high school. Dad, not so lucky, left in eighth grade to pick fruit in the orange groves of Florida. When first married, they lived in a scant cabin at her family seat, in a community where as far as the eyes could see, the land had belonged to her family—first to Great-grandfather, then Grandfather down to the grandchildren as it passed from generation to generation in ever smaller divisions. Portions were sold to whites to get money to come north and start anew. This would be the only legacy left from the harsh years of slavery—this and their richly bronzed bodies sun baked to the color of clay fields from which they came. There would be little material wealth brought to the urban ghettoes. But theirs was a long tradition of struggle, surviving, and learning to love and laugh along the way. I was born into that tradition and learned to survive as they had, making it one day at a time. The environments differed—the streets of Harlem versus the back roads of the South. But the necessary armaments to wage war were the same: faith, hope, and love that binds in trouble times.

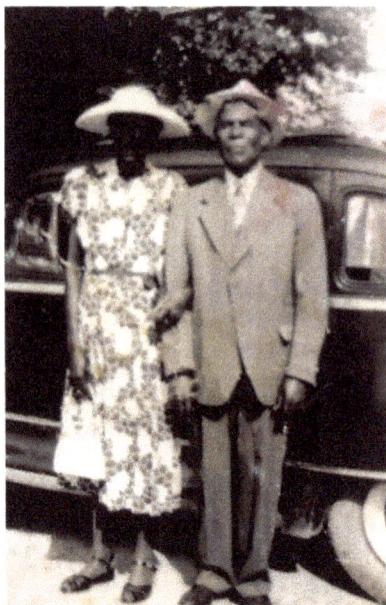

My grandmother, Fannie Rankin, and grandfather,
Will Rankin in front of their 1940s car.

This calls to mind a favorite photo of my grandparents, kept in Mom's album, which captured in monochrome and later shades of brown the essence of who they were. In the background stood an old wooden house built of loosely nailed boards weak with age, its ailing porch barely hiding the sun glinting through the rafters. Grandma and Grandpa stood together in the foreground, while to one side a shiny long black automobile had mowed the few sparse blades of grass in the otherwise barren yard. Grandma stood to the left wearing a pert Sunday hat, gloves, and floral dress that stopped below the knee and boots that seemed to come up to hide her frail legs. Grandpa, to the right, sported sagging work pants fastened with rubbery suspenders that accented his very protruded chest. A straw hat sat cocked back on his head, and a smile with missing teeth graced his face, high cheekbones showing the mixture of American Indian in his blood. It was a picture of pride! How their faces beamed up from the tinted page as they stood near the purchase of their lifetime—a 1940s car.

Daddy's origins were mixed with Indian too. In Jacksonville, Florida, the area where he grew up, blacks and Indians formed powerful alliances during the 1800s. This led to intermarriage between blacks and Seminole tribespeople. His roots can probably be traced back to such a liaison evinced by the strong features he had to show for it.

He was quite a good-looking man in his younger days. Solid and well built, he had a mane of black hair like waves on an oil slick. His skin, smooth and tan, appeared bathed in rich emollients, and never a blemish marred his face, except for a scar deeply engraved into his flesh, tracing a path from the side of his nose across the high ridge of his cheek, stopping below his wide sable eyes. It was a childhood keepsake, perhaps from boyhood mischief. A narrow mustache trimmed a broad even-toothed smile, and when he smiled, two gold-capped teeth bearing a crest of a moon and star shone brightly in front. Those heavenly imprints must have drawn Mom to this debonair sort of man.

He was a Billy Dee Williams type, but he lacked the polished speech of an actor, often searching for just the right way to put things. His voice had a slight hesitancy, yet it was firm and commanding, punctuated by large hands and arms, which he waved like a conductor's wand and dropped with force to emphasize important words. His face was strong and angular with a square jawline of the Dick Tracy kind. He wore a pinched-crown hat with a band and brim just like that. He had thin lips and eyes like oval discs that sat forward, staring. Though slightly forked, they looked at you honestly and with directness. He walked with a distinct strut that said he was "somebody." Friends called him Jack or Andy, but Mom called him Mr. Greenberg jokingly after the prominent Jewish men who owned the tenements in Harlem. Later she would change his nickname to Jelly Belly as his fine posture gave way to age.

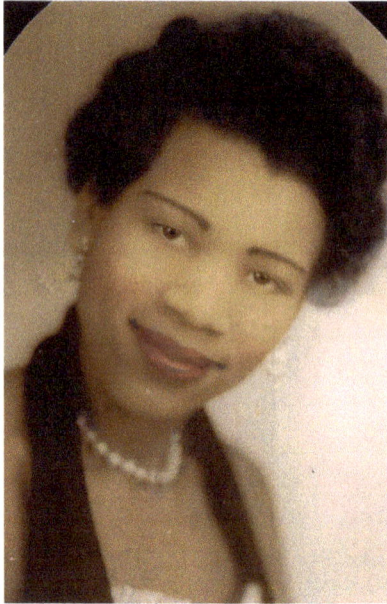

My mother, Mrs. Ernestine Farmer.

Mom was attractive too, but she didn't think so. She had short hair and wished it were longer like "pretty women," whose hair flowed to their shoulders and who had big legs. These were the women she thought caught men's eyes and held their attention. But, I am sure, in the eyes of the world, her beauty shone like a precious jewel, natural and pure. Not fond of wearing showy clothes or pretentiousness, she mocked false airs and affectations. Her adornment, like her hair, was modest and gently cared for. She had a motherly gaze but spent many hours steeped in worry, which eventually carved a heavy frown across her countenance. Mom, the burden bearer, bore us all with grace and peace, leaning on the Lord. Paying bills, rearing children, working long hours in a sweat box were duties she faithfully assumed. Her feet, roughened at the heels, stood firmly on board, anchoring our craft through stormy winds and gales. O'er the years the frown became as deeply ingrained as Daddy's scar, but the softness of her demeanor remained unchanged.

A tall woman, large boned and well proportioned, she often wore the popular shirtwaist dresses of the '50s that fit snug at the waist and fell softly to a full skirt below her knees, protecting modesty. Their V-necklines, filled with beads, pleasantly accented her pin-curled hair and oval face. But those dresses, capped at the sleeves, betrayed her long arms and large hands—hands Grandma taught to mix flour and lard to make biscuits and whip up beans and a little meat to go with it, hands taught to wash her one or two dresses nightly to wear again; big honest hands that carried home discards rich women gave her, which she thought we could use, fixed them up and made do; work hands that scrubbed floors in white folk's kitchens; hands that seasoned chicken, shook it in paper bags filled with flour, then fried it until golden brown; strong, firm hands that held us securely when crossing Seventh Avenue and 135th Street, where we lived; suffering hands, sometimes swollen and burned at the tips from picking up hot breads on an assembly line at Superior Bakery, where she worked; hands that bore no polish or paint, just a simple wedding ring, her gold band of commitment to marriage and family. In years to come, that gold would be tested as if by fire.

Mom, whose speech was impressed with the tardy drawl of a Southerner, attempted to mimic the rapid-paced Northern style. But frustrated in her efforts to speak properly, she often reverted to her comfortable down-home stride, musing, "I can't speak it, but I do love to hear it!" Her voice was a gift, perfect for old-time gospel music—a fine-tuned instrument richly seasoned by years of doing without and trying to make it. Mellowed and distinct, it seemed to well up from the bowels of her being, unfolding naturally, needing no musical accompaniment. It was a voice that knew the pain it sung about and gave comfort to all who listened.

There were times when her foot tapped or her hands clapped, or she'd rock from side to side, as the words tinged with emotion took her back to those small backwoods churches of home—churches where poor people gathered around an old piano and one sister played by ear the songs of Zion. Others clapping their tambourines sang in unison, all their frustrations seemingly swept away with song. A minister would stand and preach the Word, with the deacons chiming in "Amen! Amen!" and saints shouting hallelujah and dancing in exultation as the Spirit led them. A choir of voices like heavenly hosts filled with adoration sang,

> Amazing grace, how sweet the sound
> That saved a wretch like me.
> I once was lost, but now I'm found,
> Was blind, but now I see.
> Through many dangers, toils and snares
> We have already come.
> 'Twas grace that brought us safely thus far,
> And grace will lead us home.

Yes, Mom had a voice—a voice of sacrifice and of giving. How I loved it! Over the years, I would come to know its every inflection: up when happy, down when sad, hot and snappy when angry. Upon hearing gospel today, my thoughts go back to Mama as her thoughts went back to the South. A quietness comes; I rest and hold on. I would be strong like Mama. I would press on like Mama. And I'd have my share of troubles like Mama.

My earliest recollection of Harlem is of the apartment we had on the first floor behind a row of stairs at 260 West, a four-story walk-up not far from Harlem Hospital, my birthplace. My sister, Fay, premature and underweight, was born in Jacksonville, Florida, Dad's home, then brought on a tiny pillow to New York. She was a child of fragility. I, unlike her, was bouncy and plump, a full eight pounds with big brown eyes and coarse red hair. Harlem was to be our first playground—the fire escape, a playpen from which to view a glass-strewn world. Our first steps were taken among the rubble of a littered lot. Backs of old buildings grid with windows—many windows, some boarded up, some without glass, others having only a tattered shade—provided a veiled glimpse of lives within. The windows were connected by iron steps ascending and descending like Jacob's ladders for angels to bring blessings to and fro. They were bedecked with a trim of plants—philodendrons, ivy, sweet potatoes set in cans—whose emerald leaves entwined the bars and raced skyward. How they reached for the sun in that sunless place! The opulence of Harlem's better days was now cloaked in gray. Came times a hapless stray passed, but when greeted by a tossed stone, he wisely slipped away. Another time a mother cat brought a kindle of kittens out to play, a cherished event for us young children. Our mom, like that cat, had found a place for us, safe and protected by her nurturing arms—a four-room haven.

Two Sixty was a brownstone edifice with an elderly facade, her stoop a gathering place for warblers absorbed in idle chatter. Rusty handrails provided an iron perch for resting. The entrance led to a dark passage illumed with a single yellow bulb shining dimly. Corridor walls, marked and stained, were stippled with paint to hide their imperfections. Careful looks over a shoulder followed each denizen in and out, while escaping aromas, meeting in hallways, spread musky odorant all about.

Inside radiators whistled with steam when hot, but on rentless days, they stood as silver martyrs cold to touch. Bathrooms had great old-fashioned tubs with clawed feet standing, porcelain knobs like giant keys to turn, and curved spigots that leaked water carving a copper cascade down into the drain. Our tub, big enough for three, held Fay, Sonny, and me for a bath.

Mom, our interior designer, decorated well with what she had. Black and pink sprinkled her decor from curtains and pillows to tile on the floor. Gracing the living room, a black-and-white TV stood eminently still. This set celebrated its birthday yearly with me, for we were like twins. When I was five, it was five. When I was ten, it was ten and still working!

At the front was Mom and Dad's room painted pink. It had a glaring light in the ceiling shrouded by a rectangular shade laden with dust. The bed set was heavy mahogany with a bookcase headboard and plate glass mirror. Atop the dresser was a lace scarf, a mirrored tray with comb and brush, and a looking glass of tarnished silver. Two empty atomizers placed there were for decoration only, but the Channel No. 5 bottle smelled of real perfume, which Mom wore on dress-up days, mostly Sundays. Dad's cologne, coins, and colorful cuff links filled his tray. A plastic comb and pomades for the hair were among the other items placed there. Sharp suits hung on hangers at the back of the door, as well as Mom's nice coat trimmed with fur. Backs of chairs got tossed with wares as little could fit in the one small closet. But one yuletide, two giant walking dolls three feet high hid perfectly inside and walked out on Christmas morning to our surprise! They were white and we were black; it mattered not. We welcomed them, our playmates for many days to come.

Kids' room, to the rear, held a metal bunk and foldaway bed centerstage. These were our trampolines for nightly fun. Fay, the clown, slept below, while I climbed to the sky arena. Mom's flicking of the light signaled showtime with Fay promptly pummeling the underbelly of my bed, tossing me ping-pong up in the air to rocket down into a blanket net. We'd suddenly hush when Mom appeared at the door. "What's going on?" she'd entreat. Chirps and giggles escaped the covers; we'd hide and peek. She'd go away, but our thrashing about would bring her again. She'd shout! Silence reigned just for a little while, then we'd resume our play. Finally, late into the night, our jiggling and jostling seized. Bodies tired, we'd curl and sleep. All was well.

Our room was strewn with clothes, this here, that there, all around. Never in the large antique dresser or chifforobe could they be found. Clothes were airplanes, missiles, and jets sailing across the winds, landing where they would. We loved the game; Mom never understood. A gaping window opened onto a fire escape, where we played day after day. We climbed in and out; we laughed. Times were good then.

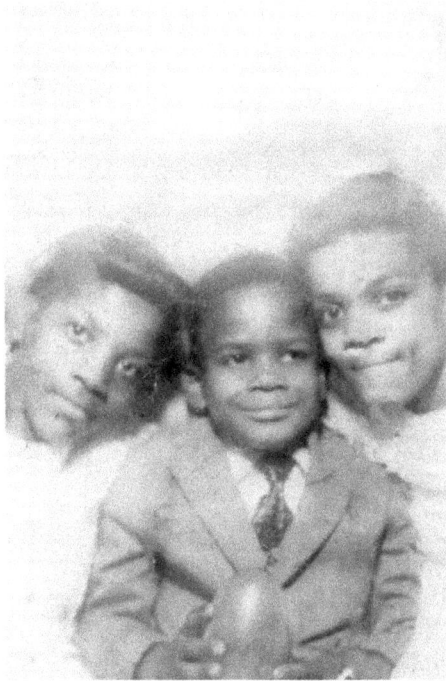

My sister Fay (left), my brother Sonny (center) and me.

Mama called us girls by name—Fay and Jean. On the other hand, Andre was dubbed Sonny Boy, a moniker reflecting the sunshine a boy brought into her life. Together we were her Three Jiggy Boogies. Dad called us dudes or stiffs, for he liked jive talk. His appearance daily from work surely brought a big happy smile coupled with an Indian head nickel for each to take to Mr. Gordon's store just doors away for candy.

On payday, he emptied his pockets of copperhead pennies for the gumball machine that stood at the storefront door holding multicolored treats inside and sometimes even a prize. Ugh! What a prize! A plastic ring? A whistle that wouldn't blow? A teeny, tiny yo-yo? Bah! But there were pretty snap beads; those we liked! Perchance, a magic turn of the key brought a stream of balls trickling down to make a bracelet to match our rings; fancy ladies instantly we'd become. Change left over bought candy sticks to paint our lips gooey red meant to turn some young boy's head. That wasn't for Andre. No way! He bought little Coke bottles filled with flavored syrup and wax that could be chewed all day.

On adventurous days, we ran to Mr. Smalls's shoeshine booth at the corner of Seventh Avenue and purchased a daily news, plunking five cents in a cup atop the counter while watching a gent with dancing brushes and rags restore old shoes to a glossy sheen. But we never paused at the number hole where adults wagered bets on the day's action. The game paid $100 for one on a straight hit, fifty cents brought $50, and one dollar $100. Folks played numbers at risk penned on small slips of paper and initialed for identification. A hit set phone wires blazing with news of the win, as if manna had fallen from heaven. Most people squandered their piteous earnings, gaining only frustration. Everyone knew which spot was the number hole, for it had items that never sold, windows never brightly lit, and a door through which traffic constantly flowed. That was not a place for us, Mom said, though she went occasionally, and so did Dad.

Racing home beneath the watchful gaze of Dad's pals—Don, the parking attendant; Tucker, a big man with a scar like his; and men in pool halls whose nameless faces peered out of doors—made us feel protected as we darted past the stores. Even winos sitting on stoops chided us lest we fall into misadventure. We knew they were Daddy's buddies, and they, knowing we were Andy's kids, became our guardian angels.

Mom's friend Ms. Bea watched, too, from her lofty perch in the window next door above Mr. Saunder's church. She was a hooting owl that cooed neighborhood news, mindful not who heard. Little went unnoticed by that roving-eyed bird. Mom was smart, seldom told her business to that old fowl, clever not to tell a secret to an owl!

She had another friend more sincere indeed. He lived one floor above in Apartment E. His name was Mr. Sherill, a whiskery gray squirrel who stored all his keepings in great shipping barrels. Having no family near, he shared his bounty with us through gifts of clothing and samples of island food. Like a rich Jamaican uncle, he attached himself to my mother and her little brood. Of course, we didn't know then, this dear kindly fellow would provide our passage out of the ghetto. A debt of love we owe him.

Our childhood playmates on that street were Robert, Curtis, Lula, Linda, Marion, and Dwight, quite a gaggle of goslings who wintered in New York and nested. Their parents, like ours, were transplants from the country, uprooted and repotted in acidic soil. They were the Johnsons—eight in number. Together we were a formidable lot, a safety measure in a menacing milieu. And what a time we had—from their house to ours, running back and forth pendulously day after day, joyous hours well spent in play. Our bonds would resist the tide of a good many years and innumerable changes.

Back then, Sunday was sacredly recognized as a rest day from shopping and work—a day to meet the Johnson kids at Mr. Saunder's church in the basement of the tenement adjacent to ours. How lean this tabernacle for the Lord was and meager in its furnishings—a mere storefront with windows covered by stick on paper in the pattern of stained glass, colorful irregular-shaped platelets accented with strong black lines meandering throughout. Superimposed, the name of the church appeared in bold letters along with the pastor's name, Rev. E. Saunders. Situated above the entrance, a humble cross lit the path to salvation, while outside life went on raging as it would. Narrow the pathway that led to this door, and few found it.

Inside the hallowed sanctuary, a modest pulpit, clothed in red velvet fabric fringed with gold and emblazoned with two gold crosses, stood on a nude wooden floor. A well-used Bible sat conspicuously on top. Folding chairs lined up in rows to greet the number of guests for the day's sermon, while hymnals carefully placed on every other seat took count. The offering plate never showed its face until that special moment when it made its way across the rows to hold the minuscule sacrifice, which it held reverently before the altar for thanksgiving. The sides of the room were naked except for steam pipes that raced from floor to ceiling in a series of linking tubes that hissed ever so faintly along with psalms. It was warm and cozy there as the Spirit of the Lord filled this temple.

Sunday school opened with several rounds of a beloved children's song:

> Jesus loves me this I know,
> For the Bible tells me so.
> Little ones to Him belong.
> They are weak, but He is strong.
> Yes, Jesus loves me,
> For the Bible tells me so!

This was followed by memorization and recitation of verses, the Lord's Prayer, and the Twenty-Third Psalm—each child having a chance to stand in the spotlight. The morning lesson appeared on picture cards depicting Jesus talking to children on His knee. Below the inscription read, "Suffer the little children to come unto me." We all liked Jesus and Sunday school but especially relished the cake and Kool-Aid served after the closing prayer.

This was called Fellowship Hour, a time for adults to chew on tidbits of gossip, while kids tried out their tapped shoes on the bare wooden floor. It wasn't long before a weary adult screamed out "Y'all stop runnin'!" in a voice rife with agitation as the tinkle of our heels turned into a thunderous romp. Halting suddenly, we gasped for breath, our tiny hearts frantic with exhilaration. One warning gave sufficient notice to cease, for not to obey meant someone was gonna "tell yo' mama!" and that was sure to bring a whack in front of people and a beating when you got home. "Don't you never do that again!" Mom would say, or she'd "turn you over to your father!" a more odious threat, for his voice had the wail of a ship's horn and his hands hit our bottoms like a bolt. The rod reigned emperor over us, adults being faithful executors of the law.

Sundays were quiet days in Harlem, no music blaring, bars closed, and night people fallen into a deep slumber, while church folk went on promenade in royal vestments. The sun shone brightly as on no other day, bathing the drab buildings in its glory, touching the pallet of the clothing, and painting a striking mosaic. Church women strolled regally in rainbow array, wearing hats with great plumes and flora. Greeted with dignity by the few vagrants who awakened to see the queenly entourage, they nodded with civility and strode past. Preachers and pimps sped off in fine caddies, faring better than most, while straggly dogs yarned at the spectacle. The queens of Harlem on that day were queens of Sheba.

The parade ended at the 125th Street Penny Arcade, which held games of chance and prizes for the lucky few. Lights and sounds mesmerized children's eyes, while delightful smells set tummies achurn with hunger. Popcorn scents and cotton candy twirled on paper cones sent nervous hands plowing in fallow pockets to scrounge olden pennies from the lint. Thrifty mothers devised clever ways to stretch the little they had. Our mom brought along a plastic pill cup made with concentric circles that collapsed to fit her purse and assembled quickly to hold three sips of Coke poured from one large drink she purchased for thirty-five cents. Coupled with two hotdogs broken in half, it provided a hasty snack for four. All ate and felt satisfied, daring not ask for more!

On days when money wasn't so pinched, we might have gone to Coney Island for rides and ice cream or taken the ferry across the sound to view the lovely Lady Liberty. But our liberty was draped in poverty and those trips so few in number.

Gala days came when all of Harlem went on exhibition in grand style, her sons and daughters parading with great pomp and ceremony down Seventh Avenue to the soulful cadence of black college bands. As marchers bobbed rhythmically to wildly exciting drumbeats, screaming trumpets sent out a gathering call to rejoice! A melodious ovation resounded from every window and rooftop. Young and old poured out onto the promenade to glance at statured men in feathered shakos and brilliantly gay attire, whose drumsticks beat out the pulse of a community in the viselike grip of despair yet energized with pride.

A corps of majestic men in uniform—soldiers, elks, cadets from the YMCA and Minisink, numerous service organizations, church groups, and followers of Daddy Grace—carried colorful banners boldly displaying their names and insignia. Ebony debutantes resplendent in lace waved atop great flotillas heralded by cute sassy majorettes. Brown shapely legs seized the eyes of male gawkers, as satin costumes shimmered in the noonday sun. Perspiration rained softly, while sky-kicking maidens curled short skirts flirtingly. Their batons flew away with many hearts!

Young onlookers gasped in amazement at black cowboys with six shooters wearing fringed riding pants and ten-gallon hats, their ornate leather saddles gird around horses of dappled gray and brown. They brought to life the Western movies we so frequently watched on TV. Swirling lariats roped our imaginations and drew us back in history to wild West days—days we never knew we had been a part. Our hearts leaped with wonderment and awe!

The gaiety of those riders bore stark contrast to the white policemen cloaked in navy straddling dark horses along the brim of the marchers, their tall boots and long billy clubs menacingly apparent, as were the black revolvers in holsters strapped ominously across their girth. Badges barely glinting in the daylight, they patrolled and controlled the chasm between the people and their pride.

With only her shell in view, the external community envisaged Harlem as just another poor ghetto with present foes and obvious woes. We saw the inscape of this neighborhood where certain persons were respected, others tolerated, but all fit as parts of a cell, each effectual in its function within an enclosed body. Residents just belonged by virtue of being black. Pompous titles and college degrees were not the best measure of station within the group, for they were the province of a select few. However, a grand showboat car or goodly apparel elevated one's stature in the eyes of many, even if acquired by illicit means.

It was a community whose life breath was often put forth in song. Musicians, being pervaders of collective emotion, became minstrels of the household, wooing us with ballads of victory and lost love. Those whose new releases topped the black music charts, like the Coasters, who sang "Charlie Brown," were greeted with a hero's welcome through the streets. Borne on the shoulders of long fancy convertibles, they emerged as idols to the cheering throng. Bursting forth like supernovas in the night sky to appear at the Apollo Theater, their pearly white teeth competed for attention with the sheen of their processed hair on billboards at dance halls and ballrooms, such as the Savoy Manor. The radiance of these bright stars quickly faded, leaving only a trail of hits to mark their passing. Though princes uptown, they were made paupers downtown, cheated of their just deserts in monetary accolades.

Esteemed highly were those who ministered the gospel to the down and troubled—preachers, pastors, and reverends. Surely, they wore the king's signet ring, entering private lives with impunity as oracles of God. Their roles were at times subverted by the few whose pernicious ways cast a dim shadow on the good works of many. Beguiling unstable souls with sweet words, they made merchandise of women especially, children sometimes being born of these illicit liaisons. But their unsavory acts in darkness often came to light, and they were purged out because of their corruption. Spots they were and blemishes!

A special honor was given to older women. We called them "Miss," as in Ms. Brown or Ms. Jones, not as a courtesy or a title meaning unmarried. It was an acknowledgment of their reaching a level of endurance in life's marathon run. Having run a good race, persevering through years of struggle and hard times with husbands and kids, they could now look back and tell the story of how they got over. Like unto a master so expert in his craft, he now sits as a learned teacher instructing young apprentices in the way, these older women became able instructors for black girls about men, child rearing, and what you had to do to get through life. By experience, they ruled as imperial matriarchs within our order. Venerable "queen mothers" taught through humor and example, having learned to look back on life and laugh. For example, one might say, "Child, a man who is already drinking the milk ain't gonna buy the cow!" meaning if a man were sleeping with a woman, he wouldn't be likely to marry her, as he is already enjoying the benefits of the matrimonial bed.

Unfortunately, black men were "kings without honor in their own country." Unable to earn adequate income to support the family, they were relegated to the position of drones in a bee colony. After serving the function of impregnating the queen, they were driven out of the nest to buzz about seeking other kingdoms, the misfortune of this being that a hierarchy was built upon generation after generation of this pattern. Young maidens, stung by charming knaves, had to turn to the welfare system for sustenance. Many families were headed by women, and many children didn't have a dad in the home.

Germane to this court were the jesters, the masters of black comedy, notably Red Fox, Mom's Mabley, and Pigmeat Markham, who taught us to laugh at ourselves. Their humor was valuable in helping us weather difficult times but detrimental because a lot of their jests were at our own expense. That brand of self-deprecating humor, which I heard as a child, often set up scenarios wherein the white man always did things well. And the black man, close on his heels trying to imitate, appeared buffoonish in his attempts to compete with his white counterpart. For example, a joke was told about a white man romancing his sweetheart in words of love: "Darling, you have beautiful eyes. Beneath your eyes the stars lie!" (Shakespeare). The black man overhearing decides to romance his woman likewise but says, "Darling, you have bull eyes. Beneath your eyes your lip lies" (Bull——)!

In other skits, black people, portrayed as ignorant and lacking understanding, did things wrong in spite of themselves or were always causing trouble. An example, a joke was told about St. Peter calling up Satan to ask if he had any room down there for some Niggers because they were giving him too much trouble in heaven. Lucifer responded, "Don't send them down here! Mine are setting hell on fire too!" Racial gibes were common at the time, but as a child overhearing, it wounded my sense of worth. I learned early to down myself, doubt myself and others like me. I became convinced of the superiority of white people and frequently felt *powerless* in my world. Mom shared jokes with friends over the phone and was careful to spell certain words that alluded to sex or were otherwise dirty so that we couldn't decipher. She and the listener would roar with laughter, and we, sensing it had to be good, filled in the details from our imaginations and laughed too. As we reached second or third grade and could put letters together to sound out words, we were getting a lot more from the jokes than she knew! With better understanding,

I determined that I disliked "snaps," as they were called. In fact, they made me quite angry. That anger in part ignited a fire that made me want to disprove those putrid remarks and prove myself—a manner of vindication.

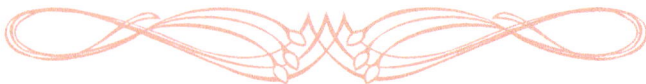

CHAPTER TWO
School Days

SEASONS passed cyclically by. Golden haze changed to crimson, ochre, and brown, to icy snow and slush, to beckoning breezes, cool rain, and back to summer's blaze again. Soon autumn leaves whispered quietly in Mom's ear, "It's time for school!" This sparked a flurry of activity as she prepared us to emerge from her safe cocoon into the outer world.

There were dresses to press and shoes to buff, and Mama had to "do our hair" with the straightening comb, as by age five, our cottony crowns had woven thick as wool. The comb was heated upon the open eye of the kitchen stove and momentarily stroked through clumps of hair dabbled with green pressing oil. As the heat wave melted away all resistance, the grease crackled and poured warmly onto my scalp. With eyes shuttered tightly, I'd hunch my small shoulders and cringe, certain the smoldering iron would leave an awful brand. Returning the comb to the flame, a strong singed smell arose as bits of hair kindled red, then quickly roasted to ash. Burnt grease and soot cooked up a murky odor that pinched at our noses, then ran quickly out into the hallway to tell all that we would soon be ready. This ritual of black womanhood I could well have done without! But Ma said we girls had to learn, even as Grandma had taught her. Dedicated to the task, she'd yell "Don't move!" while pulling at the short hairs at the nape of my neck. Paralyzed with fear, I counted the minutes until it would be Fay's turn to fry in the hot seat and I watch laughing secretly. Pondering God's reason for making me with kinky hair, I didn't feel favored in His sight. Yet I adored what came after—two pigtails tied with bright satiny ribbons, bangs in front. Preening before the mirror, I'd primp, pose, and kiss at the little girl who smiled back at me. She was really cute; so was I!

Hot grease has a smell I'd know anywhere. When I walked into a neighbor's house, it was easy to know if they had been doing hair, and I could often guess the name of the dressing used by its scent. Black hair products ranged from pressing oils and bergamots to all sorts of hair-growth creams. Among these was Dr. Posner's blue pomade with a sweet mediciny odor and Dax, which came in a choice of yellow or black. The black one contained tar to control dandruff; the other, sulfur to promote hair growth. Both smelled to high heaven! Really popular was an ointment in a brown jar we called Suffer 8. This one roared up from the hair and carried a mile away, its aroma suffocatingly sulfurous. People said it made your hair grow, so we all used it. Mama parted our thick manes into neat rows, fingered a pat of the lardish blend from the back of her hand, then carefully traced the lines of scalp. It never did much for me except gave my pillow a dirtyish discoloration and drove away insects! Aside from these, every black family kept a large jar of Vaseline handy. It served many functions as a standby hairdressing or body rub to prevent dryness and ash. We were greased from head to toe as if potatoes to be baked and readied to go.

Shiny faced and bursting with fearful anticipation, I appeared for kindergarten at the crowded elementary school close to home, P.S. 175, clad in the red dress Mom had recently bought. I waited in a hallway swarming with noisy kids, first time feeling so alone—no Fay to make this all seem funny, no Mama to say it will be all right, no Daddy to tell me, "Go on in there, girl!" I was sorely afraid.

A loud voice shouted names and room numbers, while anxious little bodies scurried in all directions. I stood watching, my nimble legs shaking in a wild marimba and knobby knees clicking like castanets. I pulled my hem down to cover up the ruckus, warm tears filling the corners of my eyes. My round-toed shoes pinched with tension as I made my way down the hall to meet the teacher. As I swung open the door in a nervous haste, my bangs rolled up tighter than a window shade, and my white anklets slid down to hide underfoot. There she was, Ms. Applebaum! She would leave an indelible impression on my memory, as I would soon fall in love with her.

She posed straight backed and trim as a mannequin cased in steel-gray attire that covered her form, but for the sheer hose that exposed her warm peach coloring. A jacket peeled off to reveal a demure nylon blouse embroidered finely and lined to prevent naughty eyes from peering beyond her dainty buttons. Quiet brown eyes matched her hair worn in a short bob, meticulously styled in a wreath of curls encircling her face. An elegant smile tinged her lips, while low sensible heels gave comfort to her feet. She had an air of refinement and speech clear and crisp as a morning breeze inviting me in. So graceful and poised, she seemed the embodiment of a good and perfect lady. How unlike the people I always knew!

The cluttered room held twenty small desks, easels, paints, books, and crayons boxes, all fighting for space. Brown-skinned kids filled the seats; I took my place among them, wishing to get lost amid the clamor. Positioned to the fore was a large desk tidily arranged with pencils, paper, chalk, every necessity in uniform order. It stood between us as a line of demarcation no one dared cross save by invitation. Ms. A. had her place. The items on her desk had theirs; we had ours. It was a peaceful coexistence.

I remember well the manicured hand that offered drawing paper, so milky white and different from mine when I reached to accept. How they looked pampered, not used to work like Mom's. I recall standing above her, glancing down at the soft curls that rest gently on her neck and remembering how Ma had tugged at mine to get them straight, how her scent was faint as dried flowers. I recall her voice, distant, aloof, as if coming from on high when reading a story. She was reachless. There was no touching, no physical contact, except a pat on the shoulder to say good job or a firm grasp to place us in line in size place order. When she extended to touch me, I'd raise my shoulders to meet her hand, needing the affirmation. I straightened my back and stood just as she did. I felt honored and special.

I decided I loved her, wanted to be just like her when I grew up. Yet I knew I couldn't for she was something I could never be—white. I could only look and long. She was there; I was here. I looked like this, she like that. Throughout my life, that dividing line I would try and cross. But I knew I was gonna grow up to be like Mama, not her! I was both happy and sad.

I, like my mother, was tan complexioned. Fay and Sonny were darker. Having tan skin yielded its benefits, as popular lore suggested light-skinned girls were prettier, men preferred them, and they gave birth to pretty babies. Black folk wanted fair children with "good hair" because they supposedly improved our race. Some women used skin-bleaching creams and dark-blotch removers to have a fairer appearance. Others deliberately sought out "high yella" partners to marry so that their offspring would be fair. I felt lucky I'd be able to use the cosmetics created for white women with tawny complexions, as darker women had little choice. There were only a few shades of powder being sold by neophyte black product companies, which looked similar to medium or dark cocoa mix. White cosmetic companies offered very little by way of products for women of color. Being "colored" wasn't easy, for no one seemed to recognize the garden of colors that we were. Stockings available were either nude for a white woman or black, little in between. In later years, other colors appeared, such as coffee and gray, but neither matched my shade of skin. I don't look like java or tin, so I just wear beige like Mama did.

For years she wore pancake makeup by Max Factor in rose beige to hide her age. Applied by rubbing the hard cake with a dampened sponge, it dried quickly, giving the face a matte look. When dry, it gave her a slightly whitish pallor that contrasted with the darker skin of her neck, creating a mask. Dark eyes peeking out, Mom resembled a geisha girl painted to perform a flower dance in spring. The wet sponge became a favored toy of mine. It felt cushiony in my hands as I squeezed it to smell its dampness. Slipping it from her dresser, I'd hide away and pat my face as she did, taking also the bright-red lipstick that matched the red paint I used at school. "I'm gonna be a real lady!" I mused to myself, smearing my lips with color and licking them after, smudging my girlish expression.

Time moved on. I adjusted to school, even liked it after a while, enjoying especially the colorful paints and crayons used to draw story pictures I couldn't say in words. Being terribly shy, I wandered off through picture books to Fantasia, a world filled with magical happenstance where the weak and vulnerable often triumphed over powerfully evil foes. As in "Cinderella," I needed to believe the hand of fate could convert poverty into wealth, all wretchedness whisked away with the wave of a fairy's wand, needed so desperately to escape to a happier place where pumpkins became horse-drawn carriages and glass slippers transformed a little waif into a lovely princess waltzing at a palace ball.

I relished all the well-known children's stories, listening ardently as the teacher read, then carefully reviewed the pictures, rehearsing in my mind until they were committed to memory: "Sleeping Beauty," "The Three Little Pigs," "Goldilocks and the Three Bears," to name a few. One fable I loved so much told of five Chinese brothers each possessing a remarkable gift, which they used to foil adversity. The first brother could swallow the sea. The second had an iron neck. The third brother could stretch and stretch. The fourth could not be burned, and the fifth could hold his breath.

But one tale was very troubling to me—the story of Little Black Sambo—being the only black character in all my books at school. Sambo was a pickaninny looking child with dark skin, red lips and a flat nose who ran helplessly to and fro trying to save himself. He didn't have a human persona in any real sense. He was mocked; people laughed at him. They seemed to be making fun of all of us. His caricature only reinforced the negative self-image that had already taken form in my mind. Is that what my people are like? I wondered. Are they desperate people, devoid of humanness; their lives a quagmire from which they long to escape? And why was he called Black Sambo as if his blackness emphasized had a great deal to do with his hapless predicament? Sambo was no Rambo. If in him was my only hope to see myself then I had no hope at all.

As a young girl being shaped in sexual identity, I looked to those paragons of beauty—Snow White, Sleeping Beauty, and Rapunzel—to hold high the mirror of femininity that I might glimpse myself in its reflection. Snow White was the nursling born "white as the driven snow," whose pristine beauty so enraged her wicked stepmother that she banished her to a forest where she lived with seven dwarfs. The ranting of a telltale mirror provoked the jealous queen to plot her demise with a poisoned apple. Death came, but the dwarfs were reluctant to place the fair child in the black ground and chose to enclose her body in a glass coffin to preserve its loveliness. She lay there in sweet repose until a prince, so enamored with her beauty, carried her off to his castle. Life returned to her, and they married. The awful queen was then killed by iron slippers as she danced at the wedding feast.

Similarly, the Sleeping Beauty, a lily-white maiden swathed in angelic innocence, fell into an enchanted sleep, cursed to rest until a man who loved her more than life came and kissed her, breaking the fairy's spell. A king's son led by visions to the sleeping kingdom forged past a thorn hedge, defeated a wild beast, and saved his love. His kiss awakened her; they married and lived happily ever after.

And last, the "most beautiful child imaginable," Rapunzel, a blue-eyed cherub with hair as fine as spun gold, was imprisoned in a witch's tower without a door. The only way inside was to sing "Rapunzel, Rapunzel! Let down your golden hair," at which time her long flowing tresses fell down the twenty-foot wall and became a rope on which to climb. In lonely isolation, she hummed a forlorn tune overheard by a handsome prince who came to her rescue. Then, exiled to a remote forest, she pined endlessly, until the desperate search of her blind lover led him back to her embrace. His sight was restored by the warmth of her joyous tears.

The powerful images these classic tales put forth came leaping out of the colorful illustrations, which were so pictorially graphic in children's books. Feeling homely by comparison to those little white paragons, I pined,

> Mirror, mirror on the wall,
> Who is fairest of them all?
> Surely, it cannot be me,
> For I am ugly as can be!
> I'm not white as driven snow.

My hair certainly doesn't flow.
My eyes are brown, not blue.
What in the world am I to do?"

Would there ever be a prince to fall hopelessly in love with me? And more important, would I ever find beauty within myself?

I began to feel like the Ugly Duckling, that gangly, gawky gray bird who was taunted and teased because he was not pretty like the cute little yellow ducklings. Hatched in a pond of geese by an unsuspecting mother, the poor dejected creature tried in vain to gain acceptance by the other birds. But in their vile dislike, they tormented him endlessly for his difference. Unable to bear their meanness, he retreated to a frozen pond, never glimpsing his true reflection in the water. One day the warmth of spring brought a flock of swans to his pond. Seeing them, he was awed by their beauty and bowed his head in shame, first time looking into the water. A strikingly lovely image peered back at him, and finally he realized he had a beauty all his own. He sailed grandly across the pond, feeling unbelievably happy.

If only tales of black kings and queens and lovely princesses with ebony skin had been told to me as I sat at someone's knee that I might feel a connection with a glorious past. If, looking around, I could have seen positive role models to fashion myself after. If someone told me I had a beauty all my own, unlike a white child's, I too would fluff my feathers, raise my head, and soar with elegance.

The images projected of blacks on TV and in the movies were wild spear-toting hunters as in *Tarzan*, docile servants, angry slaves with shackles on their wrists, or Stepin Fetchits who shined their eyes, skinned their teeth, and said "Yez, ma'am!" And of course, there were the black buffoons in the *Amos and Andy* comedy series and the fat black mammies that waited on white women hand and foot (*Gone with the Wind*). Should I aspire to be like any of these? Looking back, I saw little to look forward to. Without grounding in history, how can one pursue their destiny?

I turned to Mom and Dad for direction and inspiration. Daddy often bragged about Joe Louis, the pugilist who took on the world with his fists. Mom revered Mahalia Jackson and Sam Cook for their soul-stirring gospel renditions. However, aside from sports figures and entertainers, there was no one else being held up before me as a star who was black. Oddly, ghetto beginnings worked to my benefit, giving me something to grow against and aim away from. Although we were a degraded people cast in a dim reflection, I longed to fill in the void, sensing my view was in part mere shadows of who we were or could be, "sown in dishonor," one day to be "raised in radiance."

Kindergarten was a fun place, a place to bring what was learned at home, mix in what's acquired at school, fold in other ingredients to create a play dough to be kneaded by experience. We were so pliable, so easily molded and shaped like gingerbread children, cut out and waiting for embellishments to be put on that our uniqueness would become evident. Learning took place through childish songs and games as we playfully explored the adult world, a first opportunity to integrate and test what we knew.

As a vehicle for self-expression, the merriment of lighthearted singing encouraged our use of language as a mediator, even as we used crayons and paint to describe the world around us. Circle time was the highlight of our day, as we participated in teacher-led songs, such as

> He was going to the circus.
> He was going to the fair
> To see the senorita with flowers in her hair.
> Oh, shake it, senorita, shake it if you dare,
> So all the boys around your block can see your
> underwear.
> Now rhumba to the bottom
> And rhumba to the top.
> Then turn around and turn around
> Until you make a stop!

The game proceeded as one child chosen to be the senor/senorita danced in the center—hand on hip, the other behind the head, while everyone clapped along. The dancer swayed sassily side to side, sashayed to the floor to the call of the words, and wiggled mockingly to amuse the group. The sauciest movements won the most laughter as we flirted with our sexuality as being different, boys from girls.

When a pointed finger indicated my turn, I shuffled timidly toward the center, index finger comfortingly clinched between my teeth like Sherlock's pipe. Deathly afraid to let go, I swayed only slightly with much prodding from an impatient Ms. A., who didn't perceive the depth of my fear that I wouldn't measure up—fear so consuming I longed to retreat into my inner world to find seclusion in fantasy, holding fast to the control I felt over crayons and paints that did what my hand said do and revealed only what I wanted said. I had already developed an introverted and reserved personality with a lot of inhibition.

Imagining myself an ugly duckling when compared with other girls, I decided I wasn't prissy enough to charm the group with cuteness, or chubby enough to turn corpulence into jollity. By recoiling, I averted the jabs of their laughter and the painful sting of their jests. Very much there and a part, I experienced everything internally, while my facade was cloaked in meekness.

An integral part of the circle game is choosing who goes next. Kids left to their own devices usually pick their friends, leaving unpopular kids feeling bruised. To eliminate this disparity, kids used a song intended to randomly select players. Though childish in wording, the song was like an arrow that pierced the heart. It went like this:

> Eeny, meeny, miny, moe,
> Catch a Nigger by the toe.
> If he hollers, let him go!
> Eeny, meeny, miny, moe.

In the seeming innocence of childish games, powerfully negative messages were being fed to us like pablum.

> Row, row, row your boat,
> Gently down the stream.
> Merrily, merrily, merrily, merrily,
> Life wasn't such a dream!

Storybooks were seeds that sprouted an interest in reading and writing, which came fairly easy. Time and again, I carefully executed the letters of my first name, Loretta, in my black speckled notebook, uttering it syllabically, "Lo-ret-ta." By its sound, I thought it made a wonderful name for a cow, more seemly for something fat. It certainly didn't become a knobby-kneed girl like me. Thus, I used it only in school and preferred to be called Jeanie, having the semblance of a mythical spirit that could squeeze through the neck of a bottle.

Loretta is the kind of name that, no matter how pronounced, never sounds pretty! Attach Farmer, my surname, and the dairy label becomes firmly affixed. Kids called me, "The farmer in the dell, the farmer in the dell. Hi-ho the cherry-yo." At boiling point, each time I heard names called, cowbells rang out in my head. I'd hiccup, and my breath seemed to smell of grass, a crafty collusion of body and mind to make mockery of my dislike.

Writing evolved in partnership with pictures drawn at the easel. First, I created stories with paints, then scrawled sentences above to explain them. Most often I depicted myself as a teacher, like Ms. A., surrounded by a swarm of kids using the title "When I Grow Up!" Strangely, my mind was set almost from the beginning. It was my choice for a lifelong vocation.

After school we hurried along home to amuse ourselves outside, until evening when Mom came. She asked Ms. Bea, the busybody, to keep an eye on us as we played street games, games like jack rocks, hopscotch, clapping in syncopated beats, racing, tag, and hide-and-go-seek.

Our favorite pastime was skipping rope in variations of single or double Dutch. With jackets off, hair flying in the air and books thrown to the ground without a care, we jumped for hours on end while singing silly songs, such as,

> Grandma, Grandma sick in bed,
> Called the doctor, and the doctor said,
> "Grandma, Grandma, you ain't sick,
> All you need is a big fat kick!"

Catching the rhythm with a full-body sway, we jumped in and pumped away. Up and down with lightning feet as we made up dances in the street, jumping alone or in pairs, free of all worldly cares. Adding new steps all the while, with remarkable agility we created jump styles like the breakers of the '80s who danced in the streets to the throbbing pulsations of the hip-hop beat. We came before; we set the stage. We were the street artisans of our age.

I learned a lot about life jumping rope on city streets. First, if one wants to learn, you have to take that first leap. Once in, you have to keep moving and working your feet. One can never feel life moving and racing through their veins or their heart pumping wildly while standing on the sidelines watching. Life is best lived actively, not passively. Second, one must experience the rhythm and move with its flow. That means making adjustments to what life sends your way. Sometimes it's like hot pepper, racing fast and you don't know what's coming next. And sometimes you amble along effortlessly in little skips. Life can be as complicated as double Dutch or as simple as single. The best time is when two people can jump together and coordinate their steps to create a beautiful dance. Life's special joys need to be shared. But take heed, while you're in there bobbing and weaving, of the passing throng in their mad dash to go nowhere! Make sure they don't collide with your ropes and tie you up in their hopelessness. As you live, beware of those potentially fatal collisions that impact on your life, wreaking havoc body, mind, and soul.

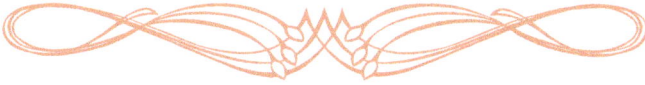

CHAPTER THREE
Family Ties

JOYFUL spontaneous moments enliven my mind with memories of cherished times past when Daddy came home and joined our play. Little brother Sonny followed along too, receiving necessary sanction from Dad's lead. Males rarely participated in girls' games, for we kept clear distinctions—what was for boys and what wasn't. Girls typically jumped rope, played house, and hosted tea parties for their dolls, while boys roughhoused, rode bikes, pitched balls, and hit strikes. One prepared for roles as mothers, and the other flexed muscles to someday rule the world.

Likewise, clear distinctions were made in clothing styles for each gender. Boys wore loose-fitting togs cut from darkly colored cloth with subdued patterning. Girls contrasted them with light pastel dresses brightened with ribbons, ruffles, and lace. Strongly held notions of femininity and masculinity were made evident by our dress—girls thought to be soft and submissive, boys rough and dominant.

Long hair was identified with girlishness too, but since I had short hair, I adorned myself with fancy doodads, bobs, and bows, much like the painter bird, not born with lovely plumage, adorns his nest with bright bits of found objects to attract attention. Black mothers, like skillful artisans, began creating plaited hairstyles of cornrow, textured designs, and beadwork, reserving the pressed styles for Sundays. But our mother had little energy for such fanciness being worn to threads from labor. She merely carved out one big braid in the top and one on either side (what you might call a "my mother works" hairdo with little barrettes at the ends).

Boys in contrast wore their hair cut to the quick, the remaining fuzz outwardly contoured by a razor's edge. To me, their misshapen heads looked like white potatoes, each having an amorphous form cast by our African past. They remind me of a toy I once had called Mr. Potato Head. The body was a plastic potato that we poked funny features on to create an amusing character. The humorous part was that no matter how we dressed him up, he always just looked like a potato. Girls luckily can hide their spuds under locks of hair.

Sex differences were carefully reinforced by speech and actions. No guy wanted to be labeled a sissy because of doing girly things, and no girl wanted to be called a tomboy, especially if she hadn't reached a stage where nature enhanced her flatlands with a few lush hills and valleys. We delighted so much in crossover occasions. Watching Dad jump, I don't know if it was funny because he was so large and had to crouch down to fit within the arc of our rope by awkwardly contorting his massive body and big feet to conform to our little game, or whether it was the oddity of having an adult male encroach upon a little girl's world seeming so ill-suited. Maybe it was just the joy of having Daddy do something with us, coming down to our level. He was so often away; when he was there, we rollicked in laughter, savoring each moment.

Unfortunately, Mom, who, when not working was busy caring for our needs, never got that overly joyous response. I suppose we took her for granted as kids so often do. We assumed it was no more than a mother is supposed to do and failed to give her adoration. We thought Dad was doing something special when he was around, for his comings and goings, like the weather were unpredictable. His time was divided between home and an increasingly active social life outside. Poor Mom, already overtaxed and spent with responsibility, wasn't up to playing with us and being silly. Her mind became a slave to worry, as Dad had begun to stray.

Weekdays Dad was suited plainly in brown khaki uniforms for his job on the waterfront unloading cargo from the tall merchant ships sailing in from ports around the world, bringing a storehouse of commodities to be sold in the United States. Items such as small appliances, manufactured goods, and electronic equipment, produced by cheap labor abroad, yielded lucrative trade on the American market.

I suspect, to Dad's mind everyone was benefitting in this exchange, except him. The foreigners bolstered their weak economies with the precious American dollar. The distributors undercut domestic prices and reaped large profits. So who lost? Dad, who put in countless hours of backbreaking labor lifting and sorting boxes onto conveyor belts, barely gleaning enough money to keep food on the table at home. It was a thankless job, under Italian bosses who were like cruel slave drivers that cursed and demeaned their workers and were not above using strong-arm tactics to control the docks.

Consequently, Dad had to shore up under a lot of abuse to support our family. Never one to complain or pour his feelings out, he faced it stoically as he thought a man should. Surely, he would not be willing to see his family go without. Like clockwork he arose, went to work every day, and brought home his meager paycheck at the end of the week. He didn't speak of the hurt he felt but locked it all up inside, then he began to drink so he would not feel the pain.

Having lost his father at age eight and his mother not long after, he joined the military with only an eighth-grade education at sixteen. He remained four years and broke close ties with siblings left behind. Now married with children and living in New York, he discovered the swirl of city life to be fast, perilous, and deceitful. Still a young man not seasoned by experience, he was not prepared for so many new permutations.

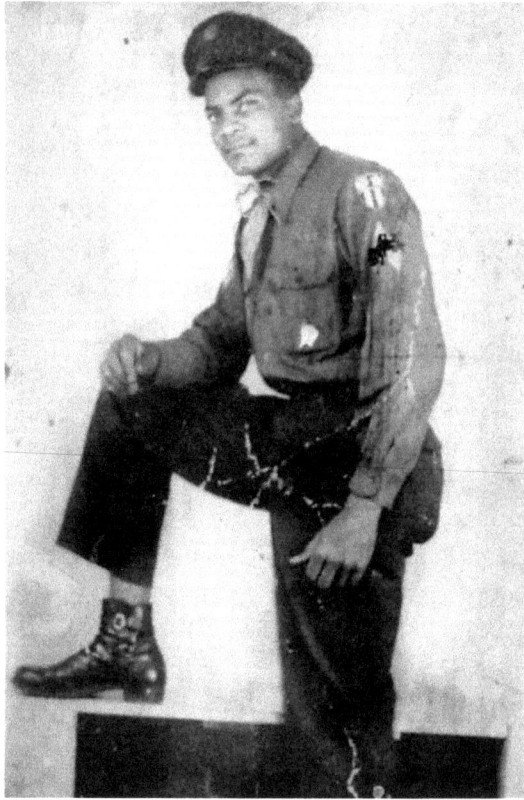

My father Sgt. Andrew Jackson Farmer in uniform.

As an army sergeant in World War II, he led a troop of men into frontline action and was quite boastful about his escapades. Always a proud man with a grandiose ego, he liked to hold his head high and have others look up to him. But there was paltry little stroking of his ego on the job and probably less at home by a wife inundated with raising three small children while putting pennies together, trying to make it.

A sense of loss and hard times exacted a terrible price, luring him away from his strong commitment to home to find liveliness and laughter outside. Drawn to the convivial atmosphere of bars, he felt comradery with those merrymakers who drank heartily, laughed loudly, and cried bitterly when it all came to an end.

B. B. King sang a song back then that said,

> The eagle flies on Friday.
> Saturday I go out to play.
> Sunday I go to church;
> I sit down and I pray, "Oh Lord, have mercy on me,
> I cry have mercy because my heart is in misery."

This was one of Dad's favorite songs perhaps because it pictured so well his condition. Dad's good looks and alluring smile led him to become a lady's man and a cool dancer. Weekends he wore playboy clothes—flashy two-toned suits trimmed with glass studs and faux gems cut well and tapered at the waist with wide lapels to accent his powerful chest. To complete the outfit, he had on a Stetson hat, a gold watch, and shiny shoes of patent leather or snakeskin. Strutting down the street with shoulders pulled back, he looked like a real Jim Dandy.

It seemed Daddy needed the nightlife, bright lights, fast women, drinking buddies, parties, lots of happenings, until the wee hours of the morning, to counterbalance the mundanity of his work. Weekdays became just a needed interval between the roll of the good times. But he was not a lecherous man and always had a way of doing things to preserve respect and protect the family.

Daddy tried to keep his other life outside our home, but it crept in surreptitiously, leaving subtle clues. The pursed lips that stained his collar red whispered of women he had met and held close. The smoke that filled his jacket was the same smoke that lurks around dim-lit bars that flow abundantly with booze and funky music that hollers out of jukeboxes dazzling with neon lights—foot-stomping music, trying songs; wailing music, crying songs; love music, sad tunes, and losing songs. The rancid odor of alcohol on his breath was eager to betray him shouting the line he must have told himself many times before, "Just one more, one more!" His massive body gave nothing away, not even a sway. But what his eyes tried to hide shone glaringly on his weary face. One awful night his other life boldly followed him home, like an ignoble vagabond, to steal away a marriage, wound a wife, and maim an unexpectant family.

B. B. King expressed it well in his song about the nightlife:

> When the evening sun goes down,
> You'll find me hanging around,
> Because the nightlife ain't no good life,
> But it's my life.
> The people just like you and me,
> Oh, they're all dreaming about their old used to be.
> I want to tell you the nightlife,
> It ain't no good life,
> But it's my life.
> They tell me life is just an empty stream,
> An avenue of broken dreams,
> But I tell you the nightlife,
> It ain't no good life, but it's my life!

Problems begat worries. Worry begat wandering, and wandering begat unfaithfulness. And unfaithfulness begat lies, and lies begat more pain and more problems coming full circle around. Pain pays rapid refunds and doesn't just write one check. It pays the father, the mother, and the kids as well. Everybody gets a check, even if they didn't submit a form.

As a young child, I didn't understand the details of Dad's dealings. I just knew Mom and Dad were the people I loved dearly, the ones from whom I was conceived, who gave me nurturance. When Dad went out, I couldn't fall asleep until I heard the key turn in the door upon his return. He moved about quietly in the darkness, finding his way to the bedroom, where Mom lay waiting too. I listened to the murmurings from their room that penetrated the wall, the muffled voices that grew louder with each passing moment, the lull of Mom's sorrowful moan as she must have cried and questioned him why.

An intense fear gripped me about the neck, wondering if they would fight or if everything would be okay that night. I pleaded with God that he wouldn't hit her. Not Daddy! Not my good daddy! He wouldn't do something like that, would he? My heart beat like a thousand tom-toms in the blackness. My ears listened keenly as I struggled to hold back the tears. I tossed and turned until they'd quiet down, but in the silence came a deadly fear of tomorrow. Would it be the same, or next time worse? And if they did fight, whom would I defend? I loved them both; I didn't want to choose. They were Mommy and Daddy, and I was just a little girl getting a giant slice of an awfully cruel world.

Mom shouted the name Pearl. I asked myself, "Who is she? She's not one of Mom's friends! Why is she here keeping us awake?" Years later, I found out Pearl was the other woman's name. "But why did Daddy need another woman when he had Mama?" That question gnawed deeply into my flesh, into the hidden reaches of my soul. It was as if he were betraying me too, my good daddy. If my father, who was responsible for my very existence, could betray me, then how could any other man come along and give me everlasting love? I felt worthless and unworthy.

Mama talked to us about it; we were the only ones she had. Those who called on the phone were just gossipmongers searching for juicy news to spread while pretending to be concerned. She told us how she was a good woman, but in spite of all her goodness, Dad had done her wrong. "Men are like dogs!" she'd say, her voice hot and angry, crying out for justice.

I wanted to fix it for Mama, to make everything all right. I didn't know what to say, but I said everything that came to mind to try to comfort her. Mama was always able to kiss my hurts and put a Band-Aid on them. I wanted to do something to heal hers. But what can a little child do but care and feel helpless? Fay, Sonny, and I were all caught in this painful web from which there was no escape. We each handled it in different ways, and it certainly affected who we would become.

Songs have a way of putting what we are feeling into words. Mom's favorite song man was Ray Charles, who sang "A Worried Mind":

> You promised me love that would never die.
> That promise you made was only a lie.
> Now after you're gone all alone I pine.

All that I've got is a worried mind.
Those happy days that we once knew,
Though long ago, they still make me blue.
And now that you've gone all alone I find,
That all I've got is a worried mind.
You have no heart, you have no shame,
You took true love and gave the pain.
Now after you're gone all alone I pine,
For all that I've got is a worried mind.

Thank God for Mondays, which brought to an end those painful weekends! Off to school again, a feeling of safety returned, the order of schedule bringing normalcy to my days. But as I advanced in grade, school also became a threatening place, a battleground where bigger, meaner kids let blood to prove their toughness and small, timid kids bore the brunt of their unkind taunts. Personally, I was the sort of kid who couldn't beat a wet noodle and didn't want to try. I felt protected in the classroom with the teacher fully in control, but I feared the madness of the schoolyard divided into mini kingdoms and queendoms by menacing overlords who ruled with iron fists. Often frightened kids fell into cliques or gangs under these monarchs, mimicking older students in nearby junior high schools marked by daily violence, fistfights, and stabbings.

Fay attended a real fortress, P.S. 119, a medieval dungeon surrounded by a great iron fence that attempted to wall out the dirt and misery of the streets. The squalor around it matched the pallor of the children's eyes, who played in her courtyard, a cemented area lined with broken windows hanging surreally like a menagerie of glass. These children had tasted penury and hunger, yet they mixed laughs and playfulness with their tears. God being good granted them that special gift. Sent by their parents with all hopes that education would unlock the gates and free them, they acted out the wanton destructiveness that poverty had wrought in their short lives.

Black teachers, funneled there rather than to better-equipped schools, worked with tremendous dedication to make their dreams a reality. Teachers like Mrs. Lawson and Mrs. Saxon taught my sister well, but their hard work was stultified by the dearth of books and supplies available to them. Systematic deprivation sounded its death knell, and all but a few were doomed to repeat the cycle of despair.

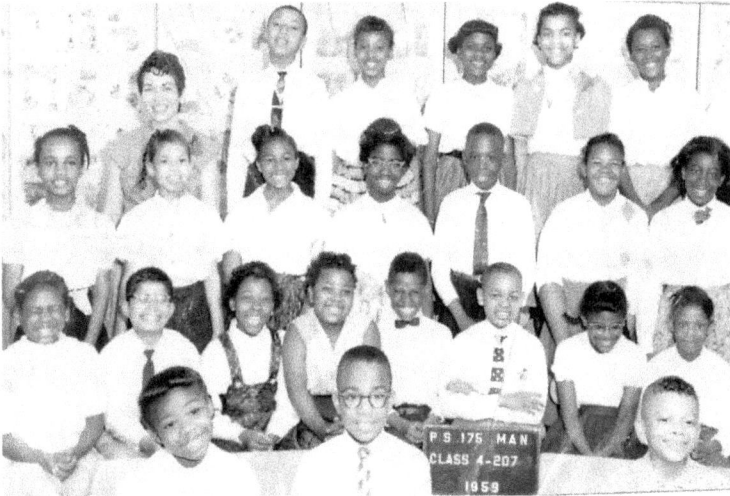

My class at P.S. 175 in Harlem.

Age placed Fay and me in school settings as different as could be, although the threat of violence loomed large at both. My school, P.S. 175, was newly constructed. Fortune had it that I marched in with the bumper crop of students passing through her doors on opening day to be greeted ceremoniously by those eagerly awaiting our arrival. Updated books were fixed at attention along the shelves and mirror glossed floors, as shiny as soldiers' shoes, lay underfoot. The closet, whose bulgy midriff attempted to hide a year's ration of supplies, contrasted sharply with the dressed pressed uniformity of the room. A contingent of new desks stood at allegiance, beneath Old Glory waving high above our heads, and a whistle clean slate board spread wide its chest, welcoming us like a proud commanding officer in salute. We, the new recruits, were happy to be there, realizing the educational advantage that was at hand.

Entry into the classroom required making it beyond the schoolyard, a challenge for me to use my wits rather than my fists. A trouble-seeking rabble-rouser and her party of insurgents positioned themselves at the mouth of the playground and badgered kids as they passed in or out. Those who let show their timidity were pounced on and beaten. Thus, the inception of my plan took shape to simply outrun them to keep away from a bloody encounter.

The moment the teacher parted the doors for recess, I leaped like a springbok into the air and sailed past the swell of students that surged through the gate. I never stopped until I reached the corner where the change of a light could save me from the onrushing crowd. In my haste, I didn't see the cavalcade of cars bearing down upon me. In a sudden spirt, I leaped again right into the path of a speeding vehicle! I was knocked to the ground, stunned, but not badly injured. Trembling like a wounded fawn, I wobbled to my feet, panicked, then darted wildly for home, telling no one of the accident. My incipience let a hit-and-run driver go free, but such is the folly that keeps company with youth. At least I learned two things that could harm me: the onsetting cars and the onslaught of kids. I am leery of both, cars and crowds, even until this day.

I timed my arrival back at school to the very second the bell rang and the wave of students crested within the halls squeezing in just as the monitors were closing the doors, offering an excuse. So convincing were my stories I was given a pass to go upstairs late every day.

It became my task to avoid all trouble spots where adults were not firmly in control, i.e., the cafeteria and the gym, by getting picked to go off and do special jobs for the teacher. At the end of the day, I gladly remained behind to clean the board, tidy up, and check the spelling papers. The job I liked best was watering the beautiful amaryllis plant whose trumpet-shaped blossoms faced the four winds and heralded each new day. Robed in fine scarlet, it stood regally near the window, beckoning in the morning sun and bidding the evenings adieu. Its petals were awash with the freshness of a rain shower, and in its bosom the wonder of nature lay hidden. I, the innocent child, was captivated by its delicateness and purity.

Looking at it, my thoughts embraced the world around me, the outer world beyond that place of mortar and stone; beyond want, destitution, desperation, and longing, dusty bricks piled high within her borders; beyond the vacant buildings, the trash, the piteous children trapped within the walls; beyond the junkies, the fast-money makers, and the white businessmen who fed like vultures on the carcasses of the poor to the pristine world that God created and surely intended all to enjoy.

I remember sowing seeds in a cut-off milk container, marveling when they grew, caring for them. It was my little portion of God's good earth, a quiet grassy place where I could run freely and be at peace—a place where the sun shone with glorious fulgence, the air was fresh, and the lilies were my forever friends. I frolicked there, played there in my mind. Time tiptoed past unnoticed. Soon the coast was clear and I could amble along home without fear.

Mom must have been frightened, too, by the problems she was having with Dad, but she held fast. Her strong Christian values provided substance to sustain her. To Mom, the commitment of marriage was a promise until death. She called it "graveyard love." In her generation, couples didn't jump to get a divorce when the going got rough. Besides having three small children, where would she go? What could she do? Go on home relief? No! There would be no welfare, just hard work and resourcefulness to keep the family going. When seasonal layoffs came at the bakery, she hired on as a maid for rich whites on Park Avenue downtown, scrubbing floors, cooking meals, nursing their sick, and bringing home their discards to fill in for what we didn't have. Dad despised "white folks garbage," but Mom cleaned it up and put it to good use, not being one to let pride get in the way of practicality.

Hardship taught Mom to always make the best of what she had. What industry helped her to acquire, frugality allowed her to keep by careful budgeting, paying bills, and planning modest meals. The large tins of oily peanut butter, boxes of cheese, and bricks of butter passed on by neighbors were heartily welcomed at our house. Each day lunch consisted of peanut butter and jelly sandwiches and a glass of milk mixed from powder. For dinner Mom cooked pig's ears, feet, neck bones, oxtail, collard greens and ham hocks, black-eyed peas and fatback meat, fried chicken, or soups made with wings, gizzards, and the like, all seasoned soul food style with herbs and spices. This was basically Southern cuisine dating back to slavery days when blacks were given unfavorable parts of meat and appendages to eat, while their masters feasted upon the choicer cuts. We kids, not being fond of Southern fare, ate beans and franks and drank Kool-Aid with our meal.

Mom stretched her dollars by shopping along East 125th Street in Spanish Harlem and along Delancey Street in lower Manhattan, where she haggled with Jews for cheap wares on outdoor stands. Dad purchased a 1959 Pontiac, black and pink with cat-eyed tail-lights. Then he drove us to a place in the South Bronx known as La Marketa, where foods sold in bulk for reasonable prices. There we bought pounds of meat and chicken in bags, sacks of potato, fresh fruits, vegetables, and dried beans.

Next day, there would be chicken feet dangling from our pots, as if some cuckoo bird had taken a nose dive and landed headfirst in our stew, which we found laughable. On Fridays, cold fish eyes stared up at us from the platter, and razor-sharp teeth captured in an eerie smile lay frozen in the grips of death. These were Dad's favorites— porgies, fried golden brown and laid to rest on a bed of onions. If Dad happened on a coon, he put the whole carcass in a roasting pan, head, feet, teeth, and all, then baked him. What a surprise to come to the table for Sunday dinner and find a snarling animal, with claws bared to fend off attack, embalmed in gravy.

Dad was a real Florida man at heart. For him wild coon was a delicacy and a palatable reminder of home; for us, it was a macabre remembrance of some poor creature who died that we might live and a palpable example of Dad's wry humor.

We liked going shopping with Dad because he could never resist a little naughtiness. Spotting juicy grapes and ripe strawberries on the fruit stands, he was tempted to pluck off a few and gobble them down quickly when he thought no one was looking. We snick-ered at Dad's apparent mischief, but he reasoned, for all the money he spent, he was entitled to a few little extras. I guess it was the same reasoning that led him to dalliances outside of marriage for "little extras." He continued to fill his wanderlust at bars on the corner, the Big Apple, and Smalls Paradise, where the music was always thump-ing and crowds jumping. He returned home, nightly, bringing his money and a woman's perfume that reeked haughtily from his person. It shouted; Mom shouted. So it went time and time again.

We ghetto kids had our first glimpse into the homes of white Americans via television, which had just begun to boom. Color sets debuted on the market in the fifties, but being hard-pressed, we could hardly afford one. Therefore, we tuned in to all of America's favorite family shows—*Father Knows Best, Leave It to Beaver, I Love Lucy, The Donna Reid Show, Ozzie and Harriet*—on our monochrome set. These portraitures of white working-class families who enjoyed all the trappings of the American dream—a house in a nice neighborhood with a car in the driveway, a dad with a good job, and a mom who stayed at home tending well-dressed kids—were in opposition to the lives we led. Material and social inequities were obvious between blacks and whites.

Feelings of resentment garnered up as we began to make comparisons. We did not have what they had, and where we lived didn't look like where they lived. Things didn't happen for us like it happened for them. We wondered why. Who was at fault? Were we to blame? I quickly surmised that we were not a part of "that America," nor were we one of "those families." I knew Mom and Dad both worked hard and couldn't understand why we didn't live as well as they did. I saw the people who had all the goodies were white, and those who didn't were not. I linked whiteness with wealth and success and blackness with poverty and failure. Television played a tremendous role in shaping racial attitudes, especially when intergroup contact languished, helping to form exaggerated perceptions.

There were many positive images projected in these shows that we wanted to emulate. They were excellent models of wholesome family life based on traditional values teaching by example, moral and immoral conduct. Parents were projected as authority figures who solved problems with humor and understanding. Children, though mischievous at times, were generally respectful and obedient. And the roles of men and women were as clearly defined as the clothing styles for each. The line between right and wrong didn't seem as hazy as it does now, making it easier then to get bearings on where you were headed and know the parameters within which you were to function. Those shows are criticized as having been too ideal, but at least they presented a standard, unlike today when anything goes and brattiness is looked on as cute.

Other TV influences were the Western movies like *Gunsmoke, The Rifle Man, The Lone Ranger*, adventure stories of good guys versus the bad guys. We traveled nightly on *Wagon Train* with frontier families as they struggled against the elements, rough terrain, and Indians to establish their settlements in the West, held together by dreams of a better life. Their dreams weren't so different from our dreams, since our parents likewise had come north looking for betterment too. What enabled them to establish prairie towns, then cities, which evolved into a fully modernized society? Who held the reins of power is what made the difference.

In the Western movies, the law was a white man with a badge and a shiny revolver, often riding upon a white horse defending the rights of good, upstanding, law-abiding, God-fearing citizens who also happened to be white. The villain, usually dressed in black attire with dark skin and scruffy hair straddling a dark mare, portrayed menacing robbers, outlaws, or Indians who threatened the status quo. I came to view whites as virtuous and good and blacks as evil and ugly.

We cheered for the white heroes and shot all the Indians down as they yipped and yelled, galloping across our screen. Somehow stirring faintly down in my gut was a sense that I was one of the Indians, not one of the cowboys, for we weren't welcomed in the camp, nor did we eat from their warm hearth. Some said we were like savages too, yet our wilderness was right in their midst, not in the far-off hills.

It seemed only white people had a right to fight for their way of life and authority to dominate others, keeping their position of power by sanction of the law. The Indians, portrayed as wild renegades, somehow deserved to be slaughtered. It mattered not that the Indians were the true Native Americans defending their homeland and the settlers were the ones who came, raped the land of gold and ore, killed the bison, and took away sacred ground.

The few blacks appearing in these movies were freed slaves, bootblacks, butlers, or handmaidens, always docile, silly minded, subservient characters ready with a "Yez suh, boss!" to do the white man's bidding. Both the Indians and blacks were pictured as sub-groups that didn't belong, but the white man, in his "benevolence," allotted small reservations of land where the Indians could be cordoned off and built shanties behind the main house for the black servants to be close enough to render service yet isolated from the mainstream of wealth and opportunity. And so we remained, even until that day, cordoned off in the ghettoes, the urban centers, on the south side of town, or the other side of the track.

The underlying message came across that the white man had inherent rights because of his "superiority," giving him authority to rule "inferior races," who like children needed his guidance and direction. He had power, both economic and political, and could manipulate the mechanisms of government, i.e., the laws, and civilian and military forces, to maintain control. He was naturally entitled to the land, its wealth, and a high style of living. After all, hadn't his descendants come here from Europe, built this country with their toil and sweat impassioned by high ideals of freedom, justice, and equality and guided by good Christian values? He exalted himself as a champion of the rights of free men and America as a bastion of liberty and good conscience.

We bought into that illusion, denied the dichotomy of the message, ignored our experiential realities, and held steadfastly to those ideals, which, by the very existence of Harlem, confounded their lofty premise. We existed in a vacuum, cut off from the mainstream yet wanted to feel a part of a society of honorable men. So we listened to what white America told us about itself through the tube and what it told us about ourselves as well. We lived one reality physically, while another reality was being shaped in our minds. This was in part because we were as much cut off from ourselves and the positive things people in our community had done and were still doing as we were from the society at large.

We children didn't know we were living in the midst of a black renaissance or that our community was a black cultural center of writers, musicians, artists, and entertainers. The white media did not promulgate that information in the way that it told the world of our crimes and violence, our slothfulness and dependency. We knew nothing of the efforts of W. E. B. Du Bois, Marcus Garvey, Elijah Muhammed, or Malcolm X to bring leadership to our people. We were too young to have read the outstanding writings of Langston Hughes, Richard Wright, and James Baldwin. Mom and Dad were not avid readers, except for *The Daily News*, which was brimming with stories of our destructiveness and misdeeds. We didn't have black publications in our home like *The Amsterdam News*, *Jet*, or *Ebony* magazine; we couldn't afford them. We were exposed to the blues and rock 'n' roll artists on soul music stations. We never saw fine performances of singing artists like Paul Robeson and Marian Anderson. We were not familiar with the struggles of the young senator from Harlem, Adam Clayton Powell, to bring attention to our problems on Capitol Hill. We had seen Jackie Robinson play but didn't understand the importance of his breaking the color line in baseball. And we didn't know just how great Dad's favorite boxer, Joe Louis, was in the fighting world. Nor did we hear of the courageous act of one simple yet dignified black woman, Rosa Parks, who refused to give up her seat on a bus in the South, starting what would become the civil rights movement.

We grew in painful ignorance to view the white man as the paradigm of goodness and truth and the black man as a dark, mysterious figure, a "boogie man," evil and foreboding by nature, making us even afraid of ourselves. And so we put leotards on our minds and flew around with Superman fighting for truth, justice, and the American way. We didn't stop to notice there were no blacks in the America that this superhero fought for. We swung through the trees with Tarzan and Cheetah as they conquered the "dark continent of Africa." We never questioned why "Bwana Jim" was able to communicate with the animals of Africa and strove to protect them against hunters and treasure seekers, but could make no emotional connection with the peoples of Africa, choosing rather to live in a tree alone.

There are Tarzans today who parade up and down Fifth Avenue, placards raised, harping about the slaughter of animals to make fur coats, toxic wastes killing fishes, pollutants killing the birds, and the destruction of the rainforests endangering our wildlife, as they step over the carcasses of broken and hungry black men lying in the streets of their cities. Can they feel nothing for this endangered species or see the blight on their withering lives?

I soon found myself hopelessly hooked on the Mickey Mouse Club, having fallen in love with the angelic Annette Funicello. In her, I saw everything I wanted to be. I longed to have a petite doll figure, a cherubic face, a button nose, twinkling eyes, an alluring smile, long hair, and white skin. I envied this little "darling of America" for the way she captured TV audiences with her mantle of saccharin sweetness. I wanted to reach out and hold her, just as I held my white dolls, dressed them oh, so prettily, and combed their silken hair. I cuddled them, cradled them, and loved them, for they were not like me. They were "perfect." I was not! To be as they were, I thought, would make my world a different place. That was seemingly impossible, so I latched on to Spanky, Alfalfa, and the other kids in the Clubhouse Gang, tagging along daily like Buckwheat while enjoying their amusing antics.

We made incursions downtown on the school bus into lower Manhattan to see how the other half lived. Kids from Harlem arrived by the bus loads at city-run clinics for free drillings and fillings. Some of the dental work was needed, the rest perhaps not. Nevertheless, every one of us got. Dentists pocketed more than a few shekels of silver for all the silver they put in our mouths. I have them to blame for my tin foil smile today, having had most of my porcelain drilled away. Said I was prone to tooth decay; I say their ethics had long since decayed because they knew the city paid.

The school caravan slipped by our somberly attired dwellings, the jumbled patchwork of tenements we called home, amid rubbish piles, abandoned cars, and broken telephones to a medley of street signs, old churches, lots overflowing with trash, greasy spoons, bodegas, and pawnshops trading for quick cash—leaving behind the derelicts who awakened with no place to go (no job, no home or anything) even though they had worked in times past, been in the Army too. Some were a little crazy now, but who cared? Who knew?

Zipping through the hydrant sprays falling like drops of rain in filthy puddles of water that raced eagerly down the drains, on past the projects and playgrounds with broken swings filled with hordes of people doing ordinary things. Peering through my window, it all just seemed so strange reaching 110th Street and witnessing the change.

There was Central Park, an island of emerald green, with gentle knolls, woodland trails, and a quiet rippling stream, across from luxury apartments with doormen standing by to greet stylish ladies whose noses touched the sky. Pampered poodles sauntered behind as they carried shopping bags from potpourri-scented boutiques with expensive-looking rags. Street vendors sold hotdogs to youngsters at the zoo, popcorn, peanuts, candy, and cold drinks too. Past magnificent museums, embassies with foreign flags, chauffeur-driven Mercedes with gilded license tags, by gushing water fountains that danced a merry jig like a ruddy Irish captain steppin' on the brig. From balconies to roof gardens life effervesced, fresh as the trailing ivies growing well on affluence, on to Columbus Circle with cabs racing every which way, to a grand hotel whose guests could well afford to pay.

There were horse-drawn carriages that looked like long ago, lovers teetering in back, whispering ever so low. But their voices susurrating softly couldn't possibly be heard above the traffic cadence and our hearts own painful words saying, "Look around you! See the luster of wealth everywhere? You are nothing because you have nothing. You people just don't care! You're marked with a brand. You're black!" As the saying goes, "Can anything good come from Nazareth? Or Harlem? No!" From those trips we brought back a lot of pain. For what we were we felt ashamed.

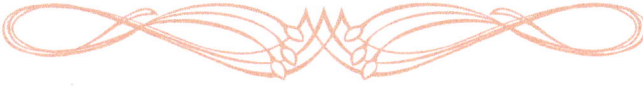

CHAPTER FOUR
A Goodly Heritage

THERE were family excursions down south to stay each summer with Mom's mother at her little house out in the country. She lived there alone, for Grandpa had since passed away. Just before our trip, the air was hot and tingling with excitement as the spirit of adventure made light all the preparations Mom would surely make. A mound of chicken was fried up, wrapped in aluminum foil, and tucked neatly in our lunch bag along with hot breads, cake, and a thermos of Kool-Aid. Its spicy aroma seasoned the interior of Dad's car, masking the staleness of the old carpet and the well-worn leather of his seats. Suitcases packed, we took off by night across the George Washington Bridge, down Highway 95, to Greensboro, North Carolina—a thirteen-hour journey. We rode cozily, three children nestled in the back, Mom and Dad in front for the long ride.

As we passed the slaughterhouse in New Jersey, effluvium from billowing smokestacks fouled the air. We jested with each other that someone had pooted and tried mockingly to find the culprit. Our raillery raised the roof and frazzled Mom's unsteady nerves.

Soon the monotonous march of road signs, like tin soldiers on parade to the constant drone of the motor, lulled us into blissful quietude. The lampblack sky was dark as tar; silence rained softly as dew. Peaceful towns and villages slumbering by the highway yawned, blinked, and snuggled under for a few more winks. Their welcome lamps snuffed out; shades like sleepy eyelids fell. Porch swings screeched owlishly in the halting still. The scene caught hold of my thoughts as I pondered on who lived there and what lives were like therein. I wondered, if we got off any exit and knocked on any door, would we be welcomed? Nah! We were but sojourners in a strange land, passing through, never to enter in.

Twenty-four-hour filling stations held vigil, like sentries keeping watch in the night, lonely outposts for wayfaring strangers traveling by the moon's hoary light to cities fire dancing in the distance as we, half sleeping, enjoyed the sight.

A panoply of luminous signs wore halos against the blackness. White streams of diamond headlights poured down from the other lanes. Their blinding sparkle outshone tiny specks of stars sprinkled, like salt, across the ebonite sky. My eyes focused on the red star fire taillights up ahead, blazing a trail as far as I could see. Yellow pavement lines hypnotically led me down this path endlessly stretching toward eternity. The restful rocking of the car put us to sleep while visions of Grandma's sun-sweet smile filled our dreams.

Suddenly, we were frightened by the rumble of a tractor trailer truck and feared this silver monster would swallow us up. Roaring like a dreadful monster going by, thrusting its mighty head into the sky, it breathed through its nostrils thick black smoke and shook the earth as we awoke. But it moved on without a peep as we, trembling, went back to sleep.

We awakened next day to a rooster's crow and saw a merry mist in the meadows. The sun smiled radiantly across pastel-painted skies. Wispy clouds rolled over hills and valleys laden with fruit trees and vines. Clay fields extended in all directions. An old plow reached back in time to days when slaves worked those blazoning fields, planting row by row as they sang of an old sweet chariot coming to carry them home. Big-bellied cows grazed lazily in green pastureland. Coifs of gold twirled on green ears of corn. Honeybees hummed a summer sonata as we arose that sun-drenched morning.

Graceful pines gathered by the roadside, like old friends chatting hours without a care, spreading wide scented branches, fanning the sweet, sultry air. Looking up, with blue-green boughs shading their balsam brows, they longed to drink from God's refreshing wellspring, wished it wouldn't stay so dry, and waved genteelly as we sped by.

After riding many hours without stopping, Daddy said we could get out, stretch our limbs, and buy Cokes at the nearest rest stop before completing the last leg of our journey along the old dusty route to Bass Chapel, the little cove in the country where Grandma lived. We pulled up to a small diner, tired, dry, and seized with cramps from the wearisome ride. We kids sprang happily from the car, charged through the door, popped up on the red counter stools, and spun around playfully as we gaspingly demanded soda from the waitress. We were too caught up with excitement to notice the hard gaze of the patrons sitting there. But as the atmosphere turned chillier than the crushed ice in the soda fountain, we felt their eyes peeled upon us.

I was sure it was because we had gotten carried away whirling wildly on the stools, so I promptly collected myself, sat straight and tall, even folded my hands, embarrassed that my momentary abandon had caused such a stir. As we glanced around the room, icy stares rolled off bent shoulders, traced us up and down, and held us in an unyielding grip. Glowering faces, flushed with unmasked hatred, defamed us without speaking. Their glimmering expressions cried out "What are you doing in here? You don't belong! Get out! We despise you!" as clearly as the handwriting on the wall.

I felt dejected and confused, not understanding what I did wrong. Could my spinning have offended them so greatly? I thought to apologize, but just at that moment, Mom came in, saw us, quickly shooed us from the seats, and sternly insisted that we get out of there, lowering her head apologetically as she went. "We will go around back and get our Cokes!" she said resolvedly, although I thought she was kidding. Following her outside, I tugged at her dress tail and inquired the reason for their anger. She told us colored people were not allowed to sit and be served at food counters with whites. For service, we had to line up at the back door, have food passed out to us, and stand and eat near an open garbage receptacle with large green flies circling about. Mom accepted this as the way things were, having grown up in the South, but I was filled with indignation. Whites hated us without reason; it was unfair! My insides churned with rage.

I will never forget that place, those people, or their vilifying eyes burning with hostility and the bitter rejection that permeated the air inside that diner. The experience seared my childish spirit as with a hot iron. My early life was shaped by those who loved me and those who refused to love me. The wound, still there today, easily reopens to seethe, fester, and ooze with pain. It's a stabbing sensation that makes me want to cry out and wrench my hands in agony. But I bear it silently, for I am not alone. It's a feeling many people of color have known in my home, America.

Some would say that was the South in the 1950s before the civil rights movement. Now we are in a new era; all of that is past, never to return again. There is no bigotry anymore, they say. We have equal rights for all, they say. We walk hand in hand into the light of a new day, they say. We hide behind colorful slogans and nice-sounding rhetoric, having learned to put a good face on everything while hiding our inner most conflicts. We try to deny the hate, which is like a consuming fire, implacable, never satisfied, and lusting to be fed. Some are active haters, and some stand passively by and say, "Well, that's just the way it is!" Both have a part in things remaining as they are.

I have looked into the face of hate and will never forget its vitriolic repugnance. Sadly, I still see it when I pass through all white neighborhoods or go in certain stores or businesses in large metropolitan centers such as New York, not to mention smaller suburban and rural communities. In some ways, it's worse now because it's not blatantly obvious like store signs posted in the windows in the Old South that read, "No colored allowed!" Rather, it lurks around or sits, insidiously staring, musing, mocking, restraining, wounding, and covering itself up in the cloak of everydayness in American life. It sits so close we can't see that it's there. We are so at home with it; it's like a member of the family. We dare not kick it out; we wouldn't know what to do without it. It galvanizes us, keeps us strong yet apart. We go on living by a tarnished rule taught to us by our parents behind closed doors that says, "You hate me, and I'll hate you back!"

If we can't hear the rumblings in our cities, can't we see the handwriting that's still on the wall? We have a lot of new legislation on the books, but we can't legislate the heart of America. What will it take to purge out what lies within its deepest recesses? We can't go back and change the actions or decisions of our ancestors, but we can make decisions to honor and respect each other now. A house divided against itself cannot stand.

Around midday we traced the meandering dirt road leading out to the countryside. My heart leapt with joy, knowing Grandma sat watching vigilantly to see the dust cloud rise from our wheels as we crossed by way of the rickety bridge, a beautiful woodland inlet, home to wild ducks, bellowing toads and songbirds of myriad colors, all joining in a welcoming chorus. Dad hailed a cheery hello honking the horn in a tune as we passed Uncle William's house, then Aunt Lillie's and Aunt Nannie's, turning in at the old church yard at the mouth of the cul-de-sac, rounding the bend hewn by tire tracks below Uncle Arthur's, stopping finally at the rural post box in front of Grandma's door.

Grandma was so delighted she jumped in a frenzy, clapped her hands, and shouted with joy, "Lawdee, look-a-here, look-a-here!" then she kissed us all, patted us welcomingly, and held us close to her breasts, affirming our belonging to her and her pleasure at seeing us again. Feeling immediately at home, we climbed up on her porch swing and savored the happy tides that filled the air as word traveled up and down the road that we had come from New York.

Cars soon filled the front yard; family members came out hurriedly to receive us. More warm greetings, hugs, and "Hi yous?" ensued until Grandma's aged white frame house nearly burst its girdling boards with uproarious laughter. Not long after, Grandma's shaky voice, frail as the gray hairs tucked beneath her net, called feebly, "Y'all come on in here and git you somethin' to eat!" That signaled the serving of the biggest feast God ever put on the table, all one could eat—fried chicken, country ham, homemade biscuits, greens, garden vegetables, potato salad, butter cakes, and sweet potato pie.

Once everyone's tummy was full and the excitement of our arrival subsided, it was time for the older folk to sit out on the porch and catch up on family news. Being without telephones gave no opportunity to keep in touch regularly. There was a lot to chat about. I positioned myself within earshot, looking wide-eyed and listening keenly as each inquired about another. "When's the last time you seen this one or that one? How's he doing?" My ears never missed the prattle of personal affairs supposedly kept hushed but told with such amusing candor the afternoon was spent on gaff and fond remembrances. They spilled it all. "Child, did you hear this about so and so? Don't tell nobody, but…!" Suddenly voices dropped inaudibly, and hand-covered lips beat like mixer blades while dancing eyes patrolled for spies who overheard, not realizing their most attentive listeners were eavesdropping from between their legs as we sat crouched at the knee. They paid us no mind; we were "just kids" becoming well informed on the way things went, listening silently with great content.

As the evening's cool approached, the chatter took a more serious turn, discussion of hard times and crisis some had weathered, persons who suffered illness or loss. Playful moths teased and chased about the dim porch light after dusk as they rocked back and forth in slat-seated chairs, looking back and remembering times past, knowing where they'd come from and how God brought them through. Someone would start an old gospel tune. Others sang along, patted their knees, and thumped the floor as sharing turned into an emotional outpouring, especially if Uncle William, the minister, was present. He was the family anchor and constant reminder of God dwelling with them. They gave each other consolation with the words "God will make a way somehow."

After the release through song and sometimes prayer, there would be a peace, a quietness that enriched the moment. Old folks had hope because they could look forward to the day they were going over yonder and lay their burdens down. Daddy loved one song, which said,

> When I get through toiling,
> Out in the sunshine and out in the rain,
> I'm going home to live with Jesus
> Oh! Won't it be grand?

In small southern towns in the '50s, even the basics were hard to come by. Prosperity hadn't yet arrived, and poor folks were leaning on each other, waiting for it to come. Families had to pull together because they were all they had. There was no government aid, ADC or Medicaid. It was family that filled in when an unmarried daughter popped up pregnant or when someone's husband up and left or when a widow struggled to raise small children or when somebody's son was under arrest. They just did what they could and asked the Lord to do the rest. I felt their bonds, saw their strength, and easily identified with what they were going through. It helped put things happening to us into perspective. I experienced oneness with them and gained a sense of family history as they told tales transcending past generations, finding humor in every circumstance with a story-teller's art.

After a fervent efflux of thoughts and feelings touching good times and painful periods, there would be a rise again in the mood, a feeling that came full circle around that somehow it would all work together for good. They said their goodbyes and went back home, ready to face life a little bit more.

I loved the elders and enjoyed their down-home style, warmth, and open hospitality. God's abiding presence with them was clearly revealed in expressions like "Lord have mercy!" "Praise the Lord!" "Thank you, Jesus!" frequently interjected in lively colloquy. His praise was always on their lips. He was as near as the little stick-handled fans from Bass Chapel found in every room of the house. Paper fans made the torrid air more bearable. Christ's presence made struggling lives more sufferable. I saw that although they suffered, they were not emotionally miserable because of their faith.

Bass Chapel was the name of the Methodist church nearby, a place of family worship central to the community. Everyone attended regularly, wanting to be guided by Christian tenets, although they didn't always act accordingly. They believed the Lord "knew their hearts" and understood such shortcomings. Not having a lot of material wealth, they were rich in experience and willing to share what God blessed them with. They lived long lives filled with hard work and honest laughter—lives as entwined as the vine-clad trees laced with threads of lush greenery, woven topiaries pruned and cultivated by the master vinedresser.

When death came, burial would be in a family plot on the church grounds. The younger generation who had slowly moved away would return to the same church for the "big meetin'," a type of yearly spiritual revival, a time when they fellowshipped with one another, recognized new members through birth or marriage, and visited the graves of those who had gone on before. In this way, continuity between generations was kept and traditions passed down from the old to the young. One day, by and by, their bodies would be shipped back home for burial and their children would have children. The process was regenerative and progenitive.

In this day, when so many children long for attention and recognition, for a pat on the back, so to speak, it is good to look back and remember the old people—how they understood the need for affirmation and unconditional love, since they literally patted us often, held us near, and gave big kisses, even to those who were a little troublesome. Looking back, knowing from whence they came gave them a strong sense of identity and wholeness so that they could teach us not to do bad things, not only because they were wrong, but also because they brought disgrace on the family name.

Today we think a big house or a fine car will bring us joy, but their joy was not connected to external circumstances. They knew how to be up and how to be down, in all things to be content, as they were close to God. Although their outlook might have been dark because of the difficult circumstances in which they lived, their uplook was always bright.

That night we slept in one plump bed in Grandma's room, a feather bed soft as down on a dandelion seed, but not before having a wash-up in an old foot tub filled with water from the well. Grandma heated the black iron kettle until steam swirled up from its great potbelly. Lugging it two-handed by its coils, she warmed the bath to a temperateness measured by her fingers. We climbed in for a splash.

A firm scrub followed with brown soap made from fat drippings and lye of our faces and hands, in our ears, across the neck, under the arms, down the back, over the bottom, hard against the knees, dipping to the toes in one fell swoop. When finished, we looked two shades lighter and smelled fresh as green grass after a dew shower. The rule was, "You couldn't go to bed until you'd washed your feet. No red dirt on sun-whitened sheets!"

She gave us each a turn on the piss pot with a chuckle and a chide, "Good night, sleep tight. Don't let the bed bugs bite!" Bemused by her admonition, I was sure not to make a slip as I was leery of crawling things. But little brother Sonny leaked all over the sheets. It's no wonder I couldn't sleep listening for the march of creepy little feet!

I lay awake, eyelids fluttering to the beat of raindrops playing pitter-patter against the roof. Soon the tapping tenor became a rumbling tympany, lightning clapped a mighty cymbal, and a sudden flash effulged in the darkness, filling the room with terrifying light. I cowered beneath the colorful patchwork quilt, pulled a pillow over my head, and cuddled close to my big sister, Fay, for shelter. For many years to come, I sought refuge with her in times of storm just as when we were little girls. She hid me behind her jovial, outgoing personality, and I supported her with my strong silence. We were most times an inseparable pair.

Grandma, hearing the squeals of her three little piglets, came in, lit the kerosene oil lamp, and placed it near our bed. Its gently flickering flame contrasted the rolling thunder cracking the sky outside. It was as quiet and comforting as the lightning was frightening. Grandma had a special wisdom, knowing what to do in every instance.

The scent of slab bacon and eggs frying on the old-fashioned wood stove called us from bed that morning. Grandma had awakened early, gone to the hen house, drawn water, peeled green apples, fried them in sugar and butter, taken down jellies and preserves from the cupboard, and brought out the jar of thick molasses to pour over the biscuits she'd hidden above the stove to keep warm. I saw the place but would need to stand on the tinderbox to reach them. A good little girl wouldn't take her grandma's biscuits, so I just sat around after breakfast, smiled demurely, and cast my eyes upward, hoping she'd give them to me. She, seeing my begging eyes, did oblige. Happily I dipped one in syrup, devoured it all in one gulp, and let the melted butter ooze down my chin as I sucked the sugary cane from my fingertips. Grandma tolerated my unladylike behavior; for that I gave her a gooey smooch. I'm sure it wasn't enjoyed equally! Somehow she managed to knead her sweetness into the bread, which I will always remember.

Heavy ironstone dishes decorated the table, but there were no glasses. Small grape jelly jars washed and saved weekly were given to us to drink from. When really thirsty, we didn't use a glass at all, just climbed up on a ladder-back chair and took a cool swig of well water from the dipper. It was wonderfully fresh and alive with good taste, a real thirst quencher unlike the trendy spring and bottled waters popular lately. Back in New York, that sure wasn't the case!

After breakfast Fay dressed and waited for a ride to town, preferring city life. I was content to traipse around the house and explore, room to room, Grandma's simple treasures. My heart was always in the country.

A speckled cat was in its wonted place in the tinderbox beside the stove. I poked at its sides, disturbing its rest to get wood for the yearning fire. He hesitantly uncurled, stretched, and scampered away as I selected a fine dry piece and pushed it through the little fire door to the stove's belly. Red-hot sparks lit the smoldering embers that cooled again to a warm glow. The ambient air, fragrant with burning wood, lent the flavor of yesterday to the hearth. I toyed with it using an iron bar to lift the eyes and see the flame. Grandma cautioned me to stop before burning my hands.

As I sat on a narrow row of steps leading to the attic, curiosity took hold. I climbed up stealthily like her old cat, counting one, two, three as I went, then opened the latch and peered into the dark abyss partially covered by dusty spiderwebs. One came out inquisitively to see who had invaded its haunt, but finding only a prying child, it crept away unoffended. Groping around in the blackness, I thought I heard a ghastly voice howl from the rafters. Did some ancient spirit dwell secretly above our heads and slip down at night for Grandma's bread? Fraidy Cat Jean wasn't hanging around to find out! I quickstepped backward down the stairs and into the small room where Grandma slept in search of other discoverables.

I found it captivating as much for what it lacked as what it held. There was no elaborate furniture, telephone, or TV—no gadgets, thingamabobs, toiletries, or finery—no carpeting or lamplighting either. She did have a single metal-frame bed whose mattress had sunk under her weight and that of her children and their children who slept there as needed. It was covered with a gay handstitched quilt that contrasted the plainness of the walls left bare except for a curio of pressed flowers under glass and a store calendar she didn't need. Her mind had its own natural almanac telling the time to plant vegetables, kill hogs, harvest fruits, and put up foods for winter.

The bed was right below one bright shroudless window. When lying there, she could feel the beams of the glorious sun shine down upon her face, look into its countenance, and enjoy intimate closeness with God. It laughed with her when times were good. Heaven wept when times were bad. She was never alone. A hand-tooled chest was positioned at the foot of the bed. On it were pill bottles, a small comb and nets for her hair, a Sunday purse with a handkerchief inside, a black velvet hat veiled in front to protect her piety, a rosary, and obituaries of those who had gone to be with the Lord.

Grandpa's hat, corn pipe, and spittoon, used when he chewed tobacco, made it appear he still abode with her. His baggy pants rested on the back of the chair. His old felt slippers (hers now) lay underneath.

One hard seated rocker marred the creaky floor where she sat up nights praying her children would not go astray, reading a black Bible with crinkled edges curled by age. In it, she had written dates of birth, marriage, and death of loved ones. Whom the Lord had given her, she placed with Him for safekeeping.

Behind this room was Aunt Josie's, Grandma's stepmother. She lived there and was taken care of until she died of old age. Her clothing, few possessions, and a tiny bed were left in place just as they had been for many years. The room retained the flat, musty odor of her snuff box and old shoes. I was sure her ghost slept there at night, even to that day, because it had a piss pot like the one in my room! Could that be who called to me from the hidden place above the stairs?

It seemed as if four generations resided in this home, great-grandparents in one room, Grandma and Pa in another, and the larger bedroom set aside for the thirty-two grands and thirteen great-grands who were soon to come. There was space for all, tying together past, present, and future generations. She maneuvered comfortably between them, knowing her place was assured in glory and in the treasure box of our hearts.

The front room was a tidy parlor with sofa, chairs, end tables, and a center rug all acquired over years of tending house for whites or selling vegetables door to door. It was a warm room dressed to greet visitors but seldom used. Guests often sat in the kitchen around the table where they laughed, talked, and ate. Grandma was not one for formalities, but she made sure everyone was fed and felt like family in her home.

While she and Mom chitchatted over coffee, I ambled on outside to see where she got the pretty brown eggs we had for breakfast. To my delight, I found two warm eggs in a lofty nest in the henhouse, but the chickens had gone out for a stroll. I ventured along the path leading to a quiet mud pond brimming with polliwogs, cattails, and flitting dragonflies. All that could be heard was the call of wild birds, an occasional splash of frogs into the water, and the shrill song of the katydids hiding playfully amid blades of grass. The surrounding scape was a serene forest, which touched the hem of a pure blue sky with the crests of its towering pines. I was enchanted by the tranquil beauty of this place and rested peaceably upon a rock, eyes riveted to the spot where the last frog submerged, hoping he would emerge again. As my long wait proved fruitless, I slipped away knowing snakes were drawn, as I was, to secret places.

I crept up by a wire pigsty where lived an old sow being fattened for slaughter at season's end. I tossed a pail of corncobs into the trough and watched laughingly as she wiggled her snout and grunted her gratefulness for the treat. Using a forked branch, I scraped dry mud from her sides while cooing silly names, making fun of her portly figure. For a moment, I was called off into the world of daydreams by the stillness that encompassed me about. Suddenly I snapped back, sought to poke her with the stick, but she'd disappeared!

Turning again, there she was outside the pen, pacing, grumbling, and warning me that she hadn't taken my waggish remarks too kindly. I panicked and took off running with the old girl hot on my heels. In a mad dash, I burst through the screen door to find safety behind Mama's dress tail. Grandma hollered, "Shoo, pig! Git! Git!" The angry hog reluctantly obeyed and returned to its pen, having proven her point to this little city slicker.

Gram said it was okay for me to go back out with a confidence that came from knowing animals as well as people. This time, I steered clear of that direction, choosing rather to practice winding the rope to lower the bucket into the well and called down to the earth spirits, "Fill 'er up!" They promptly answered in echoes from the depths below, sending up a pail of water every time. Tiring of that game, I sat and braided slender stalks of grass into dolls, naming each and tying on bits of rag to make ribbons for their hair.

Soon a mother hen crossed the yard with her breast raised in a proud strut, her brood of fluffy yellow chicks wobbling behind. I jumped up and ran, stooping with two hands outstretched to catch one of the babies, wanting only to cuddle it. Somehow I tripped and stepped on one, killing it instantly. My heart sank! I felt so cruel having snuffed out the life of a gentle, helpless creature. I had come to this lovely environ with majestic trees and animals roaming freely and became so enraptured. In my zeal, I destroyed a part of it and couldn't put it back.

I wanted Grandma to whip my legs with the switch she kept beside the stove so that I could pay in pain for what I had done. It would have been kinder than the lash of guilt I trounced myself with a thousand times over without requite. I hid, sobbed, and bore welts on the inside, unable to forgive myself. I learned that day that some things are best left alone; at times that is the most loving thing to do. It was a valuable lesson.

I sought solace from my troubles at Aunt Nannie's with her kids Henry Clay, Annie Lee, and Nina Mae. Amusingly their voices rang with a twang in draggy Southern style. My Northern lingo seemed peculiar to them too, so we parroted each other back and forth. My attempts to interest them in other childish endeavors, such as rum-

71

maging through the watermelon patch plucking for ripe, sweet melons or sitting in the graveyard whispering ghost stories, were useless.

Being older, they were intrigued with romance and sought lessons in matters of love, watching the twisted episodes of the daytime soap *As the World Turns*. They were tantalized by glamorous stars who kissed, fell in love, and married, then boredom set in and then betrayal. Sequel after sequel dramatized the perilous lives of lost souls caught up in a travesty of love with all the wrong people for the wrong reasons—people who had wealth and material goods, yet their lives were filled with woe.

This was sort of a dry run for the approaching time when they would reel out into the dating pool and try hard to pull in a prize catch. Being only eight, I wasn't interested in boys, and it sparked concerns I hadn't given prior thought to outside the realm of fantasy. Unfortunately, it set treacherous groundwork for the development of a fragile self-image in relation to the opposite sex, when coupled with the problems I saw acted out between my parents at home.

The thought of establishing intimacy with someone became fraught with fear of usury and estrangement. I turned down my emotions, holding them inward for fear that I would love someone and lose them just as Mama and I were losing Daddy. I developed a view that I could never hold Daddy or any other man's love because I was unworthy. That feeling of unworthiness plagued me throughout my growing-up years and on into adulthood.

Aunt Nannie was a woman with limited income and lots of children, a dear sweet soul who would take her heart out and give it to you if she could. She lived close to Grandma in a house barely more than a shack up the road. She came often to borrow a few eggs, a cup of sugar—small things to get by—walking barefoot with her youngest suckling, George Junior, nursing happily from the large black nipple of her exposed breast. The skin about her knees was calloused and blackened from kneeling and picking. Her toothless smile, warm as the noonday sun, graced the moment when she appeared. Life had been hard, but the Lord provided. The family pitched in to help in whatever way they could, accepting responsibility for less fortunate members. It was good to know there were others she could turn to and need not be ashamed.

Nowadays, everyone is so autonomous, self-sufficient, and aloof. Family closeness is on the wane. Each person must paddle his or her own boat, and there's no one to throw out a lifeline when we find ourselves going under. We can live right next door to someone and feel worlds apart. Though computers now connect people around the globe, we're isolated and lonely, afraid to reach out, afraid of involvement or embarrassment. So often we use the predicament of needy, hurting individuals to scorn, humiliate, and punish rather than to respond to their anguished cries. Oh, to bring back yesterday when a mother was a mother, a father was a father, a sister and a brother behaved like a sister and a brother, and a neighbor was truly a friend.

Time came to say goodbye to Grandma, for she died in 1966. Our trips south afterward were few. The many rich experiences from those years have become a part of who I am—still the child out in the country, talking to the grass, tying string on beetles' legs and watching them fly, catching lightning bugs and letting them glow between my fingers, and snapping morning glories to hear them pop; still that person who wants to be at peace, in harmony with nature, giving homage to God. Grandma left no will but a rich heritage of Jesus Christ for us to remember.

A poem was included in Grandma's obituary, which read in part,

> I am home in Heaven, Dear Ones;
> Oh, so happy and so bright;
> There is perfect joy and beauty
> In this everlasting light.
> All the pain and grief is over,
> Ever restless tossing past;
> I am now at peace forever,
> Safely home in Heaven at last.

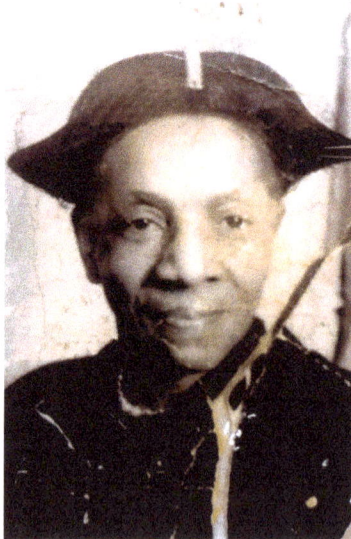

Portrait of my grandmother.

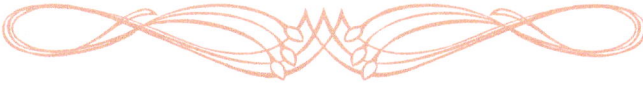

CHAPTER FIVE
Moving On Up

ON the way home, Dad always drove slowly. Why? Because Southern patrol officers watched for New York plates to stop and ticket "uppity Niggers from the North." We certainly didn't have upfront money to pay to keep ourselves out of jail.

We arrived only to find the apartment had been robbed by a trusted acquaintance with whom Mom left a key. Her fur-trimmed coat and other items of personal value were missing. Left were two large rodents seated before the TV, nibbling a snack as if housesitting until we got back. When we came in, they scurried away, wanting no involvement in foul play. Similarly, the friend avoided the taint of accusation by finding a hole for escape. Rats, being more honorable than men, only steal to fill their tummies; friends, to feed their envy. The robbery and violation of trust signalized our need for a safer place to live.

Mom's answer to this was to "work her fingers to the bone," putting in overtime on the assembly line. Dad, hired on there too, worked long hours on the same job and eventually became the supervisor. Mom started talking about buying a home and spoon-fed the idea to Dad in measured doses. He spat it out like a baby rejecting bitter medicine. She didn't give up but waited for God to open a door. He made connections supernaturally to make it possible despite our minimal resources.

Mom had nieces and nephews who were coming of age and looking for an opportunity to leave the South. They saw the dazzle of good fortune in the bright lights of the big city but couldn't see the haze that hung over the now-burgeoning black ghettoes shooting out from Manhattan into the South Bronx and Brooklyn. More than a million and a half hopefuls had migrated to the slums of New York, paying high rent for inferior housing with little chance of upward mobility. The job market offered mostly unstable, low-paid manual labor. Unemployment was twice that of whites. We slum dwellers paid higher prices for inferior goods at high rates of interest. Our chances of moving away and living where we wanted were slim. Still they came with poor education and training, wanting a taste of New York water, believing they would never thirst again. Mom took them in as temporary boarders.

First to come were Ethel, Nina, and Henry Clay, a full ten years older and in the throes of adulthood. They were eager to experience all the big city had to offer and promptly set about finding a belle or beau. I received vicarious pleasure, gazing with childish innocence as they dressed to go out on dates and lit the room at night with stories of all they had done.

During the day, they brought sweethearts over and crooned doowop and sexy love songs while holding each other close, songs like "Try Me" by James Brown, "Let's Fall in Love" by Peaches and Herb, "Yes I'm Ready" by Barbara Mason, "Hypnotized" by Linda Jones, and "The Touch of You" by Brenda and the Tabulations. I sat by peeking and snickering as they slow dragged with the one they loved, or wanted to love, and tried to see at the door when they were locked in a passionate embrace. The unction of sweet soul music soothed our aching spirits, and their liveliness brought joy into our home. Breathless air suddenly came alive with possibilities.

One doesn't remain an innocent child very long, for nature rains down a flow of blood to let you know your body is being prepared for womanhood, even if your mind is not quite ready. It happened shortly after I was nine years old—my first period. I was frightened by the downpour of blood in that private place. Mom explained it meant I could now get pregnant and have a baby, so I was to stay away from boys. I didn't understand it all, except to believe I had miraculously been given this amazing power to give life, or bring a child into the world. For me this was quite serious!

In my attempts to come to grips with changes in my body, I created for myself an elaborate dreamscape in which I acted out, through a cast of superhuman characters, the fears and insecurities these changes wrought. I added to this serial nightly and daily by tuning in and out. The episodes in my daydreams paralleled what was going on around me. Although the staging was dreamlike, I could consciously alter what went on and at times relived emotional scenes over and over again.

The basic story line centered around a family of superheroes—five brothers like the Chinese brothers in my favorite children's book, each having magnificent powers beyond that of mortal men. Not only had they special gifts, but they resembled the major races of the world. One appeared Eastern European with Nordic features and white skin. One looked more Hispanic, olive complexioned; and another had the yellow skin and slanted eyes of an Asian. Yet another was Indian with tan skin and straight black hair, and the last one was black with dark rich skin and wavy hair. None of them had the "typically Negroid" features I had been programmed to dislike.

The interactions between these supermen controlled the fate of humanity. Men and women were at their mercy, lest they use their omnipotent power to destroy all mankind. At the same time, each had qualities, such as mercifulness or charity, and interceded in kind ways on behalf of certain individuals. I suppose this was the way I pictured God, as the authoritarian father sitting on high able to judge and destroy us in His anger, yet His wrath was tempered with compassion and love.

In the dreams, I appeared in the form of a forlorn princess with ebony skin, long flowing locks of hair, and hazel eyes who lived in the gutter of a great city. Her body was covered with filth, scum, and insects. No one dared look upon her lest they vomit at the stench and sight of her ugliness. She was accursed to remain as such, until one brother's kiss broke the enchanted spell. The dark brother found and kissed her. She changed instantly from an ugly distorted creature into a lovely princess who was forever indebted to him and would live always at his side. She became his bride, but her relationship to him was that of a poor servant girl who did his every bidding while he acted with wanton disregard for her feelings and welfare. She held on for dire love of him, hoping one day to win his true and complete love. Episodes often revolved around the pain she suffered at his hand. I became the princess, and she became me as we regularly traded places in our worlds.

The movie *West Side Story* spoke to my need to understand falling in love. It was a musical performance about Hispanic kids on the Lower East Side surviving life in New York in the fifties. They'd come from Puerto Rico in search of a dream, but cultural and language barriers eked away their chances for success. Thus, they ban together in a street gang to gain acceptance, identity, and a sense of power. A group of Anglo kids forms an opposing gang to resist the tide of change sweeping their neighborhood. The gangs plan a turf war, and two lovestruck kids, Tony and Maria, are caught up in the violence. A rumble takes place, and Tony kills Maria's brother Nado. Their love is doomed by Tony's ill-fated blow. The lovers realize it isn't them, but surrounding forces sweeping them along in a torrent and angry sea. That sea—the sea of change.

I swooned as the starry-eyed lovers sang "Tonight, tonight won't be just any night. Tonight there will be no morning star." I shared the jubilance of finding love with Tony in "I just met a girl named Maria." I felt an exhilarating tingle when Maria sang "I feel pretty." I cherished the vows of betrothal in "Make our hands one hand. Make our hearts one heart. Make our vows one vow. Only death will part us now." And I cried as the lovers realized the hopelessness of their plight, "There's a place for us. Somewhere a place for us." For the first time, I had fallen in love with being in love—its magic, its mystery, its hope, and its enchantment.

I knew as a child that my parents loved me. I was clothed, fed, and well taken care of; and my education was of paramount concern to them. But there wasn't an outward display of emotional closeness wherein we kissed, touched, and caressed a lot. Nor was there sharing of feelings on a deeply personal level of our innermost selves, what was in our "heart of hearts." Our communication was turned outward to the social and political arena. Our living room became an open forum with fiery discussions about people, how and why they did things, and events taking shape in our world. As young children we were very opinionated and quite vocal on the issues of the day. We were encouraged to set goals and pull ourselves up, forge ahead, break the mold, not be like others who "sat back and collected welfare." We learned to get involved and tackle social issues.

Mom primed us nightly, much the way she used a pumice stone to scrape off the dead skin from the bottoms of her feet, hardened by years of treading barefoot in the country. She wanted to peel off the old dead image that held us back and prepared us to embrace middle-class values, goals, and aspirations. This meant brutal hours of hard work in the bakery—a steam bath both winter and summer. It also meant having little time to spend doing fun things parents and kids enjoy. We understood this was the way things had to be if you wanted to "make it." Besides, we were left in the capable hands of family members who kept the house jumping.

Somehow, I feel I missed something along the way. Every time I saw a mother take up her young child and hold it lovingly, kiss and coddle it, something twinged within me. When I saw a father pick up his kid, toss him into the air, and bring him down in his big loving arms, something hurt. Now, when I try to reach out to give a small hug or a peck on the cheek, there is a blocking of my emotions, a discomfort I can't explain. But I have learned to forgive my parents if they didn't show love for me in all the ways I needed them to in those struggling early years, for I have learned that only God's love is perfect and complete and all human love falls short. As He pours His love downward, I am learning to let it flow outward.

In the late 1950s the voice of change was heard, not only on film, but across the nation changes were in the making. Millions of black men, like Dad, served valiantly in World War II; their efforts helped secure victory for the allied front. Segregation by race existed in the armed forces, but President Harry S. Truman realized the great contribution of these men and signed a bill in 1948 bringing separation to an end. It called for equal treatment of all US servicemen regardless of color, initiating integration on a trial basis. Black soldiers returning to the States as proud men of war refused to go back to old stereotyped roles. They threw off the shackles of second-class citizenship and demanded equal participation in American life. Hundreds of thousands received training in war industries. They now had GI benefits, including education and training at government expense and government-guaranteed loans to buy homes, farms, and businesses. Better jobs and suitable housing were asked for as a right. Impatient with the system and its rusted mechanisms, they lifted their voices, calling for changes in the law and its practices. Their rumblings could be heard throughout the land. From porches, to city stoops, to unemployment lines, whisperings and murmurings became a ubiquitous and painful cry for justice.

This period was the heyday for many African Americans who showed their strength and vigor by winning recognition in various fields. Jackie Robinson became the first to play Major League Baseball. Ralph Bunche was the first to win a Nobel Prize. Marion Anderson was the first to sing a leading role in the Metropolitan Opera in New York. Gwendolyn Brooks was first to win a Pulitzer Prize.

Black entertainers excelled in the performing arts: Louis Armstrong, Cab Calloway, Charlie Parker, Dizzy Gillespie, Bessie Smith, and Lena Horne brought the finest blues, jazz, and bebop to white audiences. Sidney Poitier debuted in films dealing with racial problems: *No Way Out* (1957), *The Blackboard Jungle* (1955), *Edge of the City* (1957), and *A Raisin in the Sun* (1959). James Baldwin won critical acclaim for his books dealing with racial issues: *Notes of a Native Son* (1955), *Go Tell It on the Mountain* (1953), and *Nobody Knows My Name* (1961). Writers and poets such as Langston Hughes and Countee Cullen became known for lyrical poetry on black themes. Cullen wrote "Color" (1925), "Copper Sun" (1927), "The Ballad of a Brown Girl" (1927), and a collection of his best works, *On These I Stand* (1947).

National leaders who saw the need to end racial discrimination took to the forefront of the reform movement, lending their voices to amplify the cause. Earlier court decisions augmented their efforts. In

1940, a Virginia law struck down segregation on interstate buses. A 1948 ruling said that agreements preventing the sale of real estate to black families couldn't be upheld. A 1954 decision (*Brown v. Topeka*) ended segregation in the public schools. All white educational institutions were forced to accept students of color. The move toward integration gained momentum.

In the South, the old Jim Crow laws, which prevented us from being serviced at the counter in the diner in Greensboro, were challenged. In the North, we fought against job discrimination and pushed to move into neighborhoods of our choice. For many, these were portentous days because the winds of change sweeping the nation threatened the comfortable lifestyles and privileges they enjoyed but augured well for us because we looked forward to doing better than our parents had.

In 1955, Dr. Martin Luther King, speaking with the unctuous fervor of a Baptist minister and the eloquence of a statesman, brought the power of his faith against the Goliath of racism. A Bible in hand, he led a boycott as a protest against the arrest of Rosa Parks, the success of which demonstrated that civil rights could be won by direct nonviolent action. By 1956, it was quite perspicuous that a mass movement was underway.

More and more blacks moved to New York seeking industrial jobs, as well as persons of Hispanic and Caribbean backgrounds. As their numbers increased, whites exited to the suburbs of Long Island, Westchester, and New Jersey. "White flight" opened doors for middle-class blacks to buy homes in previously all-white areas.

Mom wanted to take advantage of that opportunity and for us to have a chance to see life differently. By then, my parents had made the adjustment from rural to big-city living. Their jobs, though seasonal, paid double time and a half for overtime work. Like many others who sought an egress from Harlem and the trappings of ghetto life, Mama wanted a home in a good residential area with better schools for her children. She wanted to "be somebody." Dad had found his niche in Harlem among friendly faces and familiar places. He wasn't prepared to move again.

Where one friend betrayed us, God brought another to our aid. Mr. Sherill, the kindly miser who lived upstairs, made real estate investments, paid cash for houses, and resold them for profit. He purchased a three-family home in the Wakefield section of the Bronx, then an Italian enclave, and offered it to Mom on affordable terms. Once in the house, two rentals would carry the mortgage. Mom was delighted! The problem was to convince Dad. Mom took the direct approach by simply issuing an ultimatum. Either he was coming with her, or she was going on without him. He came. It was the year 1960.

We rode the Seventh Avenue subway up from Harlem to see our new home for the very first time. The station at 135th Street was a dankish cavern beneath the ground, its air oppressive with the smell of urine. Our heels clopped happily as we descended the long flight of steps leading to a cubicle where a wary attendant sat. His eyes did not engage; neither was there a smile back. He nervously shoved tokens our way for the change tossed lightly in his tray. A helpless spawn in the dark waters of a reef, he cloaked himself behind the murky glass, hoping to escape the piranhas that fiercely patrolled the deep.

With a rush of excitement, we pushed through the turnstile into a silent world, wriggling like jumping beans unable to stand, unable to command our bodies to obey Mom's repeated reprimands. Finally the raging rail cars streamed into the station and roared to a screeching halt. We skipped onboard; the cars lurched forward and careened through the underground vault. Suddenly the train gave out a mournful wail, like a woman whose hour had come with great travail, bearing the anguish of her struggling black seed kicking and fighting to be free.

The coach wound its way through the entrails of the city, tossing us to and fro. Passengers staring from beneath curled brows at persons across the row wondered who would do them harm. Who would come to their aid? And who, like themselves, was vulnerable and afraid?

At 149th Street, Third Avenue, the cars emerged and ascended to the rails of the elevated track. For us, we hoped, there'd be no turning back. We were reaching toward our goal, a lifestyle better than we had known; a dream magnificent as the corona of the sun, brighter than the flood of light that gushed through the window as we climbed toward the crown; a delicious morsel, always a little beyond reach, dangling there before us like a tease. We were reaching for it again. This time stretching farther than ever before, hoping this time to clench it, hold it within our grasp, enjoy that it was ours at last!

The train meandered along the raw edge of the South Bronx, winding its way to 180th Street. Passengers shoved, bodies rubbed, and tots whined crankily in the heat. The grimace of dilapidation could be seen everywhere. On the surface, it appeared as if residents just didn't care. Like a woman once beautiful with dazzling eyes and coiffured hair, whose smile lit a room and called many suitors to her door, now gaunt, dreary-eyed her face eroded. Age has brought debility and decay. Her old lovers have softly stolen away. Scoundrels lie at her breasts and rob her wealth, leaving her languishing in despair and drinking the dregs of what once was. There is no one to succor her. No one can quiet her inner raging. She abides. She awaits death, but it comes slowly.

The North Bronx was the younger sibling who had watched the older sister wax old and gray. She still had sparkle and vitality, but her beauty was starting to fade. I knew she was getting on in years. Her hair looked mussed, her makeup heavy, and wrinkles had begun to appear. Dark blotches marked her once-white skin. Unkemptness she could not hide. Family and friends were leaving. Only the government helped provide. Her waning years will bring a slow decline. Who will stand by her in her invalidity? Will her children run and leave her in the hands of others? Or will they care for her lovingly as before? She knew the answer, because she saw black strangers standing at her door.

We came off the train onto a peaceful thoroughfare where shoppers passed time and looked. Mom and pop stores were strung along its length, like colorful beads in a two-strand necklace, which brightened the garb of the community awaiting us. The corner sign read "225th Street and White Plains Road." The noisy subway scream-

ing goodbye overhead seemed out of place in subdued, quiet surroundings. Its shrill-pitched voice pierced the calm. People sighed as
it moved along. It stood out there; so did we. Ghetto people we all
were. But we were not like her—loud and rowdy. Folks around there
didn't know that. They could only see that we were black and winced
at our coming.

A nearby deli sold culinary delights rich with Old World fla-
vors. The garlicky sauce from inside had an appetizing savor. A swirl
of aromas, sausage, prosciutto, and Parmesan cheese tinged the air
with piquancy. We didn't venture in though our stomachs panged
hungrily.

A circle of older men brought wisdom and experience to the
day's rhetoric, exchanging rapid-fire discourse in pure Italian. It
could have been something they read in *Il Progresso* that made them
wave their hands so vehemently as they spoke. Or maybe it was a
boccie game they'd played in the park, or dominoes, DiMaggio or
Marciano. I don't know! Whatever the reason they beat the air with a
choppy staccato, it was unfair, for the air had been balmy and pleasant that fine day.

The ladies didn't spank the day; rather, they enjoyed its man-
ifold blessings, milling around fruit stands, picking fresh vegetables
for dinner come late evening. Shopping bags filled, they walked
along rows of neatly tended houses with statuary of the Virgin Mary
reposed in front. Trailing grapevines from Southern Italy wove backyards into tapestries of floral greenery. In this tiny hamlet, heritage,
religion, and close familial ties blended to make a Sicilian soup pot
titillating in taste and sound.

Children gathered at the pizza man's window, waiting to sample
the hot pie they'd watched him make. With a curl of the wrist and a
twirl in the air, after rolling it out with great care, he ladled it with red
sauce, sprinkled it with cheese, baked it in the oven until its toasty
crust bubbled with juiciness. The kids bubbled with happiness.

My attention was drawn to the Italian bakery whose candied
breath sweetened the air each time the door opened. Pies and cakes
smiled from her windows. Star-shaped cookies with chocolate sprin-
kles brought an immediate twinkle to my eyes. Eclairs, tarts, twists,

zeppole were mouthwatering treats that cringed my belly. But it was the coconut cupcakes that caused my stomach to roll. In a showy place was a wedding cake adorned with lace. A bridegroom standing above whispered vows of love beneath a sugary gazebo foreshadowing the moment when wedding bells would ring for me and my Prince Charming. I comforted myself in the warmth from the oven and the smell of fresh baked bread.

One could easily read the tension in our poses as we stood there gazing upon the surface of things. A white lady stopped and asked where we wanted to go. Mom recited the address. Curiosity leading, she plied us with questions, "Why are you going there? Is it for a maid's job?"

"No, I am the new owner!" Mom retorted, pride and anger couched in her reply. Her importunity had given Mom a chance to boast. She reveled in that moment's glory.

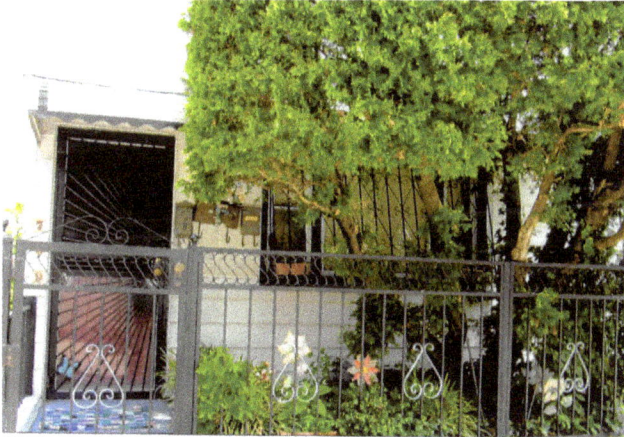

The front of our home in the Bronx.

We found our way to the house, looked it over, and loved it. It had apartments upstairs and downstairs, a big backyard with a grape arbor and an old garage similar to Grandma's barn where the chickens stayed. Next to it was a rickety old shed most suitable for a playhouse, but sort of spooky like the attic atop Grandma's stairs. I wouldn't be going in there too often! Who knew if the previous owners didn't have an Aunt Somebody hiding behind the cobwebs? On the side of the house was a lovely goldfish pond in the midst of a garden with fiery-orange lilies planted all around. Dwarf pussy willow trees grew in its L-shaped corners. Their fuzzy gray buds were soft as a kitten against my cheek. I stuffed some in my pocket to curl and sleep.

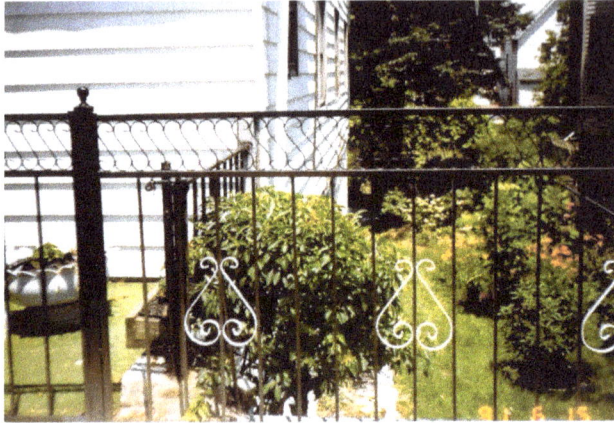

The side yard with orange lilies and a fish pond.

A lively forsythia bush pouring out of a high retaining wall secluded the yard from view as passersby walked the street above. Cascading down, a shower of yellow trinkets set the garden aglow. This would be the perfect place to meet Whimsy and Fancy, my closest friends, for hours of fun and make-believe.

How happy we were! It called for a celebration. We went home, danced the twist, the mash potatoes, and did the split, bought soda and fish 'n' chips, sang along with Jimmy James,

I Am Somebody

I remember when I was small, I saw a preacher man,
And he was walking tall.
I remember his words, what he had to say.
He said, "Hold your head high and walk in the sky,
And if they ask you why, say 'I am somebody!'
Don't be ashamed of what you are,
Wear your life with pride, don't be a scar.
The weak and the strong, the big and the small,
They have a right to be here; they too belong!
Just hold your head high and walk in the sky
And if they ask you why, say 'I am somebody!'
Stand up and be yourself, stand up and speak
Up for yourself.
In the eyes of the Lord we're all one.
What's good enough for God, you dig? Right on!
Just hold your head up high and walk in the sky
And if they ask you why, say 'I am somebody!'"

I gained from my parents that desire to work and have something. They taught us to keep on keeping on, moving step by step to accomplish more than others expect. They said put your heart and soul into things if you want to get anything out of it. Somehow they believed that equity would come.

In the following years, because of the civil rights movement, American society underwent a metamorphosis, losing the larval organs of inequality and gaining the missing adult mechanisms for full participation. As an embryonic nation that had reached full growth, it was time to go on to the next stage of life. And so, as it were, the nation crawled into a cocoon. With great wrenching and writhing, it removed its old skin and laid itself bare before the world. Gradually we were forming a chrysalis, a coat of many colors, while on the inside great changes were taking place. We hoped our structure would change and we'd emerge like a beautiful winged flower, a painted butterfly.

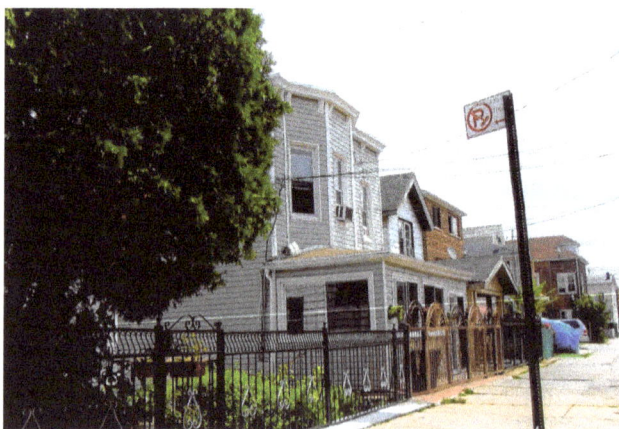

Picture of 228 Street where we lived.

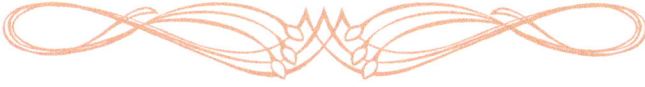

CHAPTER SIX
Displacement

WHEN we first moved into our home, white neighbors didn't snub us. On the contrary, they were very congenial, especially as they saw the type of people we were and how meticulously Mom kept the house and yard. Whites were not hostile, since they had some place to go. Having a few blacks come in didn't upset the apple cart, but when the numbers exceeded a fine sprinkling, alarm bells rang out.

During the 1960s, transformation left cities of 500,000 and over with 1.9 million less whites and 2.8 million additional blacks, while suburbia gained 12.5 million whites, but only 800,000 blacks. Most raked in sizeable profits by selling their homes to minority buyers. In the Bronx, there were no cross burnings, racial epithets hurled, destruction of property, or direct confrontations with mobs, as occurred in the South when color lines were crossed.

No, it was not a mass exodus overnight, rather a slow trickle almost imperceptible, like a leaky valve that seeps a whole system into labefaction. The face of the neighborhood gradually turned darker the way a person lying in the sun gets a tan. Most people are quite proud of a tanned complexion, but when it happens to a community, it brings *fear*. The changing face of the neighborhood emotes fear because whatever touches the neighborhood touches the people who live there. Blacks were not seen as a people with a gentle touch.

Why did whites run when blacks moved in? Why did they feel we would purloin their way of life and destroy the community? The reasons most often given for white flight were said to be economic, based on fear that if black families came into an area, crime would go up, social status would be lost, poor upkeep of houses would lower real estate value, and hard-earned savings would be jeopardized. It is said they were not bad people, just understandably human, worried about their savings, homes, neighborhoods, and children.

Whites made their prophecies self-fulfilling by running and leaving a neighborhood in transition, when it was on a downturn and in distress, taking most of the resources with them. The amount of sanitation services per person in the area went down, and things declined. Whites had the opportunity to say "We told you so!" Out went the banks, the investors, quality businesses, large department stores, and lending institutions. In came the vultures who fed on the carcasses of the poor—the agents who encouraged whites to move by inciting fear, seeking to profit off the sale of their houses; the economic exploiters who benefitted from our being on the lower end of the fiscal scale with incomes 60 percent of whites; the cash and carry stores, quick-loan businesses with high interest rates, junk stores and pawnshops; the real estate brokers who found apartments for high fees, steering tenants to landlords who charged exorbitant rents yet gave little service; and the social exploiters: liquor stores, bars, and drug dealers that offered a quick fix for our frustrations. Not overnight, it was a slow cancer that spread its malignancy a little more each day until things became just the way they said it would be. But whose fault was it?

In 1949, my birth year, the US government promised a "decent and suitable living environment for every American family." The promise was not kept because of prejudice in the housing market. The color of a person's skin still affected where people lived. Most whites were not comfortable with the prospect of having black neighbors. Their fears provided fertile soil in which discrimination grew, bias flourished, and intolerance blossomed into hate. Underlying this was the belief in white supremacy. That notion had been deeply embedded in the minds of whites since the arrival of the first black slaves in Jamestown, Virginia, in 1607. Blacks were long viewed as nonpersons by the white establishment and relegated to inferior status. Those long-held notions had proven their resiliency and had not yielded to the appeal of conscience or morality. A lot of people were locked into the prejudices of the past. We hadn't thrown out the bags of refuse filled over two centuries of slavery and another hundred years in its aftermath. Therefore, an apartheid-like system grew.

What happened when whites didn't run? In most transitional neighborhoods, there were those die-hard souls who held their ground, especially after many years of residence in one place, usually the elderly whose children had grown up, gotten college degrees, and moved to more comfortable lives in suburbia. The kids found no room in their middle-class lifestyles for aging parents. The parents, not wishing to be a burden, remained in the old neighborhood and fended for themselves as best they could. They lacked stamina to pick up and move, or resources to get a new mortgage, and they didn't want to go into debt. Besides, most felt they hadn't many years left and preferred to live them out in familiar surroundings with things acquired over time.

A very meaningful relationship developed between our family and one of those left behinds. Her name was Mrs. Mavarro, an elderly Italian woman who lived in the basement of our home when we arrived. Her husband was deceased, and her adult children had moved away. She lived in mourning waiting for her time to come. She dressed all in black, head to toe, from her cobby shoes and thick stockings to the lace mantilla that covered her silvery hair. Everything was black except the golden crucifix that stood out prominently against the dark cloth, even the fringed shawl she wore draped across her shoulders.

Lonely and isolated, she longed for attention and care. Someone always paid the rent, but not a soul came to see her. There were no friends or family to help with basic needs and no one to talk with her. It seemed she had been forgotten. Her speech was mostly Italian with a few English words mixed in. Staying alone all the time meant no social involvement in activities to give her a feeling of self-worth or to allow close attachments. Consequently, she drifted off into senility and was beset by delusions. Her speech turned to gibberish, and she was often seen talking to an imaginary person through the window.

Her only companion was a large black cat with yellow eyes called Satan. He was indeed a devil. In her need to give love, she kept him in the house and tried to stroke and cuddle him while sharing her few morsels of food. The ungrateful cat bared his claws and lashed out viciously, wanting freedom to roam the backyards in search of feline company. He scratched her arms unmercifully until they bled. Soon they were covered with encrustation and infection because of his villainy. Yet she loved him and continued to cling.

She reached out to us also, taking a portion of her monthly allowance to buy hard candies, which she passed out to us through the bars on her window. Although she couldn't really converse with us, she seemed to enjoy watching us play. Young children as we were, we understood she needed help and looked out for her in our own way. Our offers to run errands were met with an independent "No!" But Mom checked on her often to make sure that she was getting along okay.

The day came when it was no longer safe to leave her downstairs alone. She became oblivious to her surroundings and chatted more and more with unseen friends. Painful as it was, Mom contacted the relative who paid the rent, and she was finally taken away by nursing home attendants. I remember that day; it was sad and I was. She wasn't just a white lady to us; she had become our friend. Friends are always missed when they are gone.

A similar relationship based on trust and dependency developed across the street where black owners moved into a house occupied by white tenants. They lived together for years and got along well. Eventually, both the landlord's wife and the tenant's husband died. All the children moved away, leaving them alone. When he became ill, she cared for him, cooked meals, tended the house, and watched over things like a family member until his death. She resided there in the house, the last white resident left on that street, having remained through the cycle of change from Italian immigrants, to Southern blacks, to a new wave of poor families from the Caribbean. Her roots were firm, like a tree that couldn't be moved. Over time she gained much acceptance and remained active in the block association. To do what she did took guts. But when a place is your home, it should mean something to you.

Perhaps the best story of all is what happened up the street where, at first, the only other blacks on our block were the super-intendents of an apartment building near the corner. They lived in the basement of the building with free rent for performing janitorial services. Problems occurred between the husband and wife; he left her with three small children and no job. She struggled to raise the kids alone and started to work. A relationship developed between her and a Jewish tenant who lived on the third floor alone. She eventually moved upstairs into his apartment as they decided to share their lives. Although his family didn't accept her, they appeared to have a strong relationship and became close friends, whom Mom visited often.

When people of diverse backgrounds live together, there are unlimited possibilities for relationships that can form as they get to know one another individually, casting old stereotypes aside and fear of betraying their race. A mutually respectful attitude will generally ferment, and walls of misunderstanding crumble, especially when there is a balance of interests, incomes, and opportunities. Things can be worked out cross-culturally if we learn how to dialogue and cooperate.

New surroundings quickened love of natural things and roused my creative instincts. I settled into the seclusion of our "garden room," considering it my special place for easy talk with florets that attended closely and smiled back graciously as I spoke. Books taught me their botanical names, nicknames, and growing habits. Soon Mom and I were receiving plants from nurseries across the country. It gave me great satisfaction to see the plants blossom into the most beautiful assortment of shapes and colors imaginable.

I faithfully worked the garden, weeded and tended it, even prac-ticed sketching flowers or fashioning them out of paper. Fay fluttered off to meet new friends, always the social butterfly. Sonny played with our new dog, Fritz, and taught him a few little tricks. It was only Dad who wouldn't let go. He went back to the old neighborhood, to the places he knew, to a life that still detained him.

When the grapes on the vines had grown fat and succulent, honey scenting the air, we started school. I attended P.S. 21, and Fay, Olinville Junior High. At first, I feared going to class because I thought surely I would be the dumbest student in the room, having come from Harlem. I pictured all the white kids sitting around laughing while I gave stupid answers and failed tests. An intake exam placed me in 4-2 class, second from the top on my grade. In those years, classes were numbered according to academic promise. Rarely did black kids go into the one class, but I was delighted to be placed in number two, to be one of the chosen few.

It came as a surprise; I was not the class dunce. I did well despite my shyness, and the teachers encouraged me. One offered special assistance on the side teaching me to use the library system to locate books to spark my interests. I wasn't an avid reader, enjoying more the illustrations than the accompanying text. I became quite adept at arts and crafts, could turn a piece of paper into a doll, a bird, or a kite, most anything with scissors, glue, and a little thought. I took pride in my creations and kept scrapbooks at home of the projects I'd made.

I remember thinking these kids had it easy, because they were in a predominantly white school in a middle-class area. It had a good program, but there was minimal stress to achieve. In my old school, perhaps because they knew we had so many obstacles to overcome, they pushed us toward excellence, and I came away with a very solid foundation in basic skills. We tend to separate things in our minds by race and class, placing qualitative values that are not necessarily true, i.e., black ghetto school equals bad school, middle-class white school equals good school. But the fact is, I felt underchallenged in the new setting.

I had already internalized the notion that I had to work to make something of myself and do the family proud. It did, however, take some of the pressure off, and my school life became relaxed and carefree. I remained timid as a church mouse in groups, always viewing myself as less, in some way, than the others. There are powerful voices in childhood that tells you either you're ugly or stupid, which adds up to inadequate. Where they really come from, I don't know.

After school I sat reposefully by the pond, following the flaming colors as my Japanese goldfish streaked through the water to gobble down wiggle worms tossed on top. It's a wonder how they found the bait among the mud and floating leaves, but they caught them, each and every one! Dad and I bought seedlings and started a vegetable garden beside the garage. I teased him, with a last name like Farmer, he had to be a terrific gardener. What a laugh that first harvest, when his plants produced a few tiny tomatoes and pepper pods no bigger than a dime half eaten by worms! It didn't matter much. The interfacing, laughing, joking, spending time together was my chief enjoyment. You could say I was a Daddy's girl.

Life has a way of intruding in on people, just when things seem to be going well. It bursts in with a fury, storms through with a vengeance, and leaves an aftermath of pain and destruction in its wake. Devastated survivors are left trying to pick up the broken pieces of their lives. Sometimes those pieces are awfully hard to pick up— awfully hard. Only God knows!

It happened one weekend when Dad went for his usual jaunt back to Harlem for a "night out with the boys." We kids nestled in before ten o'clock bedtime. I don't know why I slept in the front parlor near the picture window, looking onto the street. I can only remember, in the wee hours of the night, being awakened by a car parked in front of the house and Mom wandering into the room in the darkness to peer through the window. Being fatally curious, I peeked too. Just then, the car door opened, and the interior light shined on a couple kissing ardently. It was Dad and another woman. That kiss shattered my parents' marriage and brought my happy little world shattering in upon me.

Mom, screaming "Jeanie, Jeanie, come and help me!" ran outside to defend her home and take her husband from the clutches of the woman's arms. She held the car door, flailed, and clawed helplessly against the reality of her worse fear come to life before her eyes, so boldly, so cruelly flaunted for all the world to see. The pain was overwhelming. Mom had suspected, accused, and been reassured it wasn't true so many times in the past. Her insides told her he had another woman, but her heart didn't want to believe it. Now there could be no more lies, denying, and hiding. What was done in darkness had surely come to light. Pearl, that person whose name had been sometimes shouted or called bitterly on the telephone when Mom was hurting and needed to talk, had come to visit. Her short stay left a scar that would last a lifetime.

I don't know if I felt sorrier for Mom or for myself. After all, he had betrayed both of us. I had been his staunchest defender. Daddy is good, I told her. He wasn't doing all the things she imagined. It was her so-called friends who wanted to take him away because they were jealous of what she had. Really, I just didn't want my daddy to get in trouble. Maybe he would have to leave. I could not admit this person who was bigger than life to me could do anything that wrong.

What could I say now to her or to myself? What would he say? Nothing, which only compounded the hurt. I wanted him to explain, to vindicate himself in some way. Mom said enough for both of them, things she didn't mean—bad words, angry words that came flowing out along with her tears. I don't think the words hurt him as much as what he saw when he looked into her eyes—a look that said, "How could you? You dirty dog!"

She didn't leave him, but there was a hardness that came over her. Maybe it was the only way she could bear the pain. For years after, he lingered in silence, continued to go out and drink on the weekends. I have the feeling it was no longer the women drawing him at that point; rather, he escaped the house to drown his shame in a bottle. He too had a look, that of a man who had lost his pride but wouldn't let down the facade. He held his head high and wore that toothy smile always.

They say time is a healer, but I say it isn't so. Not if you don't open up and deal with feelings honestly beyond surface lashing out and blaming. Pain becomes baggage that gets heavier and heavier with the passage of time. We're still carrying a load from that night many years ago. The break never mended. It's as if the marriage were caught in a limbo state. The family became like a needle stuck in the groove of a cracked record that went over and over the same words to a sad song. Dad dealt with his pain by simply imbibing more and more liquor to anesthetize himself. Mom smoked cigarettes, drank beer, and tried to talk hers out, but the more she talked, the more was left inside. Fay handled it by adopting an attitude that she would always be one up on every man so no one would ever get the ups on her, thereby avoiding hurt. Little Sonny waved a magic wand in his mind and said, "Daddy, you don't exist!" He backed away and pushed him aside, closing himself off from a father-son relationship.

Mine lies in a sepulcher deep within where it cannot be disturbed. Try as I may, I can't dig up those old dead bones and cast them out. Gloom overshadows me. I hear Mom's anguished cry for help many nights, when I toss and turn in bed unable to sleep. I wallow in agony. My heart aches. Mama's grief has taken up residence far down in my soul. It's hidden so well I can't get at it. But, God, I wish something would take the hurt away!

> An ancient spirit wanders the night,
> Ghoulish and evil she mercilessly taunts me,
> Clawing at my security, tearing at my flesh.
> She visits in pitch darkness and stays till dawn
> Brings the morning light.
> I slumber a few moments knowing she'll come
> Again and again to disturb my rest.
> Will her wandering ever cease?
> I must find her sepulcher,
> And with a silver dagger thrust her through the
> heart.
> Only then will I be at peace.

Mom's wounds gushed like an open faucet as she told the world what happened, how she had been betrayed. Her pain demanded vengeance, as ofttimes is the case. In bitterness, she smeared his name to family and friends, ennobling herself as the dutiful wife scorned. Phone conversations became a litany of wrongs she'd suffered and not deserved. How would she handle this dilemma? In light of his unfaithfulness, should she go or stay? A consensus said stay for the sake of the house and kids. Besides, she couldn't let another woman step in there and take what she had worked so hard to achieve.

Mom kept us apprised of what was going on between them. We became her closest confidants as others stopped coming around. People didn't want to hear a sad songster or get involved in problems. Most had enough of their own. We listened as she poured out her anger daily and nightly. "A black man is no good!" "A black woman has to be strong to survive because she has to take and take and take!" "A man is like a dog, not to be trusted!" "Good people get trampled on in this cruel world!" We experienced emotionally the rift between our parents and felt we had to choose sides. We all lost objectivity.

Mom's fury never abated against him or anyone who partnered with him. Scar tissue covered her very tender heart, making her a little hardened. She regularly put him down behind his back, weakening his relationships with others. Her remarks ranged from making him the butt of her jokes to open hostility and criticism of his actions and friends. Her comments affronted, challenged, or demeaned his manhood, pulling against his leadership in the home. She joked about the ineptness and stupidity of black men. We laughed along and agreed with her, becoming unwitting conspirators in his emasculation. On the surface, it did seem our men were incapable leaders since, looking around, we saw other families headed by females or who likewise had a crisis of leadership in their home.

We had no idea how our conspiracy undermined his attempts at headship and damaged his fragile ego. He bore our jabs stoically, shut down his emotions, became introverted and nonassuming of responsibility, abandoning all chores and manly duties around the house. When he got quite fed up, he blared back loud enough to shake the roof that we might know he was still "the man of the house" and countered by staying out a lot, not being around to do things with us or Mom. But he never stopped financial support, tried always to teach us right from wrong, and reprimanded us firmly when we got out of line.

It became an issue of control. "I'm not going to sit here like a sissy and let you tell me what to do!" Out the door he went. Left alone on weekends and holidays, Mom constantly complained that she had no help. A lot of emotional energy was used up fighting those old battles. Responsibility for paying bills, maintaining the home, child rearing, and making all the decisions fell to her. Dad was free to roam, drink, and come and go as he pleased. He was not held responsible for his actions. His absence and drinking gave her a great deal of power. Mom tried to content herself with buying lots of new things—new siding, furniture, and remodeling the interior. But material goods could not replace affection and companionship. She became emotionally weary and troubled, always looking into the past. She carried a patina of woundedness everywhere she went. Suffice it to say, she was denied fulfillment, as they began to sleep in separate beds and intimacy waned.

Marriage was filled with sacrifice for Mom. As Dad became increasingly passive, she became an overperformer, juggling full-time employment and household duties. It took her to her emotional limits. She was left feeling needy and empty. Her anger and sorrow never dissipated. She'd made so many sacrifices but felt Dad had made none. He wanted to "have his cake and eat it too," a nice home and family, a nightlife and other women on the side, while she shouldered all the weight. Mom was an ambitious woman with many skills. She had few interests in common with Dad. Their likes and dislikes were very different. He had drinking friends; she, church friends. Though they remained together, they were very much apart. She didn't encourage and support him; he didn't sacrificially love and serve her. Despite everything, I saw how she *persevered*.

Growing up in this environment made it difficult to get a clear picture of a woman's traditional role in a family, as ours had become so distorted, with Dad wearing the pants and Mom carrying the load. As young girls, we were being shaped in attitude by Mom's experiences, making it unlikely we would trust men to make commitments in the future. We became insecure within ourselves of our approaching womanhood, as we had not seen our mother cherished and respected in the home the way we imagined white women were.

It seemed black women were an accursed lot, downtrodden by society since slavery; used as sex machines and babymakers to fulfill the master's fantasies, which he daren't ask his wife to perform, having their young torn from their arms and sold on auction blocks to the highest bidder; used as domiciles to cook, clean, and wait on white women hand and foot. Four hundred years later, being used as sex machines, babymakers, and house mops by their own black men, never having honor or dignity ascribed to them; never feeling greatly valued, listened to, or understood; never placed high on a pedestal. What happens to many black women is that they end up shrouding themselves in the same images that society has painted, sometimes coarse in a manner, not taking anything off of anyone. This is usually a cover-up for severe insecurities in the face of very frightening realities.

In many ways, our talks with Mom were beneficial because we learned as black women we had to be steadfast, stand by our children, and hold our homes together. We had to have guts and stalwart backs to work and keep the ball rolling no matter what. We had to be fighters; but we were learning to fight the wrong people, our own black men, perpetuating the pattern of female-headed households and absence of black men in families. We also picked up the notion that black men couldn't be expected to do any better or be held accountable for their actions. You had to either put up with them or leave and stand alone. It made it difficult to believe we could take our own lives in hand, separate it from what happened to Mom, and make it what we wanted it to be. We tended to mirror Mom's biases and approached men in an insecure or cautious fashion.

Little Sonny, the sole male child in our nucleus, was particularly scarred by repeatedly being told what a black man is not and cannot do. Not having a firm relationship with Dad and lacking role models made it hard for him to develop a positive self-image as a young black male. Nevertheless, he grew up and became a family man strong in some of the areas Dad was weakest but eventually fell into the cycle. This seems almost inevitable when patterns are imprinted from an early age.

Often bitter hurt comes at the hands of people we love. I became aware of what happens when a person doesn't own up to their problem, how it hinders forgiveness and healing. There was never a release, the atmosphere was never cleared, and reconciliation never came. Blaming is like venom injected into a family's life. Yet I saw how Mom endured marital disappointment by faith and displayed outstanding loyalty in the face of his infidelity. Though in a bitter struggle, she remained committed. Her belief in God and family was just that strong. I learned from her that sometimes you have to put up a fight for the ones you love.

I feel disloyal in disclosing these experiences, in talking about the apparent contradictions in their lives. I know Mom did the best she could. If she knew how to handle things differently, she would have. And I really believe, so would Dad, if he had gotten help with his alcoholism and the problems related to it. I could never renounce my parents. It would be like cutting off a part of myself. The world without them would be a dismal and lonely place. I have so many other things to be grateful to them for. But to the end that I might pull together the many facets that have gone in to making me who I am, I share this.

> To everything there is a season, and a time
> to every purpose under heaven:
> A time to be born, and a time to die;
> A time to plant, and a time to pluck up
> that which has been planted;
> A time to kill, and a time to heal;
> A time to break down, and a time to build up;
> A time to weep, and a time to laugh;
> A time to mourn, and a time to dance;
> A time to cast away stones, and a time to gather
> stones together;
> A time to embrace, and a time to refrain from
> embracing;
> A time to get, and a time to lose;
> A time to keep, and a time to cast away;
> A time to rend, and a time to sew;
> A time to keep silence, and a time to speak;
> A time to love, and a time to hate;
> A time of war, and a time of peace.
> (The Wisdom of Solomon)

Trouble had come in season. An old Jamaican adage, "When trouble comes shell don't blow!" means you get no warning. We had gotten back in the swing of things, still held captive by the interplay of powerful emotions at home, when routine medical exams uncovered startling findings. A skin test revealed I had been exposed to TB, having shared with many others the close quarters of a drafty tenement building. In high-density areas like Harlem, TB among smokers was very prevalent. With people coughing and it being contagious, it easily spread. By age eleven, I was tall, frail, and had an incessant cough, a sickly child. The doctors feared the disease would become full blown.

Fay's case was much more serious. It began with difficulty reading lessons from the blackboard. A front row seat did not avail her. Consequently, she was referred for eye exams and later neurological testing. Results showed a growth on the optic nerve, causing her sight to fail. Surgery would be required to determine if it was benign or malignant. Mom, going at it alone, took Fay to a neurosurgeon, who performed an operation.

One day Fay was there with us, laughing and teasing in her usual jocular style; next day she was off to the hospital. Weeks later she returned home almost totally blind and in a wheelchair. The delicate operation, which involved placing a shunt in her brain to control the flow of blood, made her sight worse, and her motor skills were left impaired. She would need to learn to walk and do things for herself again. The doctor held out hopes that her condition would improve with time. Physical therapy and specialized training for the visually impaired were required for returning to school. But now, at age thirteen, she was an invalid and legally blind.

I didn't go to visit during her stay in the hospital. I knew her condition could be critical, but I was shunted off on the sidelines, watching, not directly involved with what was happening, bolted in my own world. As a by-product of the surgery, cerebral fluid backed up in her head, causing it to swell enormously. When she came home, she had a changed appearance, which frightened me. Having her immobilized in a wheelchair was equally alarming. Fate had stolen my big sister away momentarily, then given her back, but now she was different.

Somehow, I couldn't get in touch emotionally with what had happened to her. I was caught in the vortex of my own self-centeredness. I thought I was the lucky one, an attitude like "There, but for the grace of God, go I!" or worse, "Better her than me!" I felt specially privileged—better—because she was now handicapped. God forgive me for such callous thinking, for attempting to lift myself up on the shoulders of her affliction!

I stole short glances at the black threads that now ornamented her shaven head and followed with eerie curiosity the long stitches tracing the movement of the surgeon's needle through her flesh. His stitchery left permanent scar tissue, like tracks of a railway down her neck, not lying smoothly as if sewn in cloth. I was repulsed, yet I wanted to be close. I felt sorry and unfairly chosen. After all, Mom had tried to raise us with equality. When Fay was given a nickel, I got one too. When she bought her a new dress, a similar one was purchased for me. Why then had God been so cruel to her and not to me? I certainly wasn't deserving of any special favor. Sympathy and guilt danced with me for countless hours. My feet hurt and I wanted to get off the floor, but there was no retreat. I had to face her as well as others who didn't accept, who couldn't understand what she had been through, people who reacted to her disability as I sometimes did. I hated the way they stared, reminding me of how I looked at her when she wasn't looking. I saw the worse of myself in them.

Her open eyes, weak and strabismic because of uneven muscle pull, were cast with a dull haze as encroaching blindness was closing off the light. I stared in pity as she used her hands to search for things she couldn't see or held her head very close to print in order to read. Doctors prescribed thick, frosted, horned-rimmed glasses with bifocal lenses, certainly unattractive for a girl just entering puberty. Her voice tended to be louder than normal as she used her ears and speech to compensate for her poor sight (kind of like a bat sending out sound waves that bounced off objects, telling her where things were, at least that's the way I explained it to myself).

My reaction was to the external part of her experience, what I could see. Not what was going on inside, what she was going through or feeling. How could I have known the inner strength required to suddenly have a disability thrust upon you and have to live with it? Had I known, I wouldn't have been so removed. I could have learned from her.

Eventually, her hair grew back to cover the wound, but her sight was only minimally restored, leaving her fledgling spirit to wander in perpetual twilight. She faced it courageously with remarkable fortitude. Within a short time, she popped up out of the wheelchair, began to walk, entered classes for the visually impaired, and took charge of her disability. Fay just wouldn't let it get her down. Though her eyes grew dim, her liveliness shone through loud and clear. She faced this the way she faced everything else, with a tremendous sense of humor, her God-given gift. It would prove to be medicine for her ailing soul. My sister was quite a trooper, a lover of life and eager to get on with the business of living. She laughed in the face of adversity and mocked the hand that put her in that chair. Like Daddy, she never let anything get in the way of her good time.

The crisis turned out to be a blessing. We kinda held together as a family the way we always did through troublesome times. As always, the albatross of responsibility was hung around Mama's neck. Nevertheless, she continued on. Hers was not a bold strength. It was a strength made perfect in weakness. Though weighed down with troubles, she would not give up. Problems in life seemed to push her to her personal best. Added burdens fell to push the wheelchair, keep Fay's appointments, and help with home instruction. We made it through, and as time moved on, the sun began shining again.

I remember always feeling on the periphery of Fay's experience, yet unknowingly, I was very much a part of it and it a part of me. Little did I know, in later years, I would develop a disability. I look back and comprehend what I couldn't understand then—how she was able to go on in spite of it all. Growing up with her inured me for the hardships I would one day face.

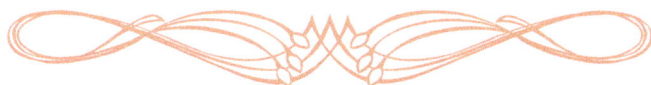

CHAPTER SEVEN
Fond Remembrances

HARD times were made easier by the good times and the special things we did as a family during those brief interludes that cushioned us from the intermittent blows of life, fond remembrances now stored up in the scrapbook of my memory. I look back on them from time to time, cherishing the tender feelings they bring to mind. I can remember…

Promenading down Barnes Avenue to Trinity Baptist Church, Mom in a big floral hat, we our Sunday best, entering the quiet vestibule, Mom resting with other saintly women on long pews. A resounding call to worship by a host of black choir voices united in song. Mom's low chords, a companion instrument, resonating finely amidst the throng…

Singing praise songs, realizing we had come a long way from a four-story walk-up to a private house—from a storefront church to a brick-front building with chandeliers, a gold pipe organ, and high arched windows along the wall that refracted gentle rays onto us all; from a minister just called upon to preach to one with a doctorate degree and fine speech…

On warm days, sunning in front of the house, Dad on the railing, Mom on a folding chair, we, squeezed in anywhere…batting our rickracks with the little red ball while watching pedestrians stroll… talking about them when they passed by…smiling to say hi…

Getting to know people on our street, their odd quirks and peculiar ways, neighbors we interfaced with each day: Mr. Cammock, the Brothers, Milton, and Don, who became strong stanchions in our lives, brightened our days with chuckles and quips and watered us so we would thrive…

Summer barbeques in the yard…hot coals…fanning exhaled smoke. Chicken brushed with homemade sauce sizzling on the fire…dousing ourselves with Coke. Counting moments until we ate…wishing it were steak on our flimsy paper plates. Couldn't wait to sink our teeth into the charred meat…sneaking a bite before time to eat…roaming freely with smoke-filled hair, knowing we'd found a place there…

Holiday parties, weekend shindigs when relatives happened by, eating, drinking, making merry. Some got a little high. Mama didn't like that, didn't like those low-class ways. She wanted us to grow up in a Christian home as in Grandma's days. Didn't allow no fussin' and cussin', which some were prone to do after they'd had a few…

Family get-togethers, foot stompin' on the living room floor, with Mom and Dad's longtime friends Lucille and Nathan…spinning records and joining in a sing-along 'cause we knew all the latest steps and the words to every song. "Y'all come on in here and dance for us!" they'd call. Their old-timey dances were from way back when—the slop, the shimmy, the rubber legs, the boogie woogie. We rolled with laughter watching them.

Music was always integral to our lives.

We created steps to "Do the Funky Penguin" and "Do the Push and Pull" by Rufus Thomas; cried the blues to "The Night Time Is the Right Time" and "Bright Lights, Big City" by Jimmy Reed; celebrated with those who made us feel good, "Shake, Rattle and Roll" by Bill Haney Jr., "Somebody's Been Sleeping in My Bed" by Robert Parker Jr. and "Pop That Thing" by the Isley Brothers; got down with James Brown in "Cold Sweat" and "I'm a Greedy Man"; fell into a groove to "Let's Get It On" by Marvin Gaye and "You Really Got a Hold on Me" by Smokey Robinson. Then we learned how to mend our broken hearts in "The Good Times" by Al Green.

Yes, music was with us all the time.

I can remember when we hung around Mama's dress tail as she cooked, cleaned, and sewed, tattling family secrets not to be disclosed. She couldn't keep hot news to herself. We were the first ones told, sitting around the kitchen table, laughing at her sanitary jokes, juicy tidbits, and funny anecdotes. Sometimes we ran to tell her what others had done to us, seeking her advice, knowing she'd have the answer because Mama was always right…discussing people we knew—what they did and why, the right and wrong of it—learning values as we pieced life puzzles together bit by bit…

Thrift stores and the Salvation Army were the places we used to shop, rummaging for "antiques" to buy for a dollar a pop…feeling very clever having spent nothing for a "priceless gem" and rushing home to display it in our home museum…

Gazing out of the back window, watching buds appear, then blossoms and fruit, apples, peaches, and pears…Sonny climbing the tree, throwing the ripe ones down. We collecting them from the ground and filling baskets. Mama gathering grapes to make wine. We sampling, sip at a time, afraid of getting "blind"…

Greeting tiny seedlings waking up from their winter rest. Chirping birds, nervous squirrels building nests. Following the seasons change as the Lord draped the windows in loveliness and knowing we were blessed with a glimpse of heaven. We had our traditions, our things we always did in the ways we did them. More important, we had each other and shared many precious, sacred, wonderful moments. No matter what that mean world was doing out there, we had a home where we could be ourselves and be accepted as we were. We squabbled over petty little things but remained glued together by love, acceptance, and forbearance. That glue became cement as the family endured over time.

Coming in off the front lines of life, family was a stronghold to retreat from battle, be filled with emotional food, and get an honest evaluation of ourselves. Within the family walls, we found safety and didn't have to be measured by the yardstick that whites used. By their estimation, a lot of our members were nothing and had nothing, but we could value ourselves where society did not value us. Together we were a collective force; we had to pull together to survive. When

Mama bought the house in the Bronx, everyone knew they had a place to eat or sleep, if needed.

Home was a place to receive sanction, affirmation, and encouragement—a safe haven where you didn't have to walk a certain walk or talk a certain talk to fit in, a place to let your hair down and catch your breath, a place to come to be replenished. Behind closed doors, we didn't do what the white man said do in the way he said do it. We developed styles and patterns that suited us and defined life on our own terms.

We had grown to a large extended family with lots of relatives who played special roles in our lives. Aside from real cousins Ethel, Nina, JoAnn, Carolyn, Henry Clay, and Earl Jr., there were play cousins like the Johnson kids we fraternized with. There was a real aunt Beulah and a play aunt Barbara. There were "adopted uncles," EJ and Finley (really Dad's cousins), Godmothers Ms. Bea and Suzy, even a play sister, Yvonne, who lived next door. All were connected in unique ways and influenced our upbringing. Each had a stake in our success or failures. We could pull up by them, copy from their models, and learn from their mistakes.

Storytelling was a family art as in the African tradition. Some, like cousin Ethel, being a natural comic, could spin a yarn on the spot, taking everyday occurrences and stretching them far beyond the truth to help us laugh at each other. Tales were passed down from way back when, recording funny things that happened as our people collided with modern society and tried to adjust to changing times and new environments.

There was one story about poor cousins in the South who lived in a time-worn shanty in the country. They had an ol' mule named Buddy-Ro tied up to their fragile front porch railing. The old kicker liked to do some railing of his own now and then. One day he tugged and jerked so heartily upon his reins that he pulled the house right down on top of them, thus prompting their move north. The self same relatives had since moved to Long Island, become "cidity," associated with white folks only, and used such proper diction no one in the family knew what they were talking about. This story was told in jest to poke fun at their attempts to take on new identities and leave the past behind. Stories were always of a loving, not intentionally harmful nature, our way of coping and passing down family history.

Since the time of slavery, societal restraints had controlled our externals, i.e., where we worked and lived. But we controlled internals, such as what we did inside our homes and how we expressed ourselves musically or in worship. Blacks were up against terrible odds in the urban centers. It was difficult to find jobs that paid a decent wage and made use of our talents. But within the family, everyone had something to contribute even if it was just their humor. Abandoning ourselves in laughter, singing, dancing, gossip, crazy talk, and silliness took some of the seriousness away from the situation and became a way of celebrating black family life and our traditions.

Stories kept the home fires burning, giving us a sense of rootedness and a connection with the past. In our hearts, ancestors remained with us—Grandma, Aunt Nannie, Aunt Betty, who died at 102. Their lives of sacrifice and humility gave us courage to carry on the struggle for justice and equality. They gave us spiritual moorings and a base on which to stand. They were our focal point to look back and know from whence we'd come. And they directed us toward a brighter future as we looked through the eyes of their faith.

In recent years, now that many in our community have advanced to a level that they can dot every *i* and cross every *t*, some of us have become so highfaluting we've forgotten the rocky roads that brought us here, forgotten that ol' time religion we learned at our grandmas' knees and those values mamas taught over the kitchen tables. Now that we've thrown off the homespuns of poverty and humility, I wonder if we aren't losing the best part of what we had in our attempts to gain access to the mainstream of America and climb the ladder to success, if we aren't losing those down-home basics that were as sturdy as the crocus sack dresses black girls wore back when they were called piccaninnies. Those solid basics helped us endure the cruel institution of slavery, the Reconstruction, the Depression, and mass migrations from the South to the northern cities. In our present condition of economic hardships, a strong sense of family and community can help us through our present woes.

In those times, I understood black family ways, but it came in direct conflict with what the world said about us and who we were. The media painted a very different picture and made me feel I needed to be ashamed of my heritage as an African American. They never described us as a principled people with good values. Rather, they perpetuated stereotypes that put us down, i.e., broken families, mothers on welfare, illegitimate births, government dependency, living in public housing, and lack of education. Negative stories about black criminals made front headlines, whereas positive stories appeared in the miscellaneous column in the back of the newspaper. Good things happening in the black belts of the South and black pockets of the northern cities were downplayed. I had little awareness of our contribution to the fabric of American life, which fostered an attitude of self-deprecation and self-doubt.

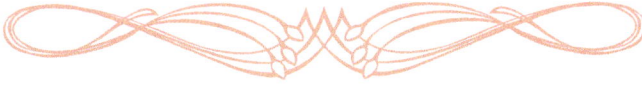

CHAPTER EIGHT
Who Am I Really?

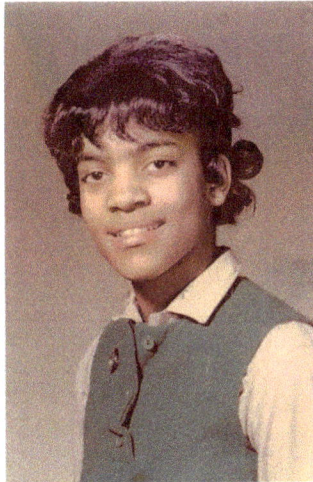

Me as a young student.

I began defining myself by what I was not, i.e., not on welfare, not a criminal, not from a broken home, not low class, not loud and rowdy, not living in the projects, not government supported, not illegitimate, and not illiterate. I couldn't define myself adequately by who I was because I didn't know who I was in the deeper sense of the word. Our link with the glorious empires of the African past had long been severed. My knowledge of black history was a pittance more than being able to name a few famous former slaves, like Harriet Tubman and Harriet Beecher Stowe. We couldn't trace our genealogies beyond slavery and embrace our African heritage. No sacred scrolls were passed down to us by our forefathers recording our trek through the wilderness of American bigotry. The pith of our experience was captured in slave songs, Negro spirituals, wailing blues, jazz, gospel, and soul—a musical history of a people attempting to become unfettered from an ignominious past. We can never put that past away; nor can white America. We are inextricably tied to one another—tied—but we do not have to be bound by the shackles of hatred forever, especially if we stop denying, come to grips with racism, and move forward. As a child growing up, I sifted what I'd heard down through the grid of my own experience and came away confused. I felt ashamed of being born black, like a nobody who had come from nothing, and concluded I would need to measure up to the socioeconomic standards and expectations of the outer culture. I felt my individual family was broken and needed to be fixed. I was deeply concerned about my parents' fractured marriage and my sister's blindness. I thought it was my destiny to be the hero who would rescue them, since grace seemed to have smiled upon me. I took on the role of "child star" who was going to do well in everything, reasoning, if I could do well enough or be good enough, it would make up for what I perceived to be wrong with us, or I could somehow heal us and make up for our insufficiencies.

Continuing in school, I tried to be the model student, got good grades, and earned the teachers' praise while fighting low esteem and lack of confidence. I was going after success to try and bring balance to the family as a way of dealing with the pain I was feeling. Fay took on the role of the clown who made us laugh, a sure panacea for any ailment. Sonny became the sacrificial lamb, whose childhood was burned on the family altar, as it seemed Dad had just put him down and emotionally left him. As Daddy became the absentee father, he became the "absentee son," present but not involved in the life of things.

Ingress into the neighborhood had not been emotionally easy. We all have sensing devices that pick up impressions and keep invisible boundaries on our communities and relationships. The border of turf yielding to integration extended from Gunhill Road at the south, to East 233rd at the north, Bronx Park to the west, and Boston Road going east.

Officially Wakefield, the hood was called Uptown, or the North Bronx, as opposed to the South Bronx. Beyond Boston Road was an area known as the Valley, almost purely Italian, stretching east to Pelham Parkway where the Jews lived. Clearly defined lines separated us and mediated our relations. Those boundary lines, seen and unseen, were not permeable and held back the natural flow of communication between groups, becoming great walls of partition that were hard to tear down.

Americans are racially sensitive and foolish about their ethnicity. Everyone wants to be of pure descent in a direct line from an ancestral fountainhead, which spewed them forth from the annals of time, to whom they owe their life's blood and cultural allegiance. Many feared the anonymity of the melting pot. Racial theory held that if you had one-quarter Negro blood in you, then you were a Negro. A drop of ink in a glass of milk changes its constitution. It's no surprise, then, blacks were ill-favored ingredients in the national stew. What could have been a pleasant gumbo in the cities was soon to become boiling caldrons of racial unrest. People of color didn't need to see the Whites Only signs in windows to know where we weren't wanted. We knew there were social as well as career limitations that were unspoken. Unconscious assumptions saturated the thinking of blacks and whites alike, stymying our progress—assumptions that blacks were lazy, incapable, jealous, and destructive, while whites were ambitious, trustworthy, intelligent, good at business, and *needed* to maintain standards and control.

Cultural bias was evident in the derogatory words we used to describe each other. In private circles, Northern whites used the words *blackie*, *Nigger*, or *colored people*. In the South, popular slurs were *monkeys*, *boots*, *coons*, *spooks*, or *watermelon eaters*. Face-to-face, they referred to us as "You people" (an obvious debasement). In formal settings, like school, the word *Negro* was used. Below the Mason-

Dixon Line, black men were called boy and a woman gal regardless of age, denying recognition of their adult status.

Soon our men adopted a style of hailing each other "Hey, man! What's happening?" and incorporated "man, man, man" repeatedly in their conversations. It was as if they were feeding their own psyches to counter the childish position they were placed in by society. Black men continued to struggle with manhood issues as forces outside our communities encouraged hate, disrespect, and anger between them, leading to black-on-black crime, acts of violence, and a high mortality rate for young males.

Nicknames for whites were Whitey, the Man, Boss, or Boss Man, and Mr. Charlie up North; rednecks or crackers in the South, indicating color and positional relation. Whites most often chose the term *American*, as if to suggest that we were not Americans, rather bastardized rejects, sired by our former slave masters, for whom there was no mother country.

We have always had difficulty selecting an appropriate name for ourselves. Generally, we used the word *colored* because it appeared on our birth certificates under race. Racial categories listed on government forms adjacent to little check-off boxes were (1) White, (2) Asian, (3) Indian, (4) Colored, (5) Other, in descending order, as if to show a digression from the pinnacle of perfection. I would always just check "Other" to take issue with their labeling of me.

We wrestled daily with mixed feelings about who and what we were. Ofttimes when speaking, one to another, we attempted to dissociate ourselves from the actions of our group with remarks like, "You know how yo' people are!" If we didn't always want to be identified with our race, when would the world begin to give us sanction?

When children are fed an acumen of shame and racial ridicule associated with their race, overtly or covertly, it becomes internalized into a low self-concept. My parents had to do a lot of talking to us to counter those negative voices carping from without and those gnawing voices whispering from within that made us feel unworthy. Mama insisted, "Don't be what they say we are! Aim higher!" Daddy added, "Don't never let nobody tell you what you can or cannot do!

Put up a fight to prove 'em wrong!" It was a message we heard again and again.

Defining oneself by color seemed natural because, in America, everyone was so color conscious and things were so color dependent, i.e., where you lived and worked and whom you married. Mixed marriages were very unpopular. Whites said miscegenation spoiled their race, or as they express it in today's language, "It's bad for the children." Some blacks believed intermarriage improved ours, as the offspring of such a union inherits the white parent's attributes. Interracial marriage has grown in the United States since more minorities have reached up to par with whites in education, careers, and economic standing, which shows some level of breakdown of barriers.

I remember an English teacher who encouraged me to look up the meaning of every word I wasn't sure of. I promptly looked in the dictionary to decipher those word descriptors used to define me. Under *Negro*, they had listed, "a person belonging to any of the black races of Africa, characterized by black skin, coarse wooly hair and a flat nose." They went on to point out that the word *Negro* had, in times past, been written with a small letter, as if to minimize our significance. It indicated, as a black female, I should correctly be called a negress, which sounded to me like someone fat, black, and ugly. A nigger, likewise, was "a member of a dark-skinned race." The word engendered such angry feelings that if a white kid called us blackie or nigger in the schoolyard, those were fighting words. Under *colored* it said "having to do with color, not black or white," implying whites were pure and my people were somehow polluted, perverted, mixed, indistinct, or tinged.

I disdained the idea of being impure, even saw my tan complexion as evidence of racial mixing in my bloodline long ago. Mama told me that my great-grandmother, on her side, was white—the kind of thing blacks spoke of proudly, as if having a little white blood in their veins made them feel more worthwhile. I felt I must have had the leaven of whiteness spreading on the inside because I was inclined toward intellectual pursuits and admired refined behavior. Surely, this couldn't stem from my black nature, I reasoned, for they said this was not intrinsic to "our kind." Deep down, I wanted to be connected to Mother Africa, not Father Slave Master.

The dictionary listed other weird words like *Negrophil*, a person who favors the advancement of Negro rights and interests. It sounded like a very sick person, like a pedophile (a child molester). One word, listed *negritudinous*, was defined as "the distinct qualities or characteristics of Negroes." We heard said, Whites thought we had characteristics like monkeys—long arms, thick necks, flattened or slanted craniums, bowed legs, starry eyes, broad noses, thick lips, and a strong odor. Some even believed we had tails! Kids made up a tease, "The other day I went to the zoo, saw a monkey that looked just like you!" to which we'd reply, "Yo Mama!" and on and on went their taunts. Evolutionists said the ape was our progenitor. But I'd seen a "Nigger fish" that had big lips. And they used to call dark-skinned people "black-a-moors" after the ones with the big poppy eyes, which caused me to wonder. Racists contended blacks were lower on the evolutionary scale than whites, thus inferior in intellect, driven by primitive passions and strong libido, and given over to violence.

My mother often gave us reminders to not go around "acting like a nigger," or we'd bring shame and be an embarrassment to our race. She said colored people were good at "singing, dancing and acting like monkeys," but we were to be more sophisticated and show we had good sense, repress all those negritudes in manner and speech that made us stand out in the white world.

As time moved on, blacks began using the word *nigger* differently from whites. It became a sort of affirmation of oneness. There was a feeling of "you and me together" in its application. I'm not certain if it was to show our bond with a sense of pride or in mutual commiseration of our lowly estate. The word evolved to mean a guy who is cool, physically adept, and can "make it" with women. It's sometimes applied to someone who "ain't too cool," "up to something," or "trying to get over." There are many creative uses of this base ugly word.

Today the media takes full advantage of the aura of blackness, highly exploiting it on film and in the music industry. Celebrities earn millions off what my mother would have considered a disgrace to the race. Years ago, if blacks appeared in commercials, whites wouldn't buy the products, assuming they were targeted at black consumers. Now we see the swaggering walk, the body moves, black hair and clothing styles, the stress on physical prowess and athleticism associated with black sexual bravado, the stare, exaggerated facial and labial gestures, street lingo and hand jive—all used to sell merchandise and imbue characters with affectations of blackness.

Artists in music videos have created a whole new visual and spoken language, which has brought the heart and soul of urban street life into middle-class homes. Much of the new imagery frightens parents but entertains their teens. Standard English has been heaved out of the window and replaced by a rapid-fire jargon and new genre of street words with nuances of meaning, often spliced together with expletives, sexually suggestive innuendos, and calls to violence. Can it be that the music of the inner city has become a vehicle for expressing many of the emotions ravaging white American youth? Have they found common ground in rap music that wasn't realized in other ways? On the surface, they may seem worlds apart, but are they really? Youth culture is being inundated with sex, drugs, and a propensity toward violence. The same cancerous malignancy is growing in both camps. Ironically, today everybody wants to be a "nigger," but still no one wants to be black.

Like most kids, we were very accepting of white kids in the neighborhood as playmates. Two old friends stand out fondly in my stockpile of childhood memories.

Debbie, a lissome young Italian girl, lived in the apartment building near the corner. I don't recall how we met, but from the outset, she was like fly paper with a tenacious hold. The cute little nudge tagged along closely wherever we went. No sooner than school let out, she came straight to our house and burst in through the door like a family member with a bubbly smile. Wide-eyed and curious, Little Buttinsky was forever in the way wanting to join in everything we did. Being older, we were charmed by our nagging little "sister" and her endearing manner. But Mama used to say she wished that child would go home.

I think she was attracted to us by our difference. Keen and inquisitive, she'd sit and stare as Mom pressed our hair, twitching her nose at the stench of crackling grease, which wasn't at all enticing, like the scent of hot oil frying chicken in the cast iron pan. Her sparkling eyes crackled to the sights, sounds, and rhythms of black family life—jumping, bouncing, ricocheting back and forth—to take it all in. She didn't despise difference; neither did she reject it. For her, it was a refreshing foray, a new experience from which to learn. Yet she didn't need to feel threatened. She came to visit, enjoyed the things we did, then skipped happily back up the street to her world. There was no penalty for crossing over the line, no losing face, no abandoning her race.

The innocence of a child is something to be admired. If we all viewed cultural differences with open, honest curiosity and acceptance as Debbie did, perhaps racial intolerance would diminish. Debbie once asked my brother Sonny, "Why do you have Bosco on your face?" referring to the dark-chocolate syrup that came in a can. Sonny was hurt by her impish quizzing, and I'm not sure if it was said in total innocence or if there wasn't a veneer of mockery applied by her family's careful coaching. At least there was a directness about her that said what was on her mind upfront where it could be dealt with. The truth about racism is that it is so often our hidden attitudes and prejudices that control us. We cloak them behind niceties of speech and practiced demeanor so we won't have to own up to them. None of us wants to pluck out those dreadful weeds growing in our inner gardens.

Debbie came and came and kept on coming until her older brother Robert, concerned that she not be labeled a little nigger lover, discouraged her frequent visits, pulling her back on their side of the line. Eventually, they moved to Yonkers. Years later, she drove up on the block in a polished, flashy red car, well dressed, and having the affluence her color had afforded her. I didn't reintroduce myself, seeing she'd put us and 228th Street behind. But I was happy to see her all grown up and satisfied with warm memories of past days.

Another friend, Johanna, and her middle-aged parents were emigres from the old country also. Her father passed away soon after their arrival, and the projects were the only decent place she and her mom could afford while putting their lives together. We met in school, and she and I quickly became bosom buddies. In the mornings, I'd take the long route walking several blocks out of my way to pick her up for school. Walking along, we chatted wildly about anything and everything, mindful of no one, caught up in girlish whimsies and fancies. Afternoons, we'd unwind the events of the day, parting only at her door with a lonely goodbye. Sometimes I'd go in to visit her grieving mom, who spoke Italian and wore black mourning clothes like Mrs. Mavarro. She welcomed me, showed no prejudice, and I, like Debbie, enjoyed the opportunity to be comfortable in her home and her world, even if for a short time.

Yes, it was always me and Johanna, Johanna and me, until puberty set in and we were forced apart by pressures from kids at school who made it seem odd or inappropriate for us to have such love for each other. In junior high school, we became very identity conscious, and the message that we were to stay within our group was made clear, especially as girls and boys paired off for dating.

My first pubescent infatuation was with John DeLuigi, a half-black, half-Italian boy in my seventh-grade class. I watched him with adoring eyes and couldn't concentrate on my lessons when spring breezes slipped in quietly through the open window and whispered songs of love in my ears. I kept my affections secret, thinking myself too boyishly built—tall, lanky, and flat chested—for him to fall for me. We never got beyond a silly grin in passing and rubbing knees under the library table when we sat on opposite sides. Actually, I don't know why I had such a crush on him; he was always getting into trouble. The clumsy, playful puppy was inclined toward mischief, but I "loved" him anyway. I remember when his mother was called to school, and to everyone's surprise, she was white, though he was black. The teacher was curt but polite to her, and the kids were all confused, but it did explain his last name, DeLuigi. I decided to be mixed was not so bad. Besides, Mrs. Loretta DeLuigi had a very nice ring to it, better than Loretta Jean Farmer.

In the 1960s the population of the projects succumbed to changing times. Government-supported racial segregation fell by the wayside, at least at that particular site. Numbers of black and Hispanic families moved in. No longer a temporary stopping ground for people on their way to something better, it became a place of refuge for large, poor families, many headed by women on welfare who would make it their permanent home. The residents were often preyed on by crime and vandalism, the buildings poorly maintained, and police were conspicuously absent.

Not to suggest all project dwellers were bad. Many successful people made their starts there, like the inimitable Bill Cosby, who came from the projects of Philadelphia, and Kareem Abdul-Jabbar, who polished his basketball skills on the ball courts of Edenwald during those years. However, for upwardly mobile whites, the downward trend of the units acted as a vacuum that sucked them out and accelerated deterioration of the surrounding area. Suctioned out were my friend Johanna and her mother, who found a cheap private alternate in a nicer vicinity.

John and his mother were not swept along with the ebb of the tide. Suburbia did not welcome a white mother and black child with open arms. She stayed and made her way in the black community. John was transferred out of the school because of his behavior problems. I believe he was placed in a 600 school, which were jail-like institutions where they placed black boys who caused too much trouble. I suppose, I am the only one who saw it as a great loss, for I lost my first love.

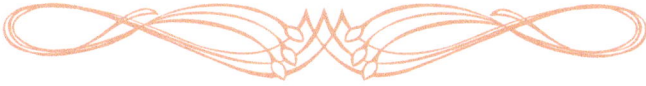

CHAPTER NINE
The Tide of Change

WANDERING waves hurried out to sea, carrying with them pearlescent stones destined for neighboring shores, sprinkling colorful shells on the once-white sands of Wakefield. Students of European, Latin American, and Caribbean backgrounds attended Sousa Junior High along with me. Roll call was like traveling to Italy, then Spain, winding around the islands of the West Indies, and up through the South. As the school population mixed in a potpourri of national minorities, conflicts arose. Each subgroup squirmed and wiggled for a comfortable spot, vying for recognition. Assimilation, even among Third World peoples, didn't proceed smoothly because of cultural and language barriers. Jamaicans stuck with Jamaicans, Latinos with Latinos, and American blacks with blacks. Each tried to retain their identities while sharing densified living space.

The funny thing about integration is that when people of various ethnic backgrounds were brought together in the same community, they tended to enwall themselves and intermingled with their own while putting up a facade for others. Whether out of fear or familiarity, I don't know. Folks seemed happier when they knew where the line was drawn, knew which slot everyone belonged in, and interacted based on the sum of preconceptions they held about other cultural groups.

Years have passed by and I now live in an integrated middle-class subdivision. The civil rights battles have been fought and won, but I still see a line or feel it's still there. I know the line exists only in my mind. Growth of closer relations between the races has been impeded by the limitations of tradition and the roots of history.

My older relatives' names were not like the kids at school. Common names changed from generation to generation. My father's last name, Farmer, was probably taken from a slave holder three generations ago and may have dated back to the days when surnames related to a person's trade, i.e., Thatcher, Taylor, Shoemaker, Miller, or Baker. His given name, Andrew Jackson, is connected to an earlier custom blacks had of naming their offspring after famous whites to give them status. For example, George Washington Carver was named after the first president of the United States. I have relatives whose names are Henry Clay and Robert E. Lee. My sister, Alice Fay, and cousin Desi Arnaz were both named after movie stars. But the new generation of black mothers tended toward names more nontraditional in origin.

In my parents' generation, common names for men were Ike, Nate, Willie, Levi, Dooley, and Knoscoe; for women, Doletha, Beulah, Aldine, Lucy Rec, and Chanie. Names of biblical origin, John, Mary, Jacob, and Ruth, were also popular. Mom's full name was Ernestine Ruby Daisy Rankin, though her friends called her Stine. Dad's mom was affectionately known as Aunt Pete. Mom's parents were called Daddy Will and Mama Fannie.

In middle school, nicknames took on powerful meanings. Adoption of a name could take you from who you were to who you wanted to be. For preteens with emerging identities, this was devastatingly important. White kids had nicknames as American as apple pie: Billy, Joey, Cindy, Kathy. Black kids had these wacky nicknames, like Pookie, Ray Ray, Ju Ju, Dupree, BB, and NeeCee. Boo Boo, of all horrid nicknames, was mine. As I grew long and lean, I was called Jean the Bean or Bony Moroni, as in Little Richard's hit song that went, "I got a girl named Bony Maroni. She's as skinny as a stick of macaroni."

I would have preferred something sweet and simple like Heidi, as Shirley Temple was called in an old movie classic. How I wanted to be like the delightful little pauper with the golden curls. I had already been well indoctrinated with a white standard of beauty—long blond hair, blue eyes, and an apple figure—growing up in the era of the Hollywood starlet Marilyn Monroe. I was particularly fond of two great feature films, *King Kong* and *Mighty Joe Young*, where beautiful, fair-haired damsels made monkeys of monstrous beasts.

At that age, girls had an overriding concern with how they looked. It was an age when kids saw every wart of imperfection in themselves and others. Normally, kids poked fun at someone who wore glasses or had buckteeth. Black girls really put each other through the wringer as they came to grips with the saddle brands of their ethnicity. Kids regularly picked on skin pigmentation and hair length, saying, "Her hair is about yea long!" while giving their fingers a gingersnap or marking barely an inch on their indexes with their thumbs. If you had peppercorn hair, you were called Beadee Head or Nappy Head. If you had thick lips, they named you Liver Lips or Bubba Lips. A really dark-skinned person was called Midnight or Smokey Joe. And if you had any combination of the above, you were not just ugly but u-glee.

During those years, girls had an obsession with fashion magazines in eagerness to try on new looks we saw in books. However, most of the models were white and had skinny schoolboy figures. We were likewise drawn to romantic novels, provocative books, and comics featuring characters with exaggerated bottle figures and beauty queen smiles. I used to try to decide if I'd be better off as a blonde like Super Girl, a fiery redhead like Brenda Starr or a brunette like the Kewpie doll Betty Boop. I loved the Breck girl and Miss Clairol commercials on TV that asked, "Is it true blondes have more fun?" longing to have flowing tresses that danced a lively reel with the wind. What always caught my eye were ads for products that gave the hair bounce and sheen. Bounce was one thing my hair would not do. It was more inclined to stand straight up on my head like dried grass.

Black girls wanted to have "good hair" because long curly locks drew many suitors' eyes. But if it was short and coarse like mine, boys didn't waste any time. Hair that fell to the shoulders was my great desire. Yet if it grew just enough to roll up in a fancy twist and comb fluffy bangs, that would have been fine! I would have loved to have had a jaunty ponytail that twirled and flipped like a white girl's or a dark mane tickling my spine bone like a Puerto Rican.

When you are a black girl in a white society, trying to achieve acceptability in the realm of beauty, you characteristically feel like you'll never measure up to the standard. You get messages flashed to you a thousand a minute through the media that you can't compete and be successful if you don't look a certain way. The stereotypical black girl was buxom and bosomy and had a big "bootie," heavy thighs, and big legs and feet, while the media pushed thinnest. It made us feel very ugly, not just on the surface, but deep down, like something was wrong with us and we were not okay. There was tremendous stress to be perfect in the way we looked, to conform to the white-doll image. We black girls were very vulnerable, having been led to believe that we were less and certainly were not beautiful. For many this led to poor self-image down on the inside.

We were like diamonds in the rough who had always been taught we were nothing but worthless cut glass. We had natural beauty but didn't know how to accent it. Rather, we ignored our beauty and tried to take on someone else's, becoming poor imitations. The concept of beauty or handsomeness, in our culture, is a very emotional issue. When we didn't feel desirable, attractive, or loveable, there was pain, which was acted out in meanest toward girls who were "pretty." Many lunchtime fights occurred when a hard-faced bully pounced on some cute, popular girl wearing nice clothes. The bully would try to claw her face and rip out clumps of her hair. The word quickly spread, "She think she cute! Who do she think she is?" Inevitably, she would be accused of trying to steal some girl's boyfriend. Lunchtime was often "punch time," with two or three fights breaking out during one recess. Fights sometimes involved nail files, pen knives, or scissors but rarely had consequences as deadly as the wild West shootouts occurring in today's urban schools.

We began to connect our low self-concept with all of life's challenges. We felt unattractive to the larger pool of men in the world and to our own black males. Proof of success for a black man, after he had gotten a good job, a house, and a fancy car, was to have a white woman swinging on his arm as if she were his crowning glory. We wanted to be like white girls, yet we joked about them, calling them "patties," saying they didn't have rhythm and couldn't dance. To us, they looked like helpless little fawns...so frail a strong wind could knock them over. Our attitude was one of resentment tinged with envy because they had what we wanted...or maybe it wasn't so much that we wanted what they had, but we desired to be recognized for our own unique qualities.

Still we knew the standard of perfection was the white woman. It moved down to other ethnic minorities, then black women, as always, were on the bottom of the pile. America recognized foreign beauties from around the world in grand pageantry. Even Asian women were placed on pedestals as lovely China dolls, with the gentle essence of the Orient in their eyes. Black girls rarely competed in contests with other beauty queens and were never expected to win.

We didn't show pride in black fashions as a people and didn't identify hairstyles such as braiding or plaiting as part of our African tradition, rather as vestiges left over from slavery that brought to mind images of bent-over women scrubbing clothes in a tub, with barefoot young'uns peek-a-booing from the tatters of their dress tails. Girl groups like the Shirelles and the Supremes tried to emulate white stars by wearing highly teased bouffant wigs, heavy makeup, and similar clothing. Whites set the fashion trend, until the sixties when designers began sneaking up to Harlem to copy the loud patterns and clothing styles worn in the ghetto and putting them on Fifth Avenue models. In fact, the miniskirt, so popular in the '60s, was an original black design.

I looked at myself through unforgiving eyes. My head was too big, body too tall, legs and arms too long—no good at all! There was nary a curve on my body nor a blurb on my chest. I was as flat as a billboard. Girls like me didn't catch too many flies, but those New York City pigeons rarely missed me with they dropped pennies from heaven.

At that age, when I was not only thinking about how I looked but asking myself the question, "What do I want to be when I grow up?" it was hard to get a sense of where I was going and be convinced I could live up to my fullest potential. I developed an overly pessimistic view that said, "There's not much of a future for me. Nothing good is ever going to happen to me because I'm not worthy!" an intense sense of hopelessness. I felt like a tender shoot trying to push my head above ground, through a rocky bed of clay, sandstone, and shale. If I made it through the levels of impediments, one day, I'd see the light. Some of the impediments were external. Others were what I felt like down inside.

It's difficult to see beyond what Mama was and Daddy was, and since they hadn't achieved highly in the white world, I didn't believe I could either. I looked around for role models or heroes to point to and say, "I want to be like that person and follow in those footsteps." But there weren't many black professionals around where I lived. Most of the teachers in my school were Jewish; some were Italians. Positions of power and authority in the city school system were held by whites, as was true in most public- and private-sector jobs. The numbers of black and Hispanic teachers were disproportionately few. Many held jobs performing menial labor in low-level service positions or doing factory work with low pay and limited benefits. Supervisory, management positions and positions of decision-making, by and large, were held by whites. They were the most lucrative, with the least amount of physical exertion. Blacks were the last hired and the first fired and had no authority. Often they were denied union membership and had no redress for grievances, whether they were discrimination or job related. If you got a job working for the city, that was considered a plum, and you stayed there until you fell numb. Unreal expectations were placed on them to be twice as good as their white counterparts in order to stay employed or get ahead.

As for professions, they used to say we had a choice between teacher, preacher, and social worker. Outside of those fields, I didn't know what else I could aspire to and reasonably hope to attain, aside from entertainment or sports, where the ball was in our court. I thought of something in the arts, since I leaned toward the creative, but wondered if I knocked on those doors, would any open for me, or would they remain like towering obelisks blocking my path? What about science or medicine? Are you kidding? I was bright, but surely not enough for that. Besides, you could fit all the black women doctors around in the crown of a hat. What about entrepreneurship or fields involving great risk? Ump! That's funny! My parents didn't have no money, honey!

Mom and Dad used to dream of opening an eatery to sell fried fish 'n' chips, which had been a popular takeout food down in Harlem. They were certain it would go over big in this increasingly black area of the Bronx, for we knew our people really like fish. But the reality was that banks would not lend money to us to open a small business due to lack of capital to put down and not believing in our success. Most blacks were considered poor business risks. With no reserve wealth or resources, no in-laws to turn to for lump sum cash, no network of friends to go in together, and no business experience, they would not take a chance on us. I never wanted my parents to come to school for fear other kids would make fun, feeling ashamed of who they were and where I'd come from.

How unlike the Italian immigrants we were, who had strong family networks, could pool skills and resources, and had tremendous experience in building. Even the West Indian workers migrating from the islands came with many more marketable skills in carpentry, electrical work, masonry, and plumbing, in part because of the difficulty our men had getting hired on construction sites or joining trade unions and the failure of the city school system to provide basic training in those areas. Additionally, for the most part, whites did not patronize black-owned businesses. From my vantage point, the prospects of owning my own business, one day, seemed nil. Besides, as a female, the thought of heading up something was frightening still.

In the vernacular of that day, we had become hip young teeny-boppers who spent our time being cool, while parents were the squares who kept the conventions. Boys skipped and dipped doing the diddy-bop walk. Girls finger popped, talkin' that jive talk. Like dance masters with natural rhythm and style, we kept the record player blaring all the while. Our steps were never off the beat, not like white people who had two left feet. We knew how to rock and how to roll, because black people had a whole lotta soul. Yeah! We got down like James Brown, when I was thirteen, fourteen years old. Didn't listen to none of that Beatles stuff. It just wasn't funky enough!

Girls "so fly" and guys "so fine" wore dark shades and leather all the time. "Hey! What's happening?" That's the way we spoke. "I'm hip!" "Be cool!" "Ain't no joke!" "Outta sight!" "Sock it to me!" "Serious!" "I'm Baddd!" Best fun we ever had, can you dig it?

Pig Latin, a silly codification, kept adults out of our conversations. It was a kid's mumbo-jumbo that made much ado about nothing. Pop-a-rop-top-yop meant there was a party going on, and if Mom would permit, we'd split downtown on the subway to join our friends for a get-together—a little soda, Ripple, and potato chips, lights turned down low, kids bumpin' and grindin' up against the wall real slow, couples practicing how to tongue kiss in the darkness. Sometimes a boy would sneak a feel as emotions began to reel. Good girls didn't fall for that deal. Oh! No! We didn't go all the way, and we told them so. Object of the game? To give a guy your number for they were expected first to call. The phone rang off the hook for Fay; I got no calls at all. I was about as sociable as a rose pattern stenciled on a wall—a Ms. Goody Two-shoes, quiet and refined, too high minded to chase a boy, too timid to grind. Anyway, I assumed a cute boy could never be mine, so why gamble and lose? Besides, I kinda liked being a prude. There were times when I was in the mood, but I was scared—real scared. And so I curled into a shell and there lay hidden very well, safe, secure, watching from the confines of the sidelines.

A lot of girls came home with hickies on their necks, as those love lumps were called, when boys bit them in the throes of passion. Think that's why beads and turtlenecks were so in fashion in those years. Fast girls displayed them proudly like victory badges. Poor me would have broken down in tears. Not Fay! She was confident, unafraid, never coy. She enjoyed toying and teasing with boys, juggling them like balls in the air. If one fell from her hand, she didn't care. She played the dating game to win. I wanted to be like her now and then. Seemed she had all the fun keeping guys in a spin.

We were like two young birds growing the feathers needed to fly—fledglings not yet plumed, fletched in Mama's teachings yet inexperienced and new, spreading our wings, getting into things. Our parents gave us freedom to venture from the nest, knowing to learn we had to be put to the test.

It was a time of relative modesty about the body. Girls believed in having a little shame, for one too loose and uninhibited quickly found herself with a bad name. It was a time when morals counted for something and honoring parents didn't make you a square. Yes, we bent the rules to savor a few enticements, but that towing line was always there, keeping us in check. We didn't speak as if parents were our buddies, understanding their positions deserved respect. If Mama and Daddy beat our tails for doing something wrong, we didn't take it as child abuse. It kept us in line, made us mindful so that freedom wouldn't become a noose on which to hang our youth.

Clothing was fun and faddy, and as always, young people set the fashion stage. Styles were not so generationally distinct and could be worn by persons of any age. Jeans and sneakers, not yet in vogue, were considered bummy clothes. They hadn't evolved into wardrobe necessities glamorized by superstars with a hundred-dollar price cards. We wore baubles, trinkets, and costume jewelry, silver earrings and bangles at best. I would have felt like a queen in a forty-dollar dress. No gold chains or diamond rings, we could be satisfied with ordinary things.

Music was not so exclusive to one age group, like rap. In our home there wasn't really a generation gap. My parents enjoyed the down-home blues; we, R&B. Bobby Blue Bland and BB King were their music idols. Smokey, Marvin, the Temps, and Aretha were our rivals. Still, we mixed it all together in a hot soul jambalaya. When company came by, we did our thing. Adults taught us the ballroom and the swing. We taught them the monkey, the watusi, the swim, the bird, the penguin, and the shing-a-ling. Music was a mediator in our relations. It spoke a language we all understood, brought us together, and made us feel good. I loved to see my parents dance closely, holding each other tight. Made me feel like everything was going to be all right.

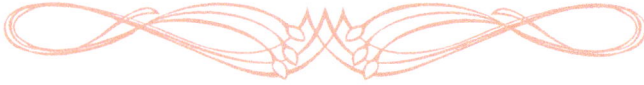

CHAPTER TEN
In Middle School

OFTTIMES our living room became an open forum in which to vent and sound off about things we felt strongly, sociopolitical issues as well as love matters. Mom and Dad made us feel our opinions were worthwhile and worth expressing. Verbal jousting, as long as it was not vicious, was welcomed as a way of preparing us for the politically hot arena we were growing up in. We confronted issues head-on and grew to be very aware of current events by following the nightly news broadcasts of Walter Cronkite. We witnessed the bilious attacks against freedom marchers in the South who had begun to campaign for civil rights and heard accusations of brutality that rang out like a booming overture against white policemen. We experienced, as if actually there, cops wielding billy clubs, spraying water hoses, and commanding dogs whose fitful snarls filled our dreams with terror. We developed fear and deep suspicion of the government, the white power structure, and the establishment.

I drew the conclusion that it was the white man's intention to keep us down for his own selfish reasons. I figured they enjoyed seeing our lives and communities in shambles, didn't want us to be or have anything. Seems to their minds, they owed us nothing, not forty acres and a mule, not a decent education in school, not a ballot in a voter box, not a house on the same block, not equal jobs in the workplace, not even a safe haven to pray, because they bombed our churches and killed innocent children.

I decided, if we persisted despite the obstacles, we'd beat them at their own game, for we were the intended losers, not winners. The whole system worked to keep us on the bottom, begging, dependent, in jail, or on welfare—powerless to help ourselves. It was a racist system so well constructed; the blame for our failures was always placed on us, when in reality the chances of making it to the top were as slim as a camel going through the eye of a needle. Yet some made it, but their success was held over the heads of others as proof, "If they could make it, so could you!" knowing full well there were many exceptions to that rule.

Although Mom and Dad were unskilled laborers, they were not lacking in drive to move up and do better. Always there was the sense we were headed for something and constantly trying to improve. Perhaps there was too much emphasis on better jobs, housing, degrees, and material items to just make us feel good about *ourselves*. But they tried to counter the messages of a biased society that said we were less by stressing self-respect and good character.

Mom sat us down and counseled us, giving words of warning and encouragement like saying to get pregnant wouldn't prove anything. We'd just make another mouth we couldn't feed and cut off our chances to succeed. Her way of strongly instilling family values was to say, "Even an ol' sooner dog can lay down and have pups! It requires no intelligence." The consequence of early pregnancy would be we'd have to leave home in disgrace, and our babies would grow up fatherless. A woman's reputation had to be carefully guarded, for society would not forgive her for sewing wild seeds the way it did men.

What pulled us through those potentially rebellious years and kept our lives from becoming a skein of knotty entanglements was being potted in rich soil. We had a good home life, although our family was dysfunctional in certain ways. There were problems between my parents, but I never felt they would really split up. They were both strongly committed to us. Mom was always there. Dad, though he strayed, always came back. If we stepped out on a rope, there would be a safety net to catch us on a fall. Yet we were warned not to take foolish chances, or as Dad would say, "Don't press your luck!"

Our parents were not too pushy or authoritarian, but they towed the line when needed. They didn't press the panic button when things happened either. Just set us free to find our way with watchful guidance after repeating the old adage, "If you make your bed hard, that's where you are going to sleep!" They did a good job of teaching us responsibility and holding us to accountability.

When I compare myself to my mother, I realize I had education, but Mom had mother wit. She understood family as a process that would all come together one day. When bad things happened, her attitude was, "This too shall pass!" Always we had a circumference of support from Mom and Dad, family, and friends. They didn't have much to give us, but we knew they believed in us and would be there for us regardless.

I was the sort of student who did my homework and paid attention in class, but the kind of education I was getting only added to my identity crisis. In studying American history, I wanted to know the role African Americans played in the development of our toddling nation. Such information was carefully excluded from the curriculum. It seemed we had been edited out of the story, except for pointed reminders we had been slaves until the Great Emancipator, Abe Lincoln, set us free, not out of moral indignation at slavery as an unjust institution, rather as an act to save a divided nation.

When studying history, it's not only important the events that took place. Who is telling the story makes a difference in what is reported, how faithfully the events are interpreted, and what light is cast on them. Since most of our textbooks were written by whites, the focus was always on the Europeans, the growth of their monarchies, governments, and kingdoms, and their quest to conquer the world. We were left at their mercy to receive an accurate accounting of what happened. Africans had a predominantly oral tradition. Much may have been lost and will never be known about our past. Not to try to romanticize what took place back in Africa, and it wouldn't necessarily make my life better now if I knew, but as the saying goes, "A man cannot know where he is going until he knows from whence he sprang."

In school texts, Americans were portrayed as a people who defended the cause of freedom throughout the world—a people who stood up against all forms of tyranny and persecution. Yet Negroes, though citizens of this country, were not free. We were still enslaved by government policies and the practices of a racist society. Racism stood like a paleolithic mammoth, defeating all foes and impervious to attack. Visible shackles had been removed from our wrists, but societal restraints kept us back from full participation in the mainstream of American life. In a competitive society that promised equal opportunity for everyone, we remained chronically stagnant. The American dream was no more than a dreadful nightmare from which we longed to be awakened. As in so many dreams, we climbed and ascended up and down political stairsteps, getting nowhere.

Naturally, in middle school, we were presented with facts about this country's great Civil War. We studied statutes enacted in the 1800s to help ensure black freedom, which was placed in jeopardy by Southern whites who moved quickly to reassert white supremacy after the Confederacy fell, through restrictive black codes and the misdeeds of hooded vigilantes who terrorized the highways and byways of the Old South: the Civil Rights Act of 1866, which provided executive authority to enforce the provisions of the Thirteenth Amendment outlawing slavery; the Fourteenth Amendment, which guaranteed that no citizen would be deprived of his rights without due process of law; and the Fifteenth Amendment, which established the right to vote regardless of race. An additional measure in 1875 decreed all inns, theaters, and other places of public entertainment must not exclude persons on account of race or previous condition of servitude.

The latter statute rang an angry chord because, growing up in a family where music was an integral part of our lives, we were confronted with the ill effects of exclusion and separation in the entertainment world. When my parents dated back in the 1940s, they were barred from attending white establishments in downtown Manhattan. And so they frequented the Apollo Theater and danced

Saturday nights at the Savoy Manor, which was the hub of black entertainment in Harlem during the Black Renaissance. It was black owned, and for the first time in New York City, whites came to a black ballroom and mixed in a social setting. They watched couples like my parents perform the swing, a lively freestyle dance with smooth coordinated movements. Whites took it back downtown, adapted it to their own dance style, and called it the jitterbug, and it became a dance craze.

Around the time I was born, a new dance, rooted in black dance halls, was born—rock 'n' roll. Its madness quickly swept white teen audiences across the country. They soon became attracted to black music stars like Fats Domino and Little Richard and looked for ways to gain access to black music and dance. TV brought black music into white living rooms for the very first time near the end of the 1950s. However, blacks were segregated from whites on the early dance shows.

I can remember waking up every Saturday morning to see black stars entertain white audiences on programs like *The Dick Clark Show*. We got our first portable color TV in 1961. I also recall tuning in on my little transistor radio to Murray the K and the Swinging Soiree, one of the only white stations that mixed in colored music. Radio stations had previously been genred either black or white. It wasn't until the civil rights movement of the '60s that blacks began demanding full integration of public entertainment. Although black Americans had rights on the books for more than one hundred years, we still could not participate fully because the laws failed to do their intended job.

In history class, I had been taught about the Revolution, the Constitution, the Bill of Rights, the founding fathers, the Boston Tea Party, the Liberty Bell, Old Glory, the Pilgrims' struggle for religious freedom, the settlers, the taming of the West, the world wars, and other fundamental themes used to teach American ideals.

Yet in discussing the American Revolution, they failed to mention that three thousand blacks fought with the colonial forces and Crispus Attucks, a black man, was first to die. They didn't refer to the 380,000 black soldiers who fought during the Civil War, whose participation, according to Lincoln, ensured a Northern victory and the preservation of the union. They never praised America's unsung heroes, the Buffalo Soldiers of the Ninth and Tenth US Army Calvary units, who fought in the Civil War, the Indian Wars, and the Spanish-American Wars, fighting bravely to protect the settlers, chasing Pancho Villa to the border of Mexico, and galloping up San Juan Hill with Teddy Roosevelt and his Rough Riders.

Nothing was said of the five thousand or more black cowboys who drove cattle through the Chisholm, Western, and Goodnight Loving Trails through freezing rain, dust storms, swollen rivers, and buffalo stampedes, contributing to the legacy of the Old West. We weren't told of black trailblazers like Edward Rose, a black Cherokee, who guided Jedidiah Smith when he discovered a wagon route through the Rockies, or Jacob Dobson, who accompanied the famous explorer John C. Frémont on his three expeditions that charted the Great Plains to the Pacific Ocean. As children, we weren't read stories of black folk heroes like James P. Beckwourth, a mountain man in the upper Missouri country known as the Black Kit Carson, who accompanied fur traders up the Missouri, was adopted by the Crow Indians, and became their war chief. Black heroes would have been so healthy for us to form strong identities.

When talking about the world wars, they never mentioned the two hundred thousand black soldiers who served in France during World War I and the all-black 369th Regimen, which served directly under the French, receiving high honors from their French commander and President Truman. No mention of the young black pilots known as the Tuskegee Airmen of the Army Air Force, who fought in the European theater in World War II, engaging in air combat over the Sicilian Islands, destroying all enemy resistance, participating in the most famous battles over the Italian Peninsula and then in Southern France, Greece, the Balkans, and finally Germany, while challenging the discrimination and segregation practices of the War Department and the nation. How much knowledge of these proud black men would have done to bolster my weak self-image. I would have looked at the photo of my father in his army uniform with a greater sense of pride in his contribution.

My dad, Sgt. Andrew Jackson Farmer, recipient of a World War II Victory Medal, an Asiatic Pacific Campaign Medal, and an American Campaign Medal, on the frontlines, was now fighting for dignity on the home front. How I wish I had understood. Suitably when he died, Dad was given a soldier's funeral—a flag-draped coffin, taps, a salute of last respect—an honor given in death that was never given in life for too many black men who gave away a part of their lives to defend this great land.

I had gone on many trips to the Museum of Natural History, the Museum of the American Indian, the Brooklyn Museum, and various historical reenactments and presentations intended to give a glance back into antiquity to the days of George Washington and the colonists. Always there was a sense that we had no part in America's history, except as ugly smudges on an otherwise glorious past. We were taken through period rooms, led by persons dressed in the costumes of the day. I felt as if I was just being taken through the motions, not that any of it really related to me. Topics came across subtly as being above our heads, beyond our understanding, and if not closely watched, we'd gladly steal and destroy things. America's historical treasures, artifacts, and antiques were for white people, who were raised with sophistication. Cultural pearls were not to be wasted on us lest we, like swine, trample them underfoot. We were quickly ushered through the exhibits and taken back to the ghettoes where we "belonged."

They didn't show us how the threads of our existence were woven into the fabric of American life, nor did they tell us we had made outstanding contributions in the fields of science, medicine, education, and public affairs. I never heard of men like Dr. Daniel Hale Williams, the first man to operate on a human heart, or Dr. Charles Drew, who set up the first blood bank. I didn't know a black inventor, Lewis Latimer, worked with Alexander Graham Bell on the telephone and co-patented the incandescent bulb. I didn't discover the writings of Jupiter Hammon, the first known black poet who wrote back in 1760, or Phyllis Wheatley, a poetess born in Africa and brought to America in chains. I didn't know the writer of *The Three Musketeers* and *The Count of Monte Christo* was black, nor had

I been exposed to other fine black writers like Paul Laurence Dunbar, Charles W. Chesnutt, James Weldon Johnson, Claude McKay, and Ann Petry. No mention was made of Frederick Douglass, one of the earliest black statesmen; W. E. B. Du Bois, who helped to establish sociology as an important branch of knowledge by his studies of black life; and Dr. Ralph Bunche, who worked for world peace at the United Nations. Nothing was said about courageous black women like Mary MacLeod Bethune, who fought for betterment of blacks through education, organized the National Council of Negro Women, and worked to eliminate Jim Crow in the Armed Forces. I didn't even know the song we sang often in assembly, which began, "Lift every voice and sing," was the Negro national anthem. We weren't exposed to black history, black art, or African treasures. It was always the white man's heritage, not ours. America belonged to them, not us. We were just here as unwelcome members of the family.

Likewise, classical music, fine painting, exquisite culinary delights, good literature, all higher endeavors were seen as beyond our scope or ability to take pleasure in. We were viewed as empty wagons that made a lot of noise without content, character, or refinement—a jivey people, not to be taken seriously. It is remarkable that this attitude persisted for so long, when history has borne witness that when our people were given a chance, they made fine contributions in traditionally European arts. A few examples, Marian Anderson, the recitalist, traveled the world giving concerts and became the first black woman member of the Metropolitan Opera House. Dean Dixon, a black American conductor, led the Philharmonic Orchestra to new musical heights. William Grant Still, the pioneer black symphony composer, wrote serious classical music for orchestras, ballets, and operas. Bert Williams became one of the foremost comedians on the American stage; Katherine Dunham was an outstanding dance performer, and Ira Aldridge was one of the great tragedians of history, famous for his acting performance of Shakespeare's *Othello*.

On visits to the Museum of the American Indian, we saw artifacts, glass beads, buckskins, deerskin drums, and ceremonial and ritual clothing. The Indians were depicted as a people who only existed on TV and in museum lore, but no longer around. We were around but not depicted as a part of the culture, like dark spirits living in a house full of white faces, present but too foreboding to be acknowledged—evil omens, symbols of a past best left buried. For to resurrect us would bring to life harsh realities that a nation whose call to greatness was its stand as a beacon of light to the developing nations had allowed one of the cruelest forms of slavery—human chattel slavery—to exist for so long within its borders. Although there had been attempts by law to eradicate its effects, we still bore the marks of slavery and its indicia. America, whose glorious raiment bears stains from the past, is yet unable to purge racism from the hearts of her people. To acknowledge this would be to legitimize our anger and perhaps spark a tide of retribution.

The black man's presence has always been seen as a threat to white people. Either we are going to do something to them, take something from them, or we are simply in their way. People used to believe that if a shiny-faced black man, like an Uncle Remus character, appeared in their dreams, he brought good luck, good health, or fortune would come their way. This is the only instance, I can recall, when a black man's appearance was seen as a good omen.

Museums, mansions, and historical archives are cultural stores where America kept tangible connectors to her past, where a person could research and perhaps trace his lineage back to Columbus or travelers on the *Mayflower*. We had no tangible connectors beyond slavery, except that the spirits of our forefathers spoke through us in dance, in song, in worship, and in shouting. Music expressed our joys and our sorrows as we pressed on to endure. Their soul was evident in the work songs we sang, when we communed with our God while bound and fettered on chain gangs in the Deep South—in hymns of praise and thankfulness for making it through one more day bailing cotton in scorching sun, or another bitter cold night in a heatless five-story walk-up; in the songs of jubilee slaves sang when they first tasted freedom; in those blues, ballads, and funky tunes we played in black bottom joints and honky-tonks on sultry Saturday nights when we let off a week's working for Mr. Charlie in the only way we could, taking on new identities as the Smooth Operator, the Hip Undulator, the Fast Talker, or Cool Walker, as Superfly, Red-Hot Mama, or Ms.

Sweet Thang. Nights when our spirits were set free to soar and swing, clap and fling, bop and slop and lindy-hop, boogie-woogie and shake our booties—whatever felt good for a time, 'cause come Monday morning, it would be back to the grind, "hitting that slave" with little satisfaction. All our passions came alive in the form, style, rhythm, and rituals of our rich musical repertoire.

Celebration through joyous song and dance, playing instruments, and wearing of showy apparel was an instinctive part of our African heritage. But even that was discouraged, when blacks taking on the worship style of Western Christians, were discouraged from beating on drums and dancing in the spirit, being told they were irreverent and filled with impiety. They were to sit and worship quietly like white folks.

In an attempt to relegate us to the mentality of slaves, all vestments of our past were systematically stripped away, leaving us naked and ashamed. We were branches broken off from our family tree, no longer connected to our source. The sap couldn't flow through to us to give us life, nor could we be engrafted on the new American stock, because of bitter rejection by a society whose laws were invidiously discriminatory. We were forced to thrive on our own and continually rejuvenate our own life force. By junior high school, I was refusing to pledge allegiance to the flag of the country I knew intuitively had disrobed me.

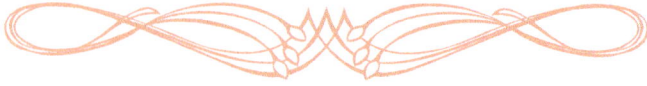

CHAPTER ELEVEN
Our Badge of Shame

THIS brings to mind a book assigned as required reading entitled *The Scarlet Letter*, a beautiful narrative rich in imagery and metaphor. It is a sad tale of a woman, Hester Prynne of Old Salem in the days of the Puritans, who, because of an act of forbidden passion, was forced to stand on a pillory in the public square for three hours and thereafter wear a badge of shame emblazoned upon her bosom. The letter was not only sewn onto her garment but seared deeply in the fleshy breast of her spirit and couldn't be taken off. She was visibly marked and set aside to public infamy and scorn. As the wearer of the scarlet letter, Hester had an intense awareness of being scoffed and looked down upon by her community.

For the sin of adultery, she bore a long and lonely penance on the outskirts of town, living in dreary isolation, eking a bare subsistence by the talents of her hands. Even the daughter born of her secret liaison seemed possessed of an evil and devilish nature, betokening the transfer of the mother's iniquity into an impish spirit come to life in her child. And so she struggled on in bitterness of heart under a weight of great sorrow and rejection. Life for her was like hanging from the edge of a craggy precipice, a deep chasm awaiting her inevitable fall. Yet the coldness of the grave would have been preferable to the frigid earthly damnation to which she had been consigned.

Worse than death, she wandered among the living, cut off from the nurturance of human kindness.

In her penitent heart, Hester became a woman of great compassion, giving to the poor and hungry, sitting at the bedside of the infirmed, comforting the dying. Her own experience with suffering made her feel pity for others going through hardships. In her function as a sister of mercy, she was able to help and sympathize with others while asking nothing for herself, nor did she look for gratitude for her deeds. In fact, her benefactors often spat upon her after receiving her assistance.

Meanwhile, Rev. Dimmesdale, pastor of the church and, unknown to his parishioners, father of Hester's baby, carried on as a pillar of the community while refusing to come forward, confess his shame, bear the ignominy with Hester, and acknowledge their love child, Little Pearl. He continued his ministry with guilt gnawing away at his conscience while his health was being consumed by fiery inner turmoil. He was mercilessly hounded and tormented by Hester's true husband, Roger Chillingworth, who kept his identity a secret, posed as a friendly companion, and lived in the same house. Brought to the point of death and concerned with the final resting of his soul, he made peace with God and man by taking his rightful place on the public pillory with Hester and Pearl, confessing to the astonished crowd his complicity in sin. Upon the death of both men, Little Pearl received her inheritance, yet in another society.

Evil, sin, and repugnance are represented by blackness in this story—black weeds growing from a sinful heart, a black forest shadowed with gloom where witches and enchanters met at midnight to conjure up wicked deeds with the Ugly Black Man, a type of Satan. From my reading, I easily connected being black with being bad.

Just as Hester Prynne bore a mark of disgrace or shame, the scarlet letter, I bore the stigma of having black skin, which also attracted society's scorn. I, like Little Pearl, am an illegitimate child, not of pure stock. My mama's (mother's) mom was the daughter of Ol' Captain, a white man who, like Rev. Dimmesdale, stole the pleasures of a woman's body in bonds to serve his longing, then held his head high before his compeers so as to protect the sanctity of his good name. What was created in the dreadful admixture of his sperm, in lust for power and dominance, and the slave woman's seed of suffering forbearance, was a nation of half-breed children raped of their pride and cheated of their rightful inheritance. Instead, we became a reproach, detested by others, viewed as bad by nature, possessed of a "black and troubled soul," the sins of our father visited upon generation after generation.

When will America come forward to expiate its wrongs, expose the dark secrets of its white soul, display itself "black and filthy in the view of men," and uncover the evil of its past? When will it climb the black weather-stained scaffold in the public square and confess to not only having enslaved the black man but also having defiled his marital bed by lying with his wife with utter violence and malice of heart. Every penile thrust of rampant desire pierced the spirit of black manhood and discharged hate into our relations. Will they go on forever feigning innocence and looking pure as new fallen snow?

Why won't they acknowledge us, the black babies they fathered and left to grovel and scrape an existence in the fields, while our all-white siblings feasted abundantly from Daddy's table? Give us our indemnity and set our mothers free from a four hundred-year penance! How many white men slink around with hand over heart to conceal a telltale letter burning luridly from their pinkish flesh? They fear the horror of exposure, even now, looking askance with guilt-ridden faces but blush to be held accountable. The malfeasance America committed in the storm of adolescence cannot be hidden. Bad memories live on.

The malignities of their sins decry them from dark shadows of old shanties, from the marshy swamps of the bayous, from musky back rooms of old mills and factories, and from maids' quarters behind marble stairs. The black man agonized because he couldn't protect his woman from being used as a sperm receptacle for the white man's seed. He looked into the faces of his children and saw a likeness not his own. He was imbued with anger. His soul yearned for revenge, but he had to bridle his wrath under a cloak of meekness to provide for his broken family, being satisfied when their mirthful glee lightened the yoke he carried on his shoulders. The black woman bore the pain of being violated, degraded, shamed, and left alone. She was made a mockery of and not treated with respect by society.

I understood, at that point, why the media never portrayed black women as beautiful or desirous. It would have made the white woman too fearful of what was going on at the office between her man and his attractive black female employees, while she sat home in pampered splendor watching TV. She was put on a shelf, kept out of reach of any possible involvement with a black lover, lest she be dethroned and the black man lynched. To assuage her fear, they painted us in the image of ugly toads that not even a bullfrog would bellow at. Interestingly, now more and more white men and black women are coupling and forming their alliances—the white man providing means and access, the black woman, strength and substance.

Both blacks and whites would like to see a better day and look back with great consternation on our painful past. Yet we cannot cling to its irrevocable record, bandying back and forth hate for hate, acts of violence for violence suffered. We are a free people—free to face the consequences of our virtues or our vices.

To bring about healing, we must take hands in the market-place, acknowledge our bonds and the contiguity of our experiences, thereby affirming our mutual right to share in the bounty of this nation. It's time for honesty and forgiveness. Let us walk with our backs to the past, turning toward the future. If we live in the past, it is hard, with its pain and regrets. If we look to the future with our fears, we lose hope. We have to rise to the challenge of the moment, faith in God being the foundation of our endurance. From it will come strength to overcome the past. Let us hold on to the progress in our country bought with the blood, sweat, and tears of those who came before us. Reject the idiocy of violence rooted in anger, despair, and hopelessness. We must go forward, building on our heritage, standing on the promises of God, enjoying the miracle of His continuing grace. Let us remember the many lessons on forgiveness found in His word. Hate, though directed at others, is inevitably self-consuming.

Over the years the black community has been a lot like Hester. Though she had become a type of shame, she did not revile her persecutors; rather, she committed acts of kindness and human service. We've done this too, shared what we have to help someone who is down. Even needy outcasts of other races have received our care and acceptance. We've opened our hearts and doors to many unfortunates, giving food and sup when they had no place else to turn. Some, like the Puritans, spat on us in return when they got on their feet and found themselves able. Yet we went on making room for them in our communities and responding to their needs.

After black neighborhoods in New York came under siege of drugs and violence, community activists like Rev. Al Sharpton attempted to use the notion of the scarlet letter to bring social ostracization on people who openly sell crack, cocaine, heroin, and drug paraphernalia on city streets. In concert with the police and the Nation of Islam, they marked the doorways and windows of Harlem's crack houses and drug dens with a large *X* painted in red indicating they were condemned by the firm foundation of the community, the majority of decent people who lived there, exposing their locations so that law enforcement could move in and close them down. This was an effort on the part of civic and religious leaders to set up a unified front to rain retribution on those negative elements of the community who were causing our ruin and made them anathema to our residents. The black community, as in past times, began to accept responsibility for itself, not leaving it to police or outsiders to control us. We've found that fear, secrecy, and covering up aid in the success of the drug trade. We do not want the stigma of drugs to tarnish the image of pride we are now trying to project.

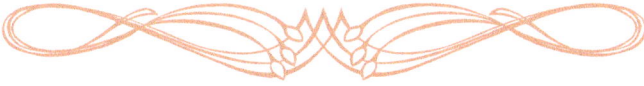

CHAPTER TWELVE
Crossroads

THINGS were changing; nothing ever remains the same. My thoughts were changing. My sense of who I was or could be was changing. My body was growing and changing. My school and neighborhood were in transition. Our country was moving into a new era. The world was being transformed. Change rarely comes without much turbulence.

I had grown to resemble a large brown water bird, lank and lean with strong graceful movements. My arms, much like the wings of a pelican, could extend over an expanse of space far beyond my narrow frame. My fingertips were able to touch tall doorways. Why, I could almost reach up and catch the sun between my fingers! So I thought. My head (big as a honey dew melon) sat atop a slim pod-like body. Jean the Bean had become quite an appropriate appellation for me. I had the legs of a grasshopper, and my hands and feet were outsized like Mom's. I walked like my dad, shoulders back, head held high, with a measuredly restrained gait. I was stick figured. Being the tallest girl in class with a low-toned voice, I didn't feel very cutesy. By this time, I'd become convinced I was a girl trapped in a boy's body. It felt abnormal.

A girl in my class named Pat looked the way I thought girls should. She was small, dainty, long haired, and fashionably bedizened. I never took my eyes off her, always comparing in my mind our physical differences. She was quiet but knew how to draw attention by making noise with her good looks and faddy dress. Girls encircled her like swarming bees, hoping the brightness of her radiance would enliven their dull appearance and deflect male attention onto them. She was Ms. Popular, and I was her most envious admirer.

I was now a teen standing at the crossroads, on the one hand a child, yet moving toward adult interests and experiences. Though curiosity beckoned, I was not ready for sexual experimentation. I was an avowed "goodie-goodie" and would blush to look at anything depicting the naked body because it made me feel fresh and bad. I was inquisitive, but chicken. I wouldn't dare do anything risqué for fear of getting caught and tarnishing my well-polished reputation. There were a few innocent trysts with boys, nothing serious. I tried to circumvent real life by experiencing things vicariously through my active imagination.

Romantic novels and lingerie were powerful stimulants that sent me off into a world of fantasy in which I created imaginary encounters with a handsome suitor and pictured falling in love, quiet walks along tree-lined streets, stops for a tender kiss, vows to make it last forever. I resurrected my dream princes often to work out problems in relating to others, then carefully laid them to rest until conflict sparked the desire to pick them up again.

Once in rambling through my mother's dresser drawer, I found a tube of jelly, which became a potent fetish unleashing wild imaginings of what went on in the bedroom between my parents. That subject, to my mind, was very taboo, and I quickly chided myself for the mental invasion of their privacy and breech of the filial respect I held for them. Mom and Dad did not embrace or show affection in front of me. I grew to associate sexuality very much with privacy, not linking any other negative inhibitory thoughts to it, except that it was to be sacredly kept within the confines of the bedroom.

Mama continued to warn against getting P-R-E-G, which she'd spell rather than utter the words. We had lots of talks but never got down to the real thing because parents and kids kept a certain distance, especially on the topic of sexuality. Mom had a way of talking without going into detail. What she didn't say our minds elucidated for us, and we understood what she meant. That way, she balanced the need to communicate her fears about precocious sexual involve-ment and her need to keep her position as mother untainted by unclean talk. Anatomical information I scavenged for in books.

On warm days I'd come home from school capering along in my mind, still quite childish in a lot of ways, loving to whistle and talk to myself, rapt in my own world. I was really my best friend because only I understood me. I spent a lot of time alone tending the garden while laughing at things I crafted with my dauntless imagi-nation—dolls, animals out of twigs and bits, birdhouses, funny little drawings. Yet I was steadfast and stable, not given to caprice or sud-den whimsy. Who we are is really so flimsy at that age, that develop-ing stage. I would often be found sitting cogitating over issues I felt strongly about while showing nothing without.

At home I could be quite vociferous and loved to battle ideas, strong willed when it came to getting things that I wanted. But in school, I was shy and easily abashed. I was always mortified that someone would call on me, that I'd have to step up to the plate, stand, and deliver. Was sure I couldn't follow through and would make a fool of myself. More comfortable with adults than kids, I liked to match wits with them one on one. With my peers, I felt inse-cure to let myself be counted, always feeling either superior or infe-rior to them, never on the same level. Mostly I delved into myself and busily gathered information about plants and animals. Happily, I did my schoolwork and spent long hours on special projects. I could get into work easier than I could people.

Although a good student, I wasn't nerdy. I knew what was hap-pening but chose not to get involved. Uncertainty and lack of confi-dence held me from letting myself go. I didn't roam without restraint or speak without much thought. Active only in my private world, I wore a mantle of quiet reserve. I had developed the sensibilities of an artist, a passionate love of beauty in nature, easily bruised by peo-ple. I felt safest and most secure with older folk with whom I could exchange ideas yet not be in social competition with them.

Because of my physical appearance, I dabbled in athletics, but tryouts for the girls' basketball and track teams convinced me I was not apt to be a sports person. The call for fair hiring practices for minorities echoing from the civil rights movement pushed the school system to transfer black teachers into previously all-white districts. As a result, a young Afro-American instructor was assigned to our school to teach physical education. Being hip and realizing the growing trend toward black consciousness, she started an African dance class in the downstairs gym. None of the white girls joined; for once it was just us.

It wasn't a hate thing that made us glad they weren't included. We needed the opportunity to develop an awareness of our own cultural heritage. What better avenue than through creative dance exploration? She introduced new ways of expressing ourselves—ways that seemed tailored to our movement styles. It channeled the frenetic energy that came along with puberty and left us tingling with a sense of pride.

African dance class was a lively experience. For the first time I didn't feel like I was barging in unwarrantedly on somebody else's culture. My body seemed right for it, not awkward and ugly. We put bright dance skirts on over our black leotards and wore head wraps of Kente cloth, a Ghanaian fabric. As we pounded out barefoot the beatings of Olatunji's talking drum, our slumbering spirits came to life. Bells around our ankles jingle-jangled, filling the hollow gymnasium with polyrhythmic revelry. A gaggle of giggly black girls had become an African dance troupe. Our performances were as festive and colorful as we were.

It was so unlike the May Day festivities held in the schoolyard and the International Day assemblies where kids suited in native costumes, put on little vignettes about children in faraway lands, focusing on the Italians, the French, the Dutch, the Germans, the Swiss, the Jewish, somehow never getting around to people of color. If a skit were presented about Africa, it probably centered around a little jungle boy living in a hut with wild beasts roving across his front yard. For kids growing up in the asphalt jungle of New York, many from the projects where they had no front yard, saw few trees, and couldn't keep pets, there was little experiential linkage or identification with the character. At best the sight of a half-nude boy with only an animal skin covering his personals whipped up a froth of laughter.

Regrettably, this didn't give us an appreciation of the ethnic diversity and rich cultural range of languages, foods, dress, and religions to be found there. Negative images of Africans as spear-toting savages were still being perpetuated.

I imagined myself in another place, another time, as a wild creature, free and uninhibited, not shy. I just let go and for once made my long arms and legs work for me. I twisted and contorted my body to match the pulsating beat and gradually opened up like the petals of an exotic flower blossom. I wouldn't say I was a great dancer. I would say I found in African dance a vehicle for self-expression I desperately needed at that time. It helped me realize true beauty is not superficial, but it emanates from the deep recesses of the soul. Everyone has beauty, if we can just reach down and let it flow.

Thank God for a black teacher who could see the importance of building our self-concept through artistic expression. I developed a love for the arts in all forms, responding well to things that stimulated my eyes and ears, that I could do with my hands.

A male teacher instilled a love for creative writing by reading the classics to our English class. I remember very clearly sitting close to his knee, listening with rapt attentiveness as he read from John Donne's *Devotions upon Emergent Occasions* published in 1624:

> No man is an island, entire of itself; every man is
> a piece of the continent, a part of the main.
> If a clod be washed away by the sea, Europe is
> less, as well as if promontory were, as well as if a
> manor of thy friends or thine own were;
> Any man's death diminishes me, because I am
> involved in mankind, and therefore never send
> to know for whom the bell tolls, it tolls for thee.

Those words fell on my ears like fresh rain on parched ground. I listened so closely nothing else going on around me mattered, not boys blowing spit balls through straws, not noise from the halls, nor girls gabbing in the background—not even the bell announcing the period's end broke my attention. The words were so satisfying it was as if I had just eaten a fine meal and was now ready to kick back and relax. I didn't fully understand what the selection meant, but I could well appreciate its beauty. I recall repeating it to myself until the words were overlearned and stayed with me.

Thank God for a white teacher who didn't condescend and limit his instruction to what he thought was on "our level," realizing that a person must develop an appetite for something good before they begin to crave it. That introduction sparked an appreciation for fine writing on a higher level than I had known before. A desire to write took root at that time, but I suppressed it because, as always, I doubted my capability.

My love of literature was never actuated. I found intense reading and book work cumbersome and had difficulty locating books of interest on my grade level. I didn't know how to use the library system, would get befuddled as I walked through the door, and thought I'd look stupid if I asked for help. I did pen stories with illustrations to share with family and classmates but shied away from reading them aloud.

As ninth grade neared and a choice of high schools had to be made, I tried to assess my talents and skills. My strongest pull was toward art. On recommendation of a teacher who had seen my drawings, I chose a specialty high school for art on Fifty-Seventh Street. Not believing I'd get in, I applied just as kind of a fluke. After all, I had to go somewhere and didn't want to end up in my neighborhood school. So I prepared a portfolio and went for an interview.

As hap would have it, I was accepted for the college-bound program with a major in fashion illustration. I couldn't believe someone had found me worthy! I was both challenged and afraid. The balance of the term, I was a bundle of nervous excitement. This would all be so new, riding the subway downtown to the heart of the city each day, mingling with the artist set. Poor little me would have to step out into that big threatening world. I didn't feel ready. But soon I would come to enjoy the new freedom while holding on to the security of my parents' home.

By the time I graduated in 1964, John Kennedy had been assassinated, the war in Vietnam was escalating, and the civil rights movement was in full swing. A contagion of social unrest spread across the land. America's ideals were called into question, and everything she stood for was being challenged. Young people, breaking free of old restraints, sparked the sexual revolution. More adults and kids got involved with premarital sex, as moors and mores about sexuality loosened. Long-held values began to erode, and the nation went to war with its traditions.

Out of that soil, wet with idealist porosity, sprang the flower children, taking on the establishment with its hypocrisies, dreaming of peace and love in a new world order. Those years, characterized by civil disobedience, riots, sit-in demonstrations, and antiwar protests ended our feeling of safety as Americans. Inner turmoil bred doubt and suspicion about the federal government, the CIA, the Pentagon, and the FBI. People under thirty thought everyone over thirty were antiquarian relics who needed to be tossed aside so that a new age could be ushered in. Members of my generation called the baby boomers are now having to look back on what we once thought was so right and so radical. Back then, we had our causes. Now we live with the effects of our reshaping of America. We are often not proud of the changes we wrought.

For black Americans, time was ripe for confronting the racist nature of our institutions. We banded together, mustered our courage, and cried out in one thunderous voice, "No mo' Jim Crow!" Newton's third law of motion states, "For every action there is an equal and opposite reaction." We had been pushed enough; we were ready to push back. That groundswell of emotion, billowing up from poverty and despair, did not abate until the walls of bigotry crumbled, and the foundation of the nation shook in a rumble heard around the world.

At fourteen I wasn't old enough to attend the Freedom March on Washington on August 28, 1963. I watched from my living room as two hundred thousand Americans converged on the nation's capital, singing, "We shall overcome" and demanding an end to injustice. Martin Luther King, our black messiah, having assumed leadership of the nonviolent movement to achieve racial equality, spoke eloquently from the foot of the Lincoln Memorial, like a modern-day prophet calling the nation to repentance. The powerful reverberations of his voice vibrated a chord in my heart. That chord, once touched, revibrated with every inflection of his tone. Like a hammer, it pounded at the portals of my being, causing my eyes to tear. He had given voice to all our hopes and aspirations.

There were tears in his eyes, too, as he gave his "I Have a Dream Speech" behind all the fiery passion. Maybe he knew, like Christ, who had come before him, that he was hopelessly speaking peace to a people hell-bent on violence and hate, suffering from hardness of heart. He spoke of a vision, but many with sight cataracted by personal prejudice couldn't see it. The clarion call was for my generation to be stirred to action and forge a bulwark in defense of human rights. Just how we'd go about achieving that goal was uncertain, as some favored direct confrontation and others peaceful means. My mind was focused on the struggles that lay ahead.

During this time, a great boxing champion rose from our ranks, the very embodiment of our fighting spirit. He was a black braggadocio who blinded his opponents with fireball punches and lightning speed. His name—Muhammad Ali, a young, gifted, and black man fighting his way out of the ghetto, holding forth with Howard Cosell on national TV, proclaiming himself "the king of the world." His brassy limericks would have seemed foolish had they not been backed by sportsmanship, agility, and boxing skill.

I thought he was a good-looking man like my father. He and I used to sit in the parlor on the edge of his bed watching the fights on Friday nights. He'd swig beer and throw punches in the air while I rubbed the TV set, trying to touch that handsome face, calling Mom to come and see him, asking if she thought he was cuter than Dad. I liked playing devil's advocate, hoping to spark a twinge of jealousy in him, to prove his love for her. She would, of course, seize the opportunity to say Ali looked better, to which he'd dryly retort, "Aw, that big mouth. If Joe Louis were around, he'd flatten him!"

Dad's superstar retired from boxing undefeated in 1949, the year I was born. He too had been a sergeant in the Army and donated the purse from his two title fights during the war years to Army and Navy relief. Mom sometimes called Dad the Brown Bomber, Joe's nickname, when he strolled the house bare chested, showing off his powerful pecs.

Joe Louis won the hearts of Dad's generation; Muhammad Ali, the hearts of ours. *Muhammad* in Arabic means "worthy of all praise," but to me it meant victory. He came to prove himself, not only an able fighter, but a man of religious commitment and moral fiber. To my mind he'll always be the greatest.

I saw him again on TV after thirty years looking heavy, slow, stifling to walk, and stammering to find words to accept an award for his illustrious career. The alacrity of his youth was gone, his body but a shell of the man he used to be. Sickness had dealt him a powerful blow; time had taken its toll. It was a painful reminder of one of life's most positive and tragic truths. Nothing remains the same. Only God is immutable. As we try to come to terms with changes in our lives, it is only His unchanging hand that can steady us.

The killing of President Kennedy was one of those watershed events that left a benchmark on our culture. I had followed the Kennedys with hungry fascination: the president addressing the nation, "Ask not what your country can do for you, but..."; Mrs. K. graciously hosting state dinners; both parents on board their yacht at Hyannis Port gloating over Caroline and Little John at play, living lives so pampered and guarded. Broad-smiling Jack with the Hollywood looks, and Jackie, so cultivated and refined, were national treasures to a people enamored with the rich and famous.

We didn't go to the shore often, except to Orchard Beach to bathe in waters spoiled by wastes floating across from the city dump and polluted by the exudations of teeming thousands who flocked there on hot days to rinse off the toil and moil of city life. By then, my parents had given up sweated labor and taken on jobs in the community that didn't pay much. Dad traded in his black-and-pink Pontiac for a little doodle bug that puttered him back and forth to work at Bronx State Hospital. Occasionally, we all piled in and went to City Island for our favorite fish 'n' chips, but the chips in our pockets were fewer than the french fries on our plates.

Lots of poor girls wanted to be like Mrs. Kennedy—rich and stylish. She was every woman's woman—at her husband's side, mother to her children, a regal hostess, and goodwill ambassadress. While her husband and Nickie Khrushchev decided the fate of the world, she decided what type of pate would be served at the upcoming function and how many times the sheets would be changed daily in the White House master suite. He was like a modern king, she a modern queen.

I remember the day of JFK's assassination, November 22, 1963. Around midday school was let out early. His sudden death shocked the world. Mournful days followed as I watched the play-by-play on TV, from the killing of Oswald by Jack Ruby to the passing of the flag-draped casket and funeral entourage through the nation's capital. Whatever security I felt as an American was shattered that day. The political turbulence I had only read about in small countries had now come home to rest on American shores. Little did we know the violence would escalate, claim the lives of a few great men, and leave the nation without a sense of hope.

On the world stage, the US and Russia had begun the nuclear arms race. The US exploded the first hydrogen bomb in 1952. Russians launched the Sputnik in 1957, and the US launched its first satellite in 1958. The two countries had formed a nuclear balance of terror. By 1960 Khrushchev was at the UN, with his shoe banging on the table, protesting US U-2 flights over Russia. Cold War tensions were high in Europe, in Asia, and on the doorstep of the US in Cuba. The US sponsored an invasion of the Bay of Pigs, nearly setting off World War III.

In 1961 East Germany put up the Berlin Wall, and Yuri Gagarin made the first flight around the earth in space, followed by John Glen Jr., an American. By 1963 the USSR and the US had set up a hotline between the White House and the Kremlin, in case of accidental nuclear war, by pressing the button. Fear and intrigue loomed over us as Hollywood bombarded us with "What if?" films depicting the horrors of a nuclear incident. The threat of war was eminent.

I was a frightened kid emerging into an even more frightening world. It was uniquely fitting that they chose for our graduation song a West African chant "Kum Ba Ya," which invoked the Lord's presence in succeeding rounds as somebody sang, somebody cried, and somebody prayed. It is translated approximately "Come by Here."

> Kum ba ya, my Lord, Kum ba ya,
> Kum ba ya, my Lord, Kum ba ya,
> Kum ba ya, my Lord, Kum Ba ya,
> Oh Lord, _____ Kum ba
> Someone's singing Lord,
> Someone's crying Lord,
> Someone's praying Lord,
> Someone's learning Lord,
> Someone's hoping Lord.

I was always hoping—hoping things between Mom and Dad would get better. They never did. Their marriage was wrecked by a slow leak. Home became an emotional quagmire where hurt festered and anger grew.

I didn't experience all the fights and foul language other children of alcoholics have gone through. It was more Dad stumbling in, tripping over furniture, the strong smell of alcohol accompanying him, putrefying the air with its presence, crawling in bed, sleeping with him instead of Mom. Our "problem" returned home nightly, and no one knew what to do about it. There were times when Mom lashed out with a few choice words, but mostly there was silence, ungodly silence that held us breathless until daylight came and things went on as usual. Slipping out of bed, I'd rush to move the furniture or catch things before they fell to protect the family from breaking and to keep Dad out of trouble, covering for him, not letting him take responsibility for his actions.

I always wanted him to be more than just an "alkie." It hurt when Mom called him "You old drunk!" and when others said similar words. I'd created in my mind my "good daddy," to protect myself from facing what he was, being blinded by childish love. Wanting the family whole, I took up the task of getting their marriage back on track. Jean, the rescuer, was faithful and protective as Lassie and Ol' Rin Tin Tin. Trying to put my parents' marriage back on track was like trying to repair a broken teacup. The more I tried to align the jagged edges, the more mix-matched they appeared. I ended up with many deep cuts in my emotions and got bonded in a gluey mess.

As a young girl playing God, I needed the wisdom of Solomon to determine who was right and who was wrong. I concluded we three kids were the real problem. After all, if she didn't have us, then she could be free of him. All her suffering was for our sake. We were *responsible*.

For Mom, the issue was his unfaithfulness and disloyalty. Trust and intimacy were never restored, no apologies were made, nor was forgiveness given. They never got down to the root of the problem, which I believe was alcoholism itself controlling Dad's thoughts and lifestyle. Being caught in the affair only pushed him away more, as he couldn't face the blaming and sense of failure, especially since it was treated as a round-table topic of discussion for the entire family. No longer just between the two of them, everyone was involved to complicate matters, taking sides, deciding whom to uphold.

As time passed, Dad drank more often to take away the loneliness and ease the pain. Yet it was the drinking that was controlling and destroying him. He couldn't admit he was wrong or talk about his weaknesses. He asserted positively he could handle it and could put the bottle down at any time. Mom suffered so much from the strain of this relationship. It consumed all her energy and attention. Regurgitating her hurt daily to those who listened, she set herself up as a lovelorn lady running a telephone advice column on "What a man will do if you let him." She felt violated, disrespected, and probably deep down inadequate to hold her man. Mom's shame led to deep contempt.

She carried a clenched fist for all black men who collectively had done her wrong, continually telling Dad he was rotten and no good, which fed more into his desire to escape. Often she'd make comments like, "They should take all black men and string them up by their balls!" Or she'd say, "If I could find a man with even half a ball, I could do something!" A tough skin had developed over her broken heart.

No one knows what Dad was wrestling with. If it was uncontrolled lust, I don't know. He didn't seem to have a pattern of affairs, although he frequented bars and night spots. I think he sought out environments where liquor was in abundance and the guys made him feel like a big cheese. The bottle itself became his woman.

So caught up in their affairs, I alternately blamed him, blamed her. Secretly I felt if she were more of this type of woman or that type of woman, Daddy wouldn't have strayed. Then I'd change and want to spank Daddy and say, "Why are you such a naughty boy?" It was always easier to find fault with Mom than to accept Dad was what he was and not what I wanted him to be.

Yet despite his faults, I still feel Dad was a good person, and there is a lot I appreciate about him. What he did for us and gave would be too innumerable to tell. Many things he said during those years flitted by like insignificant flies but are now part of the precious memories that allow me to feel his warmth again. He was so down to earth and easy to relate to; no one was a stranger to him. By socializing freely, he'd developed a keen perspicacity in dealing with people and had a frankness that made them want to respect him. He wasn't a wanton, reckless person. He felt one's life had meaning and people ought to try to stand for something. In the end, maybe it was a feeling he couldn't live up to his own standards that undermined him. None of us ever got deep inside enough to really know.

For one thing, he always had answers to life's tough questions. Even if they weren't the answers I wanted to hear, at least I could confide in him and know he had heartfelt concern for my well-being. His answers were as simple and basic as he was. "There's no easy way in life! You have to look it right in the nose! Stand on your own! Earn your keep and be independent! Bide your time, hang in there, and you'll make it!"

In his view, there was no sense harping and complaining about this or that. It was all part of life and you just had to go ahead and deal with it. Like a ship's captain, you were to hold the helm steady, come what may. Plot your course straight ahead. Don't worry about what others say or think! You had to tell people some yeses and some nos and not let them ruffle your feathers. For me, the flaw in that philosophy was that it didn't take into consideration how my actions affected others, but it helped develop strong determination.

The fantasy world that I often retreated to didn't provide answers either to my family life overshadowed by alcoholism, Dad's unfaithfulness, and Mom's desperate reaching out for someone to rescue her from a difficult marriage. I always felt terribly *inadequate* to handle the momentous problems tossed my way.

Now that I am an adult and I know that I have blown it and I have failed, it is helping me to be more forgiving when I think about my parents. Hurt people hurt people! I understand a lot of what Mom and Dad did was just acting out the hurt they couldn't effectively communicate and didn't know how to resolve. My hope is that we who go on living won't do more hurting because of it. The evil that we do lives after us. Pain is not interred with our bones.

Dad died at age sixty-seven, just as I began to write this section, the results of three crippling strokes in a two-year span. Pain rankles down inside more than ever now. I spent so much time trying to heal, trying to save, trying to put Humpty Dumpty back together again. Grief is but an adjunct to what I've struggled with since childhood.

It seems he'll go to his grave, but the problem will live on in me, through feelings of guilt and a disquieting sense of failure. I prayed so hard for God to fix it and jumped in and tried to fix it myself. Neither worked. It seems death was the only "solution." Mom will be free, but I fear I'll never be free of the burden of their relationship, never be free of wanting my good daddy, never be free of the conflict I feel toward her, never be able to have a sense of closure in my relationship with him, since all those issues from childhood remain unresolved. I dreamed of the day it would all change and Mommy and Daddy would live happily ever after.

There was a poem included in Dad's obituary that read in part,

> So often we like flowers dwell,
> Too deep within our human shell,
> And pass through life "not understood";
> Nor making all the friends we should.
> (Tony Pettito)

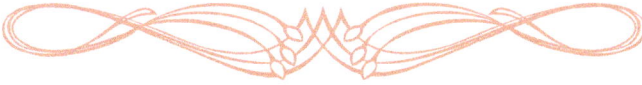

CHAPTER THIRTEEN
Rites of Passage

IN earlier grades, my shy personality protected me from having to make demands to be recognized and heard. But as I moved through my teens, I felt called on by the times to take a *stand*.

I was growing up against a backdrop of racial unrest raging in cities and towns across America, watching news coverage of unfolding events, as the yearnings of our black nation spilled over into violent confrontations with the white power structure. Blacks put on a show for the world as they stood with dignity against the segregated system in the Old South—marching, carrying placards, singing freedom songs in the midst of angry mobs.

1962: University of Mississippi. James Meredith attempting to register at Ole Miss, met by Gov. Barnett and members of the white Citizen's Council, turned away at the door. Molotov cocktails thrown. White passions whipped to a frenzy. Federal marshals sent in to maintain order. Thirty-five marshals shot, two killed.

1963: Birmingham, Alabama. Seven hundred marching schoolchildren attacked by police dogs and water hoses ordered by Mayor Bull Conner. More than two thousand put in jails. A white armored tank patrols the city streets.

1963: Jackson, Mississippi. Medgar Evers shot and killed in an ambush after leading demonstrations against downtown merchants. The KKK holds highly visible rallies. Grand Dragon gives news conference espousing hate.

1964: Freedom Summer. Thousands of freedom riders from up north pouring into Mississippi for voter registration of rural blacks, encounter fierce opposition by angry crowds. Eighty workers beaten. Thousands arrested. Three workers found brutally murdered on a farm.

1966: The March Against Fear. Marchers coming into Jackson, Mississippi, attacked by guns and tear gas. People crawling around, choking and crying. Others on the ground being kicked and hit with rifle butts. Blacks and whites fight in the streets. All normalcy is destroyed. Fear reigns.

1968: Birmingham, Alabama. Four flower-laden coffins borne by tearful pallbearers. Anguished parents, overcome by grief, sing "We shall overcome" as they bury their young.

Faces of hate raced across our TV sets. Hellish scenes are forever etched in my memory. Blacks had become emboldened to pursue equal rights, placing in jeopardy their lives and livelihoods. Fear and intimidation could no longer impale our quest for freedom. Blacks were rising up, refusing to accept being called colored or Negro. They wanted to be called black and were now mature and proud to be members of the race. Crowds thundered "We want black power!" at massive meetings and rallies.

I sensed the intimidation of the mobs as they hurled bricks, bottles, and racial epithets at men, women, and children praying and singing. Recalcitrant whites, comfortable with their privileged positions, would not yield without a fight. Nonviolence seemed nonsensical to me. Seeing snarling white bigots spit at peaceful marchers proved their hatred and contempt. It was like herding innocent sheep before vicious wolves, I thought. I felt incensed that injustice was so entrenched. I wanted to cry out, "Fight back, you fools!" not under-standing the battle or who was leading the struggle. The battle was the Lord's. The marchers were just positioning themselves to "shake up Jesus." He would grant the ultimate victory.

Most victories were bittersweet. Blacks grappled with whites and won in tiny increments, desegregated schools and public facil-ities, voting rights, and some job parity at the cost of lynchings, blood, sweat, and tears. It brought forth assurance we had power. Like toddlers exercising muscles needed to stand, we wobbled, fell, hobbled to our feet with unsteadiness. Finally, we stood against a mighty foe, trying to fling a stone that would strike the fatal blow. What is more important, we believed we could have an effect, could change our world and our circumstances. There was a feeling in the air that *change* was coming. We, the young people, would be the cat-alysts to make it happen.

I entered high school in the tenth grade in the year 1966. I was tested and placed in an advanced English class. The teacher was a dour Jewish matron; I was the only black student there. She didn't feel I belonged and assumed it had to be a quota that caused my placement in her room. She resented me. I became her scapegoat for most of the year. Whenever tough questions were asked, she called on me, hoping to embarrass me, sure I wouldn't know the answers. My written assignments had to be copied on the board so that she could teach the other kids from my errors. Her tone of voice with me was agitated, commanding, as though I was doing something wrong. I shuffled around and tried to please her, but inside I sensed her hos-tility. She didn't feel I deserved to be in there with her smart Jewish kids and looked for ways to prove it.

Near the end of the term, tenth graders took the SATs. She was certain the tests would yield evidence of my ineptness. We were tested at various sites around the city, and the scores sent back to our home school on long computer printouts. Ms. —— called us up to her desk one by one to see our score. When she reached my name, she spoke with the same ire in her voice that had been simmering there all year. She was confident she possessed proof positive. Her eyes sizzled with intensity as I slowly approached her, head down, shoulders crouched. Brimming with anticipation of a long-awaited victory, her finger quickly perused the list for my score. She looked up incredulously! Among the highest in class, higher than the kids she expected to do well. Angrily, she fumbled through papers, searching for backup lists, even called the office to check its correctness. Her voice crackled with rage as she shouted, "Somehow you must have managed to sit close to someone and cheat!" knowing full well the tests were tightly monitored and students were placed two desks apart. It didn't jibe with her *perception* of what I was capable of and what the other kids were capable of that I should have that score. I savored the moment knowing our little tryst had left her wounded. It made up for the misery I suffered all year. I set my shoulders high, stepped to my seat with a bit of impudence, singing,

> Can't let nobody turn me around,
> Turn me around, turn me around,
> Can't let nobody turn me around,
> I'm marching up to freedom land!

It was then I realized, if I wanted to make it in the white man's world, I'd face battles of my own with prejudice, would need to stave off attempts to discourage me, and have to prove myself time and again.

Being a sensitive girl, I feared the rejection and disapproval of people—thought I needed to meet all their expectations to be "okay." I was bound up, acted like I didn't have any needs, but I was very much needy.

At Art and Design, I found myself with talented young artists, the creme de la creme from all five boroughs. A motley set of Bohemians of the beat generation who rejected conventional dress and proudly adorned themselves in thrift shop castaways, old jeans, work shirts, and wire-framed spectacles, wanting to project an image noticeably different from parents' darkish straight-laced garb worn to nine-to-five jobs in the business world. They were the avant-garde, gifted with creativity, taste, and imagination, ahead of others in new ideas, style, and design awareness. Kids who approached the world through their senses, having by nature a delicate capacity for feeling and responding to things around them, quickly touched by something beautiful or sad. Crazy dreamers carrying the accouterments of the trade in large black portfolios that made them teeter-totter as they walked. Each with a green knapsack flung across his back. Each fuzzy head filled with visions of success in the fickle art world.

I met two new friends early on, Alice and Carol, from the Uptown Bronx, just as I was. Being of the same ilk we immediately latched on. Reared on *Leave It to Beaver*, we were each eager to learn about the seedier side of life. We became faithful companions, riding the trains together back and forth to school. Three innocents—Winkin, Blinkin, and Nod—though not above a bit of mischief now and then.

Sometimes we'd sneak out of school and take the D train to Greenwich Village to stride amidst the hippie crowd: the libertines who went their own way and cared nothing for the older generation's rules, unwilling to conform to traditions they felt were repressive to individualism and liberality; free thinkers, holding loose opinions about everything from religion to sex and marriage; misfits, who abhorred the workaday world—the turned on and the tuned out.

Or it was off to Forty-Second Street, the seamy underbelly of the city, to lurk around the creeps and vermin, both human and animal, that slunk out of crawl spaces, tacky adult bookshops, and X-rated movie houses. Once we slipped in to see a porno film and brushed quickly through the rows to find seats without being noticed. One of us accidentally swiped a man's raincoat from his lap, exposing him holding himself in hand, to our utter mortification. We hit the doors running, wailing like frightened banshees for the death of our innocence had come, though we hadn't expected to have it wrested from us so abruptly! There's a problem seeking wisdom by dredging through society's dross. You can't do it without getting filth on your person, dirt most difficult to wash off.

After that day, we settled for more innocuous haunts, quiet niches selling tie-dyed garments and handicrafts, modish boutiques hawking "way out" fashions to identify us in with the in crowd. Dress that announced we were students of the aesthetics, not mindless clones marching to the mindless drone of materialism. Bangles, strands of colored beads, carpet bags, pea jackets, and a pair of Clarke's shoes were the basics of the look. We matched them with bric-a-brac and this-and-that from Army Navies and secondhand shops. Everybody seemed "hip" to us, except fuddy-duddies like our moms and pops.

And so we chased an elusive image and did foolish things to gain acceptance, like going into import stores, picking up little what-nots, and simply walking out, to see if we could get away with it. The one who came out with most won the game. It wasn't stealing, we said, just liberating what should have been rightfully ours. Funny how we used the trends of the day to justify what we knew was wrong.

If we had a few bucks, we'd go in record dens that sold Marley, Havens, Simone, Dylan, and Hendricks along with snaky water pipes and drug paraphernalia. Our attraction was to the look and voices of the '60s counterculture, not the life. We didn't get high, attend pot parties or love-ins, hang out at concerts like Woodstock, or run off to Haight-Ashbury. Our brief skirmishes with mischief never took us far across the line. Mama's raising held us. Mostly we had fun zig-zagging in and out of that maze of iron and filth called the subway, experiencing the press of human flesh, squeezing in cattle cars, riding escalators, treading up steps. Once on the surface we'd traipse across Fifty-Ninth Street, the hub of Manhattan, where everyone went to shop, browse, or be seen in the crowd. Traffic was bumper to bumper. Car horns honked, tempers flared, neon lights glared. Hordes of people moved in every direction at a maddening pace. We went with the flow and kept our wits about us, lest we fall victim to the predators who pounced on easy prey.

We got a little tough ourselves—learned to scrape, scrap, and elbow our way to get where we were going, learned to respond fast and recognize the face of trouble. It was a life studies course in the sociology of survival. The mean streets of New York are a fascinating human laboratory with enough gutter rats to conduct a million studies.

The straphangers we rode shoulder to shoulder with on the rush-hour train were gargoyleish-looking characters, twisted, ugly, and profane—caricatures of city life itself in all its gross exaggeration.

We pointed and tec-heed at the circus of frowning faces, vowing never to become like that. Never to end up fat, with slumped carriages, turned-over shoes, red bulging eyes, bad breath, and a humdrum job we couldn't stand. We'd change the world before conforming to it or being broken by it. With youthful enthusiasm, we prepped a fresh canvas in our minds, painted on peace and love, dabs of harmony, then spattered it with freedom, justice, and equality. There were no dark clouds in our pictures, no gloom or doom. In the world we imagined, there was no war, no violence or hate.

Inevitably, we'd wander into Bloomingdale's, hoping a dip in a spending spa for the rich and free sprays of musky aromatics would hide the rankness of street sweat or that nearness to furs and exotic perfumes would lend us the elegance of the caviar set. Yet nothing could mask the deep feeling we were not "supposed" to have nice things because of our minority status.

Once settled in high school, it was time to think about earning money for carfare and clothing. At that time Mom was on lay off and filled in by doing maid's work for wealthy whites. As a start, she arranged for me to assist an elderly convalescent suffering with diarrhea. My first assignment was to wash her up and change her diaper. The washup went well, but once the diaper came off and I was faced with stinking reality, there ended my career as a maid.

My first job was down on 125th Street, the heart of Harlem. In the early sixties, Harlem was still a colorful, vibrant community unreeling a symphony of images, desperate by nature, of those who dwelled there in—pimps, players, fast-money makers, ramblers, gamblers, flimflammers, dreamers, schemers, political extremists, druggists, muggers, young lovers, unwed mothers, out-of-work pops, hungry tots, I-got-soulers, and Holy Rollers, all strivin' and jivin' in one captivating dynamic—young and old alike being put through the sieve of the black experience in a community unmatched in flavor and resilience. It was a community rankling because of the insult and injury done to its members by a biased and segregated society. Whites had turned away, heedless to the cries of her needy, hungry, naked, and imprisoned. Life was bare to the bone, down to the real nitty-gritty.

Many jobs for teens were created in depressed areas like Harlem as a part of President Johnson's "War on Poverty." The federal government, under the Economic Opportunity Act of 1964, sponsored antipoverty programs that stressed vocational education and training for disadvantaged youth. I was employed at a community action agency known as Haryou-Act, Unlimited. Their goal was to match talented young apprentices with experienced black artists and musicians willing to share knowledge and expertise. These symbiotic relationships provided incomes for both and ensured outlets for their work to be exhibited in black neighborhoods.

I was placed under the tutelage of Mr. Norman Lewis, an abstract artist, well-known in downtown art circles but little known to the black community at large. Many black artists found themselves caught in the same travesty. To bridge the gap, Haryou sponsored numerous community projects, giant murals painted on playground walls, refurbishment of old buildings, art displays, and street fairs. They were instrumental in founding the Studio Museum of Harlem to exhibit black artists' work.

My tutelary friendship with Mr. Lewis grew to a keen respect for him as an artist as well as a person. Our daily conversations veered from art to people, places, things, life itself. I'd sit close, gaze at the heavy wrinkles around his eyes, and want him to fill me in, tell me all about this thing called life. I was given a look through the eyes of a bent browed cynic. To him, everyone and everything were tainted and a little suspect, except perhaps a wide-eyed fawn like me silly enough to sit by an old man's knee listening to his musings. He'd seen many ills in the haunts and hollows of his years. As he spoke, he sometimes sought refuge in the icy silver flask carried in his coat. He was a lone wolf, no wife or kids. There was just me, the string bean who always wanted to hear what he had to say and was always most impressed. I was well warned by him not to be so trusting and gullible, lest my unguarded belief in the ideal lead me into a fatal collision with the real.

Now I had two alcoholic "dads" in my life. Neither I could really understand. Both seemed to have all the answers yet needed liquor to distill the pain of their existence. Guess I didn't realize how much hurt life can hold when one gets older and dreams you've dreamed have not materialized. You look back and see there's not much left but emptiness.

Poverty programs have been highly criticized as wasteful rip-offs of public coffers that sent the wrong message to ghetto youth, implying society owed them a handout. I feel they were of great benefit, because they gave us jobs we otherwise would not have had. In addition, they gave us a place to go, learn, dream, and aspire to reach our goals. At Haryou, I learned about artists like Charles White and Claude McKay, as opposed to Rembrandt and Piaget. This fostered a sense of hope that I could become an artist if I worked hard at it. I was not incredibly talented in drawing. But I was a very creative person and needed to find where I'd fit. And I was going through a crisis of identity that only a dunk in a sea of blackness could ameliorate.

Harlem was a spawning ground for movers and shakers of black consciousness. It was our home base, the community of all black communities, the center of our collective being, the place we all originated from or passed through. We couldn't go back to Africa, but we could all come to Harlem and feel at home. It was a place where blacks responded viscerally to white America with clinched fists and angry voices, but to one another with a brotherhood salute; where a rank growth of hair and Afrocentric dress became physical statements of black pride and awareness of our roots; where vendors sold items to accentuate the soul look and black hands in back kitchens made the very best cooks. It was a place where R&B became the rhythm of the streets and everyone walked with a rocking beat; a place where tears often fell like rain, rueful smiles attempted to cover up an awful lot of pain, and slumlords made rapacious gains off the least fortunate.

An unseen force, like that which moves an ocean tide, was sweeping through black neighborhoods, pulling our people out of their inertia—a desire for pride and dignity that would only come with self-sufficiency and determination. We began to look back across the portals of history, searching for our identity, for the soul of blackness tossed from slave ships into icy waters on long journeys across the sea. We looked back to what was once ours—our names, our family tree, our traditions—longing to snatch them back from the hands of time, make them ours again, and restore wholeness. We reached back to our motherland, embraced her like a child once lost, who had come home at last. A thousand conga drums beat in our hearts as we looked forward with joyful anticipation to leaving the sweltering ghettoes of the North and stepping out into a land of promise. Once freed from the shackles of racism, poverty, and ignorance we'd don the dress of kings and queens, robe ourselves like royalty, and shod our feet with sandals like our forefathers wore when they walked the desert sands of the Nile Valley in the dawn of civilization. We tried to put on blackness for the reason actors put on stage dress, so the audience knew immediately who we were and what we represented. The American psyche would be our stage, and we put on a grand show.

For four centuries we had been judged by white standards of beauty. Whole generations had come and gone and never learned to love themselves. Now black had become "beautiful." Our aching spirits were lifted by the movement for black pride. Previously blacks had been taught to mirror whites, to identify and assimilate. But like water and oil, they just would not mix. Now we no longer wanted to "fit in." As the movement grew, we began to accept ourselves as we were. Black groups banned together calling for a national black agenda, serving notice on white America we would soon be "coming to dinner" and wanted our fair portion to be put on the family table. Black artists and writers exploded with a wealth of expression of this new nationalism. Intense political debate waged over issues such as economic parity and disproportionate levels of unemployment among blacks. Many minority candidates ran for public office and won.

By 1965 the civil rights movement had begun to lose steam. There was a sense of euphoria, freedom, and rebellion in the air as people took to the streets and black anger erupted like volcanic ash. Those impatient with the political process called for revolution. "Right on" became their popular slogan.

Black nationalists, notably the Nation of Islam, stood on street corners in Harlem distributing materials that set our hearths aflame.

They rejected Martin Luther King's philosophy of nonviolence and advocated a more militant approach to solving our problems. From their ranks would come one crying in the northern wilderness with fiery rhetorical style. He raised a tumult that would not be quieted. From the grave, his voice still speaks to black men today.

Little had changed outside the South. Migrant farmhands who came north seeking better opportunity found bias as unyielding as clods of clay in dry fields had been to their pickaxes. They were stuck in decaying neighborhoods where conditions were overcrowded and dirty. Urban wastelands had become bastions of hate because Northern whites hid behind masks of liberalism and weren't forced to confront their prejudices. Since the Civil War, the North had been thought of as a haven for blacks to find jobs, shelter, and security, in reality, a fleeting illusion for all but the best educated and skilled. Housing and job discrimination, fertilized by fear and hatred, grew as rampantly in hard asphalt as it had in moistened clay. Leaders' call to end slums and create jobs fell on deaf ears.

In the South, entire communities could be mobilized to fight segregation. They could easily pinpoint their enemy and set goals. In northern cities, it was hard to organize people into a cohesive group. The white man told us our problems were our fault. There were no clear Jim Crow rules and segregated stores. Racism in the North was more subtle but very present—as present as a glass door that prevents one from leaving one area and entering another or a glass ceiling that stops one from moving to a higher level.

The voices of leadership that had been a strong gale blowing across the South lost their intensity against the cold winds of Northern indifference. There were other voices, equally as passionate, competing for our attention. This period was a hotbed of issues, school integration, jobs, housing, the Vietnam War, equal rights, the draft, challenge of traditional roles and values, women's roles, the pill, and sexual freedoms.

From this compost pile, laden with catalytic energy, sprang the greatest firebrand of our time, El-Hajj Malik El-Shabazz, or Malcolm X. His incendiary remarks excited our thinking and presented a challenge to act. His was the voice many urbanites listened to because it was gritty and defiant like folks from the city. It shook the granite walkways of black neighborhoods and the invisible walls that held us within their confines, awakening us from our slumbering sleep.

He had a hard edge, caustic and abrasive, like folks who had to scrimp and scrape to survive; hard like factory workers' lives; hard like landlords' hearts when you couldn't pay your rent; hard like not having five cents; hard like the Almighty Hawk, Mr. Wind, who whistled around street corners, turned at any address, and charged right in past the plastic taped-over windows; hard like standing in line for welfare or unemployment, looking at eyes that look back, saying you are dirt or averting you altogether to infer your insignificance; hard like billy clubs used to bust black men's heads against the pavement; hard as having a baby when there's no one else but you; hard as the labor that comes on strikingly, forcing new life through. His voice was similar to the rappelling drum that called the early colonists to war in revolt against the British. A call to brotherhood, to stand firm against injustice, not by a foreign power, but by America herself, which had become our oppressor. The same spirit of indomitability and belief in liberty led the founding fathers to establish this nation and draft the Constitution. Malcolm said that document had given us the right to bear arms against the established order because it was breaking its own law. He wanted to bring the issue before the world court and let public opinion judge our case.

Some whites felt blacks ought to be beholden to them for bringing us "out of the jungles" to "the greatest country in the world" and giving us whatever opportunities we had been afforded. My parents felt the same way. I remember my mother and father saying, "I haven't lost anything over there in Africa! I am an American, and this is my home. If I can't make it here, I can't make it anywhere!" They didn't understand the notion of reclaiming our roots, connecting with our past, going back in order to go forward.

Malcolm called black men to rally their manhood and assume leadership of their families and communities. He emphasized self-respect and self-reliance, realizing education and economic empowerment would be key to breaking the bonds of racism. As important would be changing the way we characteristically behaved. He said it was time to stop shuckin' and jivin'. This was radical talk both in terms of the white man and the black woman who had grown accustomed to domination and rule. Malcolm had clear insight into the problems urban blacks were suffering.

He taught that we were born with rights and must exercise those rights to be treated like human beings, to be respected, to know our real names, to know our real past and who our forefathers were, to fight for our personhood and pride. He expressed all those gut-wrenching emotions that poured out when we were angry and hurting about our situations. They were so intense we didn't want them to surface, because when they did, it was with the fury of a storm. Their strength made us feel strong and powerful, when deep down we were weak and vulnerable. They imbued us with a sense of power to take control.

It was easier to listen to the clamor for revolution than to buy into Martin Luther King's "turn the other cheek" philosophy. Use of force always seems to make more sense to Americans than peaceful means. We are a warring people. Violence is very much a part of our tradition, intrinsic to daily life in our society. Fighting doesn't always help us get any further than what we are fighting over, but it's the alternative we choose often. Voices of insurrection always sound good, until we begin the body count and weigh the loss of life and property against what has been achieved. The scales never balance.

In Barabbas's day, he saw the needs of the people and called them to arms against the established order. But victory was not his, because he didn't count in the Lord. It is He who upholds one nation and brings another down that incurs His righteous judgment. Martin Luther King did not believe arms would bring victory, but the Lord Himself would see us through to the promised land, if we held on.

Malcolm told it like it was; Martin, how we wanted it to be. Both were necessary in the process of our becoming. I listened to Malcolm at every opportunity, but kept it from others. I felt as if I were committing an act of treason, giving an ear to someone who advocated black autonomy, community control, and the right to armed self-defense. Anything that contradicted what I had traditionally been taught seemed terribly wrong, and I doubted its voracity.

After all, if his teachings bore any truth, wouldn't the major networks support him? Wouldn't the sage instructors whom I admired in school expound on his philosophy? Wouldn't my textbooks be filled with these ideas? Were these the rants of a fool, or was I reluctant to acknowledge him because I'd be forced to ask and answer the question, "What am I personally going to do about it in terms of my own life choices?" I attempted to dismiss him by saying all black nationalists are a bunch of troublemaking extremists. A side of me wanted to respond and take a stand, but I was sorely afraid of what I had to lose—afraid of the cost I'd have to pay for dignity.

Struggle with evolving racial identity unleashed a torrent of such intensity my emotions became hot buttons easily pressed. Like a sponge over the years, I had soaked up bad feelings, hurtful remarks, and little indignities and cached them deep inside. Images I'd seen on TV or in books were now written across the marquee of my mind. Once I read an account of how a slave master long ago had taken a small black child, made him curl before his chair, and used him daily as a footrest. The imagery was so powerful I could actually envision myself as the frail child lying under the burden of the cruel master's feet. It impacted me so much that I really started to dislike feet, anyone's feet. Couldn't stand anyone putting their feet on me, not as a casual gesture or for any reason, not even on furniture near me. It felt belittling and threatening, made me uneasy and annoyed.

I began organizing things in my mind along racial lines, i.e., ways of interacting and responding to whites differently from my own people, which I am sure I was doing all along, but now it was more focused. I wrestled with feeling the need to prove myself as good as they. I reasoned, "Whites are against me, so I must strive with them and try to measure up to prove my worth." On the other hand, I'd see blacks and say, "They are like me, so I must side with them and love them, even if I often don't like them." There was a tendency to lump everyone into categories, black or white, and label one good, the other bad by nature.

Reality then became what existed in my own mind, what I told myself to be true regarding race. Whatever experiences came along that tended to support the archetype or blueprint I had drawn up in my head, I clung to. Those that controverted it, I brushed aside. Things said around me, black truisms like "You know Whitey don't want us to have nothin'!" fed this perception of us as saints and them as devils trying to keep us down and hold us back.

My parents never taught me to hate. But when from an early age you have heard that whites say you are inferior and have done all sorts of bad things to your people, it seems natural to want to hate them for what they've done. It seems like the black thing to do, almost as an act of self-love. If I love myself, I must hate them, at least that's what we deluded ourselves into believing. Maybe not hate really, but harbor bitterness for the injustice we've suffered.

Yet I had been taught to love, that God is love, and had even seen pictures of Christ depicted as a white man with long blond hair and blue eyes. I was angry and confused. How could a white man in heaven be all for me when white men on earth were all against me? I decided to pull away from "the white man's God."

Before long, I stopped chumming up with white kids so as not to be called an "Oreo," black on the outside, white on the inside. Still those who influenced me most at that point were white teachers whom I reached out to for counsel. I was emotionally torn, being pulled in two directions. It seemed the only way I could make it in *their* world and become successful was to learn to walk, talk, look, and act like *them*. Yet I had a burning desire to express who I was. I felt conflicted between wanting to express my blackness and be comfortable with it and wanting to be accepted in the white world and have credibility in their eyes.

When I looked at my people, sometimes it was through the eyes of shame and self-loathing and sometimes it was with a wanting sense of pride. My identity was so fragile as I regularly beat up on myself and "US."

My sentiments were with the peace movement, and I spoke out vehemently against the war. Folk songs by Dylan and other socially conscious artists rang from my lips. My heart fluttered passionately in tune. One favorite song, "The Times They Are a Changin'," became a classic. It was the song that moved our generation.

Dissenters were expressing opposition to the war in ever-loudening voices that reached a crescendo in the late '60s. The conflict became more bloody and difficult as the administration lost sight of its objectives. By then, 180,000 troops had been sent to Vietnam, many of them black. I questioned Uncle Sam's right to require us to fight and die in the rice fields of Southeast Asia, when we held second-class citizenship here at home. And why should we fight Third World peoples who, like ourselves, struggled against white rule? The cream was being skimmed off the top of our communities. Those able to pass tests and in good physical health were put on the frontlines, in the line of fire. This posed a threat to the leadership of our families and neighborhoods.

Although I echoed the cry of the hippies, "Make love, not war!" I felt we could never really be as one because they could take off their bummy clothes, trim their hair, and go back to being white. Their poverty was by choice; ours wasn't. White kids could always join their daddy's firm and climb the economic ladder. We couldn't. There was no access for us.

Besides, all the talk of peace and love hadn't changed things much in the inner city; neither had school desegregation. Merely sitting next to a white kid in class didn't put us on equal footing or force us to live in the same world. Issues involved not only race but also class. Social, cultural, and psychological unification of blacks and whites could not be achieved by the institution of laws or the integration of schools and the workplace. There was tremendous political backlash for white candidates who supported the liberal agenda.

The nation itself was beleaguered by a spirit of violence and anarchy. Anarchy was at the same time taking place around the world in France and China. In the midst of all this social upheaval, many young people were caught in a riptide. Free love, sex, and drugs became the order of the day. Value systems that had been around for centuries were thrown out of the window. Behavior that was before unthinkable now became fashionable. I foolishly ignored Mom's warning against sexual experimentation and wandered curiously into the danger zone. It was a season of violence as war raged on foreign shores and within our borders.

I became one of the young zealots riding the zenith of euphoria, adamant about bringing forth *change*. One weekend I could be found down in Washington, DC, at the Pentagon, protesting the war, being tear gassed and trampled. Next, I'd be at Howard University watching the new black home coming queen wearing a pompom-looking Afro assume her throne, caught up in the spirit, as fist waving crowds dinned, "Ungowa, Black Power!" I shuttled between cities on Amtrak and between movements in my mind.

I was angry that my generation was being called on to fight a war we had no emotion for and couldn't understand. I was even more incensed that white kids could beat the draft, being of the more privileged class, but blacks had no way out. We were first in war, last in peace. Looking down the barrel of soldiers' rifles brought me face-to-face with the awesome power of the government to squelch and destroy dissent. A bone-chilling fear passed over me as I realized how easily I could be annihilated just like a peasant in a rice patty if I came up on the wrong side of the system. The powers that be had everything under control, so it seemed.

My friends and I made our way across 125th Street daily amid a splendid profusion of sights, sounds, and madness to catch the subway. Bouncing along, we spoke solely of goals and dreams. We talked up big plans about what we were going to do. Actually, it was more talk than action. We were dripping with eagerness and enthusiasm about the future. An aura of expectancy seemed to lighten the impure air as we assured ourselves we would "make a difference." We felt we had the bull by the horns and could conquer the world if we wanted to. We were ready to take on issues and initiate happenings.

We went about renovating old tenements, scraping muck off their faces to uncover treasures of hidden beauty and richness. To me, those structures symbolized the black community itself, encrusted with years of decaying debris caused by poverty and neglect, while below the surface, potential wealth and resources lay untapped. Only those willing to look past the obvious and dig a little deeper found the storehouse. We who dug deeper into ourselves saw beauty amidst the rubble of too many bad experiences, too little hope, and too much discouragement.

We began covering those towering monuments to urban blight with strong positive images in colorful murals of our heroes, Malcolm and Martin, and faces of the children reaching for a brighter tomorrow. Sadly, those street paintings became backdrops for drug sales and street corner shootouts by fourteen-year-old thugs in the eighties.

Heightened interest in arts and culture led me to check out books on ancient civilizations that covered languages, customs, traditions, art forms, folklore, dance, and ceremonial dress. I made the rounds to art museums noticing similarities between the masks created by primitive artists and works of European masters. It appeared they had stolen the recognition due us and achieved fortune and fame. They basked in what should have been our glory. It angered me that in order to rediscover our African past, we had to go through them. They separated us from it. How could we rely on them to tell us the whole truth? So we attempted to define ourselves, for ourselves, by peeling off successive layers of our collective personality, down to the pith, our essential parts. Self-pride could only evolve through experimenting, exploring, and analyzing what we thought blackness was all about, not what had been imposed on us.

Black artists came forth with a spectrum of powerful new images of black life. Some of it was spiritual, meditative, and reflective or angry and reactive; some spicy, alive, piquant to taste; some cool, laid back, and mellow; some as down-home and basic as the blues. And some of it was pure survivalism captured by one artist in a monochrome portrait of a black child smiling up from the gutter where he sat licking an ice cream cone, heedless of the virulent organisms breeding in the cesspool where he played. Other powerful images sprang forth, black Madonna, Jesus, and Santa Claus.

Soon I was ready to throw off my "slave name" and assume something more reflective of the essence of true black womanhood. I'd have chosen Nefertiti, black queen of the Nile. But of course, that wouldn't go over big with Mom and Dad or with white teachers who questioned why we wanted to be called anything besides Beulah Jones, Willie Jackson, or Loretta Farmer. Those who took on new names in an effort to assert black pride were mocked to scorn. In light of that, I just insisted everyone call me Jean, obliterated Loretta from my record. That, to me, was a modicum of progress.

A new song caught my heart's cadence:

> I wish I knew how it would feel to be free,
> I wish I could break all the chains holding me,
> I wish I could say all the things that I should say,
> Say it loud, say it clear for the whole wide world
> To hear.
> I wish I could be like a bird up in the sky,
> Remove all the bars, I'd find out how to fly,
> I'd soar to the sun and look down at the sea
> And I'd sing 'cause I know how it feels to be free!
> (Nina Simone)

Sifting back through our human experience, I found flecks and nuggets of gold sprinkled on the sands of history by our black ancestry. I also found many bug-a-boos hiding in the family closet we'd need to be rid of to get ready for full acceptance by the mainstream of society: unprofessionalism in business dealings for want of better business sense; tardiness and unreliability; deficiency in using the resources of the black community to support the black community; not having public deportment; drinking or eating then throwing refuse on the streets; rowdy behavior and loud laughter; noisiness and blasting music; accepting dirt and sloppiness where we live; not demanding high standards in services provided to us; defacement and destruction of property; too little civic involvement; not getting out to vote; shortage of mechanisms for solving our own problems; lack of stability and consistency in our homes; not enough time spent teaching and relating to our children; robbing or ripping each other off; low personal standards; the pall of crime, violence, drugs, and alcoholism cast over our neighborhoods; and the scourge of AIDS.

These problems are not unique to the black community, not by a long shot! But under the dense and stressful conditions that they occur, their potency intensifies, serving to continually undermine our attempts to move forward. Social ills and the stigmatization that accompany them have been the bane of our existence. Still our ancient songs of sorrows were filled with hope and belief in a God who is no respecter of persons.

I saw my world was changing at a dizzying pace. My grand-kids will know nothing of the world my grandparents lived in—will not have the pleasure of drinking well water, making grass dolls, or soaking in a foot tub bath, nor will they see the body of a black man dangling by the neck from a tree, having been lynched. For them, it will be a better world, or will it? Hate is still around and flourishing quite well. In fact, I hear it's on an uptick.

Childhood is a struggle—the quest for identity, but one of the many facets of growing up. I continued my search for roots, delving into the past to ferret for gems of knowledge to reflect light upon the present. Actually, I felt betwixt-and-between, often reluctant to identify with my people because of embarrassment about a lot of our ways. Yet a strong esprit de corps showed itself when in a group. I grew queasy about relatives too, viewing them as country bumpkins, not highly educated and lacking city savvy.

In perusing the distant past, looking to recapture pride, I over-looked the positives we had going at that point of time to feel good about. Blacks were so emulous of whites, wanting to be like them in every way, changing to make ourselves acceptable. I feel we threw out the baby with the bathwater—got rid of those qualities that were our strengths and provided stability.

Now that many of those things are extant, like the strong sense of family and community, and that old-time religion that was the basis of the traditional beliefs and values we once held, I look with longing and cling to what vestiges remain. They stay alive in me, pop up time and again. I am a repository of history. A new understanding and fondness for old stories, ways black people did things, and how they spoke back when has grown—makes me feel good inside, like I'm okay. Funny the cycles we go through.

Sometimes I feel I don't belong in either world. I'm not all that gung-ho black, black anymore. Yet I have feelings of nationalism about my roots. At times, I find it very hard to relate to that black person who is on the bottom, but I feel responsibility toward them. Issues are never as simple as black and white.

By eleventh grade I'd nabbed a steady beau named John Louis Steptoe. Sexual experiences soon followed as his sunny presence filled my lonely hollow. Our relationship at its zenith was much like Batman and Robin, a dynamic duo crusading into the art realm to make our mark, though his natural talents far overshadowed mine. John was truly a prodigious teen. By age sixteen, he had written and illustrated his first children's book, *Stevie*, in black English. I tagged along, sunning in his glory, accompanying him to publishers, meeting bigwigs, visiting posh residences in Westchester.

As he teetered along the edges of success, it seemed he'd found his key of admittance, but what about me? I warmed in the air of expectancy yet hadn't found my niche. Fashion illustration proved not to be my calling. I wasn't bent for the world of glamor and glitz. It went against my earthy nature. I sought a vehicle to express my creativity that wouldn't compromise my integrity.

Dreamily, we walked around with reels, turning in our heads, showing us fast-moving pictures of how things would, could, and should be. For a while, puppy love was as sweet as sugar candy. Then came the day I had to ask Mom to take me to the doctor. Why? Thought I might be "PREG," that terrifying word she always spelled because of the authority it had to wreck young girls lives and because it had done so to too many of our own especially.

I remember well the burdensome fear that loomed over us the way thick black smog hung over city skies that day, as I slumped in the office chair, waiting to be called, and the great sigh of relief Mom heaved when I tested negative—remember how I thought I'd let her down and how courageously she stood by me and didn't lecture. How I promised never to let it happen until I finished my education so I'd make her proud and not end up like scores of other girls on the public roll. How in the time that followed John and I drifted farther and farther apart, and when we reached our nadir, an awful introduction I had to his new love who turned out to be a he. My idealism and my heart suffered their first crushing blow. I kept it secret so no one would ever know my hurt and shame. I found out life is not a Cinderella story. My prince turned out to be a toad.

It's said blood is thicker than water and partying helps the blues. At family affairs, Fay, Sonny, and I became three dancin' fools, poppin' jive, slappin' five, spewing heptitudes. In their company, I knew my identity; there was no doubt I belonged. It was a comfort just to sit around listening while the family talebearers rattled off the same old stories, added new ones, and mixed in a few lies to make us laugh. Several generations gathered as our numbers grew and the family machinery chugged on. Cousin Ethel married Bill. Soon two girls were born, then a trio of boys ambled along. Cousin Henry fathered two more. His sister Nina added a girl to the score. Aunt Beulah relocated with her three. JoAnn married John, Carolyn married Billy, and Earl married Effie. New marriages meant new families being established. It was certain we would pass on love to all future members.

We nourished our traditions of time spent together during holidays, eating big dinners and celebrating noisily into the night. When the world outside seemed topsy-turvy, togetherness lent a feeling of security, made everything all right.

Never was there a more popular family member than Fay. She had all the dance moves, all the funny jokes; attention swirled around her. Her gift for unrehearsed humor drew peals of laughter. I sat drolly in the shadows, watching her jest. Jean, the dry intellectual type, depended on facts and figures rather than style and humor. Fay fared masterfully in social situations, while I, at best, managed to interject myself now and then but quickly retreated into quietness. The family accepted it was her way, not mine. The outside world was never quite so kind.

Feelings of inadequacy continually infected me at school. I began to get good at solitude. I just couldn't come out of my shell and let my hair down in a group. When you don't feel adequate, people don't treat you that way. Others were able to read my low esteem. It became a ruse that hid my ability even from me. Yet I liked assisting others; I wanted to do something for someone else. I had a special love of children and felt no impediments in relating. I always had a tender spot for their needs.

Those were days of rambling dreams and wanton freedoms—a period when torrid emotions, like the Caribbean winds, arose with great passion then quieted to a balmy breeze blowing out to sea. That period of time when I knew adulthood was just over the next ridge. I was filled with anticipation of what lay ahead. My internal juices were stirred up, fast flowing, readying me to do something, be something. What? I didn't know. I wanted to lift up freedom's torch, go to the battlefield for what I believed in. A giddy sense of power befell me. I was invincible, or so I thought.

Though my head bobbled with youthful expectancy, it was modulated by the notion I could only go so far because of my ethnicity. The sky was not my limit. Having ingested the old staples for years watching TV, Andy, Perry, Dr. Welby, Jack Benny, George Allen, and Gracie, I knew their episodes like the back of my hand. But looking at their world was a lot like looking through a peephole from a dark room into a well-lit room. Everything appeared so bright and glittery, but reaching it seemed an impossibility, unfeasible as squeezing my long body through the narrow viewer and coming out on the other end. I could see a better life but didn't feel I could access it. Growing up in a community trying to live on hope, struggling under self-condemnation as well as societal condemnation, I found it really hard to love *me* and people like me.

Waveringly I pressed on, finished my courses. In June 1967, graduation day crept along, that much awaited ceremony marking my emancipation from childhood, setting me free to make my own decisions and be my own person. To accept my diploma, I wore a lace-trimmed mini angel dress of bleached linen and round-toed shoes like when I first started school. I looked pure and innocent, but I was not. I was more comfortable in a child's world.

I had grown to like my slender physique, since the white fashion model Twiggy had come from England and made having a bean pole figure a fashion craze. People used to say black girls had big behinds like horses riding up high on their backs. Short skirts were not supposed to look good on us. White girls were known to have cute little apple figures, with the flat rear ends, so I decided to strut my stuff, shimmied my little flat fanny across the stage for all the world to see. I was proud as could be that I had finished my education and that at least in some ways I was the same as they. My hemline was way, way up! My spirits likewise were way, way up!

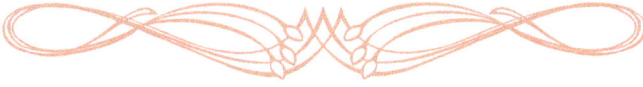

CHAPTER FOURTEEN
Emergence

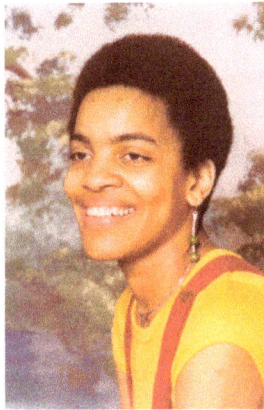

When I went Afro.

DURING that time Nina Simone sang a jazz song whose plaintive lyrics asked with great poignancy, "Who am I? Who am I?" Its deep questioning mimicked the inner bleating of my soul. I was eighteen and newly unincarcerated from youth. I no longer wished to be under the aegis of ruling parents. I wanted a free rein to do what I wanted to do as an adult. I pondered a way to say to the world, "I'm free and I'm me!" Being one with a visual orientation, I sought to make a strong visible statement.

Next day, I went down to Harlem to an Afro barbershop and got myself a short freedom cut to unveil the natural beauty in me. A frothy exuberance bubbled over inside. My narrow frame could hardly contain my glee as she snipped, clipped, patted, and sprayed oil all over my crown. The blunt cut left mere peach fuzz above my hairline. Easing the drape from around my neck, with a flick of her wrist, she shook years of hair growth atop a matted pile of wool on the floor, probably belonging to the girls who'd come before. With a grandly affirming smile, she tapped me on the shoulder and said, "You're done, sister!" while handing over an oval mirror in which to see. Oh me, it was just as I'd suspected! Hidden beneath that phony processed mess was an authentic black queen! Like a jolly jumping bean, I popped up from the chair and rushed out carrying my pik and a can of Afro sheen.

A whir of pleasurable ruminations whooshed through my mind during the long ride home. No longer would I be demeaned by feeling unlovely just the way I was, no longer ashamed of having kinky hair, no more feeling I had to be mixed with another race to be beautiful, no sitting in parlors for hours letting a sweaty overworked woman sizzle my brain or burn my scalp with lye. Dash away chemicals and their awful smell! My hair now had the scent of a juicy coconut, tropically sweet and ripe for the picking. I could shampoo, shower, and just go out. Say it loud; I was black and proud!

This was my first important decision. Mom and Dad couldn't stop me. It was my hair. But I tied on a scarf so the new me wouldn't come as too much of a shock. Home was the place I harbored my heart. I didn't really want to hurt anybody. That evening Mom and Dad were reposed in bed before the TV set. I stood at the door as we chatted on matters of little consequence. Mom, noticing my hesitance to uncover, inquired, "What's under the scarf?" I pretended not to hear and raved on about this and that, until at her insistence I doffed the wrap, pulling it off with a ginger snap. Mom took one look, turned over, and whimpered into her pillow. All that thick hair she'd nurtured and fought with for years had vanished in an instant. The suddenness overtook her.

The Bible said a woman's hair was her adorning. She was not to cut it off. Dad, looking past furrowed brows, said to me, "Now see what you have done to your mother!" then to her, "Don't worry, Ernestine. They've all gone crazy!" His summary remarks encapsulated the problem with our entire generation.

There are points in our lives when we are not the same, benchmarks we can look back on that are points of turning. There are times we wrest away the old, put on the new, and lay aside things that are hurtful and limiting. It was my time of emergence as a "sister." I put on a different look, dressed Afrocentrically in handmade things—hoop earrings, long skirts, gele wraps, and leather garb. My musical tastes broadened to include jazz, Afro-Cuban, and Latin music. I started to dig Mongo Santamaria, Eddie Palmieri, Miriam Makeba, Hugh Masekela, and Olatunji. My readings included the Last Poets, Amiri Baraka, Nikki Giovanni, Richard Wright, James Baldwin, and Kahlil Gibran. My new haunts were Latin clubs, jam sessions in city parks, and art fairs where community artisans sold batik wares, African prints, colorful dashikis, and flavored incense.

In those yearning years, white kids veered off into Eastern religions, mysticism, and transcendental meditation, while black kids embraced Islamic and African religions, Afro-Cuban lore, black arts (hoodoo, voodoo), the Yoruba gods, charminism, and astrology. Small sacks filled with potions were worn around our necks for protection reminiscent of slave practices in the Old South using "roots" to ward off evil. Strands of tiny multicolored beads appeared inside collars and cuffs, symbols of obeisance to the Orisha gods, Ogun and Orishala. And of course, there were the familiar peace signs or shapes of Mother Africa painted red, black, and green on leather strings. We reached back for spiritual artifacts from our past to recapture that which seemed so irretrievable—our myths and rituals of worship. Feeling orphaned by history, we clung desperately to bits and pieces of our cultural heritage to gain a sense of belonging somewhere.

Our new way of greeting one another was "Hey, brother!" or "Hey, sister!" A surge of kinetic energy flowed through our communities, moving us forward, though much in fighting and debate arose on finding the right direction. The country remained highly politicized and racially divided.

Simultaneously, America was passing through her season of rebellion, the one movement feeding into the other. Society underwent cataclysmic social upheaval. The younger generation, holding little with holy reverence, ridiculed long-held norms and traditions. Old verities like faith, honor, morality, and sexual restraint were becoming as outdated as high-button shoes. Chaos, violence, and insecurity were rampant. Mopheads wearing psychedelic rags were raising a new voice in America. Drug use became a recreational sport. Kids got turned on and tuned out. Premarital, extramarital, and homosexual sex was deemed okay between consenting adults. A "new morality" took hold.

The pill helped usher in new freedoms for women. So did radical feminists who declared, "A woman needs a man like a fish needs a bicycle." They suggested the only way a woman could find personal satisfaction was to leave home and compete for jobs and salaries in the workforce. Women began to burn their bras as hostility toward men grew. The Beatles came along and said they were more popular than Jesus Christ. A popular atheist wrote a book, *The Passover Plot*, declaring Christ a hoax. Others said God was dead and cast doubt on His existence. Theological confusion took hold. Large segments of our generation left the church to follow their own way. Black congregations were over 70 percent women. Black men left the churches in droves.

Popular slogans for the times were "Look out for number one!" and "If it feels good, do it!" Popular music greats, like Sinatra and Sammy Davis, were singing "I Did It My Way" and "I Got to Be Me." We became known as the "Me" generation. Black people took a wrong turn in the '60s. Living in a society and surrounded by people espousing the "Me, myself, and I philosophy," we latched on to it and began to let go of what had been at the core of our endurance, a strong faith in and dependence upon the Lord and on the church, His agency on earth, which had been our way station in troubled times. We stopped believing, as Grandma's generation had, that it was what you were and what you believed that made you somebody.

For our generation, as the doors of opportunity squeaked open and we began to slowly climb the economic ladder, we let go of concerns with our inner man and became superficially and externally minded. We were no longer worried about being like Jesus, no longer looking for power in the blood to transform our living conditions. We aimed for education, position, and economic power. We began a process of renewal, i.e., new homes, cars, and clothes. We stopped singing "I looked at my hands, and they looked new. I looked at my feet, and they did too!" Character, integrity, and moral fiber were put on the back burner.

We shed those things for the new because we assumed they were better. Our priorities began to change. We started looking for God in things acquired, degrees held, and positions attained. We transferred the focus of our lives to things and money and lost spiritual moorings. A collision of values and philosophies took place in our homes. Our family structures weakened.

The welfare system, which expanded in the '60s, aided in the decline by encouraging separation of black families. Women with children could get a monthly check and Medicaid cards only if they had no man in the home. Black women could live better without men, and so they decided, "I don't need a man to help me do bad. I can do that by myself!" They began to depend on the welfare system. Black men were made to feel they had no role or value, without a job or financial security for the family. Male leadership waned and accountability lessened. Their absence markedly weakened the family infrastructure. In our efforts to pull up by our bootstraps, priorities were getting misplaced.

Like others, I was greatly concerned with moving ahead. Born sandwiched between a popular older sister and a baby brother, I'd have fallen into obscurity, except for doing well in school. Therefore, doing well became my way of getting attention and dealing with self-rejection. I scored high in academics and reasonably in art, so I applied for a scholarship to a design school in midtown Manhattan. Mom and Dad disagreed with my choice. They advised me to take a brief secretarial course that would lead to a secure job. A black girl casting her lots in the art world, to them, was a foolish risk. This caused a breach between us. I went ahead anyway with my plans.

A haughty headmistress who was not especially overjoyed to greet a black applicant conducted the interview. She had a snobbishness about her that seemed to say, "Dear, dear! What makes you think you would fit in here?" as a smirk ran off the end of her nose. She asked point-blank why I wanted to be an artist and not a maid, let's say, adding that in her opinion it didn't matter what you were as long as you did your job well. "If you are a maid, be the best maid you can be. That's what's important!" she said. Something bristled inside of me as I mustered up the confidence to reply, "But I don't want to be a maid. I want to be an artist!" then I left, certain never to hear from her again.

An inevitable surprise came weeks later stating I'd been granted a scholarship. Perhaps it was an act of conscience or the pressure of the federal government on all-white schools to open their doors to minority candidates that forced her hand. However, the interview cast a pall of gloom over my experience there for the next two years. I was fearfully overwhelmed and consumed with feelings that I didn't belong and couldn't measure up. I got bogged down in negative self-analysis. My work suffered and grades went down. I was just too tense to relax and be creative.

The other students, many of them European, behaved well and didn't treat me like a token Negro. Remarks that are racist and mean-spirited are most often said when we are among family and acquaintances, not to strangers. That is where we affect those we know intimately, while putting on a good face in public. I remember one Swedish boy in the elevator who asked if he could run his fingers through my Afro, said it looked very "tactile." People were very touchy-feely in those years. I reluctantly obliged for the sake of making friends.

I did make one friend, a girl from Seoul, North Korea. On weekends I'd visit her home in New Jersey. We'd play out in the rain and jumped over earthworms for fun. Though from opposite sides of the world, we were real soul mates, she and I, confirming culture and race were not insurmountable barriers.

In my second year, I crossed paths with a neighborhood boy, Clinton Barrett, whose interests in music and art made it seem we had a lot in common. We took an immediate liking. He listened and provided support at a time I found myself faltering. Soon we were hanging around each other all the time. My parents became deeply alarmed, warned we were getting too serious and it would affect my education. I guess I'd become so tired of being told what to do that even if what they said was reasonable, I just didn't want to hear it. Consequently, many battles and conflicts arose.

The winds of rebellion beguiled me into believing I didn't have to put up with it anymore and secreted me out of the house to do my own thing. Clinton's mom, a Pentecostal minister, regularly rained fire and brimstone down on him too because of his willful ways. He and I parlayed our needs for independence into an excuse to run away together.

Thus, we took off, two wildlings, clothes in a shopping cart, not knowing whence we were bound but following foolishly along. We left our parents' table to go sit at the world's table and (I dare say) to drink from the cup of folly. Fay left the nest the year before, married her high school sweetheart in a lovely home wedding. Since I was hot on her heels trying to do everything she did, that provided added prompting.

For a while we reveled in our newfound freedom. Good friends who had a cubby hole in the South Bronx put us up. At first there was music and merriment, but as days wore on, our welcome petered out, and reality slowly seeped in. When the food dwindled, so did the fun.

Mama didn't like the idea I was living in sin, "shacking up" so to speak, and had been giving me the cold shoulder. I thought getting married would solve the problem. Clinton woke up one morning and said on a whim, "If you want to do it, come on let's go!" I foolishly followed. There was no trousseau or parents' blessings or family guests, no fancy dress, no wedding ring, limousine, or anything— just a five-dollar license redeemed at a local church before a dutiful minister and a cleaning man holding a filthy mop who'd been asked to stop and stand while we joined hands.

From there we were off…to the welfare office. Where else could we go? No jobs, no money…so…there we landed! They gave us just enough money to rent a little nook on 170th Street, a dirty place with not much heat and a few food stamps so we could eat. They called it an emergency check and told us not to expect to come back for more. We figured we were all set, I guess, decided to do the best with what we had. And so we roamed the streets and collected things from garbage heaps to furnish our honeymoon suite.

Days passed; friends came by. My husband and they got high, smoking pot and beating on drums, creating sultry rhythms. Where was I? In the kitchen burning heat, trying to make something out of nothing to eat, learning how to survive, keep myself and him alive.

Frightened, alone, and faced with problems that I had little resources to handle, I began to seek refuge in my fantasy world—the place I had always found safety as a child, the place I had gone to so often to work out conflicts. In an atmosphere of African chants, incense, and driving rhythms, I was bedeviled by marauding spirits that serpented my mind into inner regions where reality and fantasy become conjoined and one has little ability to separate one from the other. Bizarre faces, frightening thoughts, weird sounds, and pungent scents regularly invaded my psyche, keeping me in a state of confusion about my surroundings. I became unable to separate dreams from reality and unable to share what was happening with others for fear of appearing insane. On many occasions, I imagined myself as the poor black Indian princess of my dreams, put on her costume and long hair, and talked to myself in despair, wrenching my hands, praying for a prince to find and kiss me—free me from my lowly estate.

One time, when left alone, I was summoned out of the door by a haunting melody that led me to a dark dangerous park at night to sit on a high wall, music raging in my ears, faces grimacing at me from the trees, something telling me to jump, pulling me down into a nearby stream, torrents swirling in water that should have been a babbling brook. Snapping out of it, I suddenly ran for my life back to the apartment to sit in the chair and wonder if I had really gone anywhere, then seeing the evidence…a trail of mud…tracked in on a rug. I'd made a mistake and knew it, but there was no escape, not even in imagining.

We desired strongly to carry on, but four evictions came along, tossing us out of one place after another. Our nests, made in the crannies and rookeries of the South Bronx, were crowded, dirty, mean tenements where poor families lived like packrats amid the squalor, where it was hard to get your hands on a dollar and everyone was black collar.

Many hot nights I couldn't sleep for the cry of hungry babes, so I stayed up and watched cockroaches put on parades. The smell of piss and sweet perfume minced the gloom of my somber room. I'd open a window for a waft of the breeze, but voices and music sailed in when I tried to get down on my knees. The scream of sirens pierced the night, pulsating the fear and rage that hung like an invisible backdrop to this hellish stage. My days were filled with boredom, emptiness, nothing much to do but sit, worry, and wonder how I would make it through.

Poor neighborhoods in those years were like concentration camps. Blacks and Hispanics were socially barbwired in, and Whitey, barbwired out, except that he still held the reins of power and authority. He could decide if you earned a living or could withhold that right. He decided who ate and who had a place of rest at night.

In 1968, Dr. Martin Luther King was struck down by an assassin's bullet in a crime so heinous shock waves rippled through the black community. Our wounded spirits erupted with pain and bitterness. Many blacks decided nonviolent resistance would not alter the conditions in the slums and resorted to more militant approaches to solving our problems. There were calls for separation, and every political issue became a bone of contention picked clean by either party. We, the young radicals, thought surely "the brethren" would rise up and be his nemesis, avenge America for the death of our fallen leader. Surely, now was revolution time.

One issue came to a head in Harlem over a vacant lot that had been chosen for the site of a new state office building supposedly to bring renewal to the area. Community activists saw it as a takeover, an encroachment that signaled greater loss of community control.

My husband and I had been hanging around with squatters, who set up a tent city on the site. There were nightly meetings around camp-fires as we chanted, sung, and talked of the showdown we would have with *them* if they ever attempted to take over "our land." We would die on that spot rather than yield another inch to their control.

On cold nights, the brothers heated the air with fiery oratory beneath a banner of red, black, and green (red for the blood shed by our fathers, black for our racial bonds, and green for our mother Africa) proudly erected above our outpost. We were *all* going to take a stand for this hallowed ground, defend it with our lives. Surely, the revolution had come!

It had been announced that around noon on a certain day, a wrecking crew would come to break ground and start the project. Newscasters warned a confrontation was anticipated. Everyone was fired up and ready. This was a test about people who were *serious*. Frankly, I expected a miniature Armageddon to take place right there in the middle of 125th Street. But when the day came, barely a handful of ragtag participants cowered beneath our flag, shouted a few epithets at the wind, and quickly dispersed, leaving the midday crowds going on with business as usual—in and out of stores, shop-ping, scurrying quickly back to work.

What happened to our revolution? I learned that day, when people are given a choice between ethics and earnings, they most often choose the latter. Taking a stand on what we think is right comes with a high cost—high enough that most refuse to pay it.

Before long I found out (you guessed it!) I was P-R-E-G. Almost simultaneously Clinton decided anywhere away from me was where he needed to be. I'd suggested getting a nine-to-five job would be nice, but he said no dice, said working for the Man would com-promise his manhood, something I never understood. What would become of the tiny life inside of me? Didn't take much to see that it would be totally my responsibility. I had blown it royally! Oh, he was *sorry* things didn't work out and promised to do "the best he could," but that wouldn't do the baby and me much good. He began staying away night and day. I had no one to talk with and didn't know what to do or where to go next. Everything seemed so *hopeless*.

I felt like a stupid fool, like I should have known better—Ms. Smarty-Pants, Ms. Go-Getter. How could I have let this happen to me? That pivotal event changed my course. But not before I fell into a deep emotional pit and had to make the climb back up to stability. I was all grown up but still not "developed." Life had to apply more intense pressure to bring me to maturity.

It was the Aquarian Age, in the era of bell-bottom jeans and mood rings. I didn't need a mood ring to reveal I was in trouble and didn't know how to face it. A baby certainly wasn't a pet rock. It would have to be provided for and taken care of. I wanted to reach out to someone for help, but I'd strayed away from the family and lost their support. I went to the welfare office, and they told me I'd have to go to court to force him to provide for the baby. Fighting was not my forte; I didn't want to go through that. I decided literally to throw in the hat and take my foolish life, end the conflict that raged inwardly.

Life seemed to implode in on me. My insides attempted to regurgitate the distress, but it wouldn't go away. I was ejecting green vomit with the taste of bitter gall. One lonely, despairing, and desperate day, I decided to end it all. Making my way to Seton Park, behind the junior high I'd attended seemingly like eons before, I scrambled in the dark to a high precipice and stood on a ridge, from which I could see the spires of tall buildings looming all around me, like monuments of doom bearing my effigy.

Suddenly, I must have jumped, although I don't remember it, only the feeling of falling into a deep chasm and lying immobile as if asleep, then strangely awakening to see morning light peeking past the trees. God had given me a reprieve and left me in the land of the living. For what, I didn't know, but I knew it just wasn't my time to go. I'd have to pay for my mistake and learn the hard way. As Daddy used to say, "If you make your bed hard, that's where you are going to sleep!"

What followed were hours of vomiting and wandering with reels flickering in my mind. Eerie images, as in the creep shows and sci-fi movies I'd watched in matinees, played horridly inside my head. I made my way down to Harlem, the place that cradled me lovingly as a suckling child, to the office of a fatherly black obstetrician who, when he discovered I was bleeding, admitted me to the hospital for fear I would miscarry.

When my prior history with TB exposure came to light, I was quarantined in an isolated room. I ate on disposable plates, from a disposable spoon. There I lay dreadfully alone, looking at white coats and people wearing masks going in and out, feeling something was terribly wrong with me, sure the baby or I would die. In an odd way, I liked it there, since I felt safe and every day I ate three squares. Four major holidays I spent hospitalized: Easter, Mother's Day, July 4, and Thanksgiving. The kindly doctor admitted me each time there was a show of blood or perhaps because he understood I really had no place to go. He feared complications and told me of a strange parasite that fed on fetuses in the womb. I was horror struck at what might be going on in my inner sanctum.

As the baby grew, I could feel it moving and kicking. I wanted it to live, not die, stopped thinking of myself only and thought of him, for I was sure it was a boy. He was someone I could hold on to and feel strong. I'd have to be strong to prolong his life. After my last release, I went to stay with my sister, Fay, knowing time was near. Soon my bundle of joy would be there.

There's nothing like knowing a baby is on the way to snap you back into reality and help you focus on what's really important. No longer was the peal of a trumpet in my heart calling me off to war. No longer did I dream of a Nubian nation rising up to claim its glory. The voices of insurgency were like the wind rumbling against the windows of my mind. When I opened the window, I found there was nothing there but noise. I no longer listened to overtures made by radicals, nor was I pulled along by the sinuous whims of youth. Following a winding road that led where it willed was too treacherous. I wanted safety and security.

While out there on the highways and byways of the black community, I took a long hard look at my people. I saw the good, the bad, and the ugly—lots of ugly, a lot I couldn't be proud of. My discovery was they were just people, no better or worse than others. I lost my giddy sense of euphoria about blackness. Trying to worship the black race, as if there was something inherently good in us (as opposed to the white man, the devil, or the pig) didn't fly. I came to realize the same thing that was wrong with the white man was wrong with the black man. Our people increasingly were losing their sense of family and community, as we became more self-absorbed and greedy. As a minister once put it, "The problem is not skin, it's sin."

Those foundational cracks have the whole black community now teetering on the brink of annihilation by its own black sons. We're engaged in social suicide, killing ourselves off. Many of our young people don't value their lives and have no sense of hope for the future.

By Christmas I was fat as a tick, but the baby didn't mosey along until New Year's Day, when a spat with grits and eggs compelled him to vacate the premises. Still, it took thirteen and a half hours for him to complete his tardy arrival, making his birthday January 2, 1971. The pain of childbirth let me know I didn't want to go back that way again. It helped change my direction. I immediately checked his earlobes to see what color he was going to be. Colorism had infected me.

I remember vividly sitting on the edge of that hospital bed, holding the little bunting someone had given me to bring the baby home in, weeping bitterly, deathly afraid I would not be able to handle motherhood. The thought of taking that fragile tiny infant and having to make all the right decisions for its well-being caused me to shutter in my shoes. I felt I had blown my life and didn't want to be responsible for blowing his.

A sudden flashback surfaced of the previous days when I was wandering the street pregnant and wanting to prepare a layette for his coming. I resorted to shoplifting tactics of high school years when we put small items in our school bags and simply walked out of stores. I'd gone into Woolworth's and tried to lift a pair of blue satin baby shoes and got caught. I was so embarrassed and humiliated looking into the manager's face as he berated me, saying, "Didn't your mama ever teach you not to steal?" It was then I knew taking care of a baby was for real, not some childish game of chance you play. How could I keep food in its mouth and clothes on its back? My high dreams had met with an unkind reality. I was homeless and penniless.

At that moment the nurse came in and announced the baby wasn't quite ready to go as he had developed a high fever. Thank God for a slight respite to think, plan, and decide my course. What alternative was there but to call my parents and ask if I could come home. Their answer, a resounding yes, under the condition I put the past and my husband behind me. I gratefully agreed, made space for the baby, and slept on the settee. What happened to the child's father? I didn't care! I was certain he would find a lair and get his comeuppance.

My next task was in choosing a name. Many young women of my generation abandoned traditional names of European origin and denominated their children with West African names, some they didn't know the meanings of but liked the way they sounded. First names and last names didn't always match, like Adeosi Johnson or Abeoke Williams. Others formulated their own Africanized names by incorporating American patterns with borrowed elements from African languages. Names such as Shanese Wilson and Danika Coles demonstrate this cross-cultural blending and the desire to create something unique while holding on to our past.

To Africans, the meanings of names were very important because the words by which a person is known becomes his identity. I wanted my baby's name to signify the struggles of the past and present. After scribbling down dozens of tries, I finally settled for Malik Chaka Barrett—Malik in honor of El-Hajj Malik El-Shabazz (Malcolm X), who articulated the anger of Afro-Americans in the '60s, and Chaka, a South African warrior who led his people in fighting to preserve his Zulu homeland from British rule during the colonial period. His name symbolized a new generation who would have pride in their blackness and know their roots.

Malcolm's three names were descriptors of where he was at various stages of his self-awareness as a black man. He went through transformations in the persons of Malcolm Little, the street hustler; Malcolm X, the incendiary radical; and El-Hajj Malik El-Shabazz, the learned world traveler. I wanted my son to have the heart of a warrior and the mind of a great teacher like Malcolm. I prayed his strong, manly spirit had been reborn and the struggle for dignity would live on. Thus, I penned his name to the birth certificate with guarded optimism about his future.

The period of idealism ended for me when men of great social conscience and commitment were smitten by death: the Kennedys and our beloved leaders Malcolm and Martin. All the passion that had caused my heart to pummel and burn with anger simmered to a quiet inner rage tinged with helplessness to effect real change. Air slowly leaked out of my big yellow balloon, my hopes deflated.

I wanted to believe in peace and love but found out it was white peace and love. Blacks weren't included unless we could become what *they* wanted us to be and fit where *they* said fit. We were only being accepted as tokens within their groups. There were still many taboos against race mixing and limited cross-cultural interaction. Very little honest dialogue and openness took place between the races about our problems; therefore, there could be no reconciliation and forgiveness. Bias and prejudice seemed etched in the granite of our national persona. Flower Power became basically a white agenda, militants were pushing the black agenda, and the Manson family was trying to trigger a race war to throw the entire nation into helter-skelter.

The black movement had broken down into factions, fights, and feuds as various militant groups came to the foreground and vied for allegiance. Like most people, I was frightened by their extremist rhetoric and methods. When I saw what they seemed to represent, I no longer wanted to be a part of it. I came to realize anyone who attempted to take up the scepter of leadership in the black community was put down, derided, or met with a violent death. We were always left with pat little excuses that absolved the government, the police, the FBI, and the CIA of any guilt.

I suspected white America would never let 22 million blacks organize behind one leader. It would be too much of a threat to their security. When young whites went off the deep end, like Patty Hearst, they were spanked and sent back home. Blacks usually ended up in coffins, as did Fred Hampton when he rebelled against the social order. The brothers in Attica prison gave a shocking eye-opener of what the criminal justice system was for us. I perceived in the actions and policies of the government, the planned genocide of young males, in order to control our growth as a people. Concluding it unsafe to take up the gauntlet of political activism, I decided to abandon the national movement in favor of individual effort to affect just the little sphere around me.

I had become a new person, no longer Loretta Jean Farmer, now Jean F. Barrett. The name change by marriage meant a new identity, not as a wife, but as a mother. Malik immediately became the love of my life. Most of my attention centered around him. I wanted to do all the little things necessary to ensure he would survive. My overriding passion became to make it for his sake. Something about having blood of your blood and flesh of your flesh clears the mind and gets your values in place. I had been raised on family and faith. Knowing my child depended on me impelled me to put up a better fight. I began to discover my inner strength. He gave me the surge of energy I needed to go on, although I wasn't well.

At my doctor's recommendation, I sought professional help to pull the pieces of my life together. I visited a therapist daily at the height of crisis, then weekly for counseling and encouragement. Meanwhile, along with tuning in and out, I was blacking out and coming to. Consequently, I was referred for evaluation by a neurologist. Tests disclosed the episodes were a type of seizure that caused short interruptions of consciousness. Medication was prescribed that sparked a near-fatal reaction. By grace it was reversed in time.

In a sudden rush, a sequence of maladies assailed my weakened body like wild dogs after a sickly calf. Severe anemia necessitated my taking potent vitamins and undergoing weeks of painful shots. Seething boils in both armpits had to be lanced five times, and for a long period I wore bandages and a sling to drain them. Loss of weight and a heavy persistent cough alerted doctors my TB might have become active. Preventive drug therapy over the next two years required regular trips to pulmonary clinic for constant monitoring and x-rays. I was such a frequent hospital attendee I felt like an employee.

Then a chance visit to my dentist's office uncovered a malignant growth underneath my front teeth. After I started turning blue, it had to be removed too. Additional dental work required eleven root canals and crowns, numerous filings, and two molar extractions to remove impactions. Then there was the inflammation that required a fifth hospitalization. It's no wonder I was so weak and down under!

Malik remained in the hospital's infant unit as it appeared I was not ready for child rearing. Daddy suggested I put him up for adoption, but I couldn't consider that option. And so, when the nurse called, I mustered my strength and went to get him. From that very day, Dad exhibited a special kind of care to let us know he would always be there. As the only father Malik ever knew, he did all he could to pull him through. Wherein he seemed unable to bond with my brother Sonny, he did with his grandbaby. God gives second chances in such instances.

When not keeping medical appointments, I was at the social services office on Tremont Avenue. Within that airless tomb the stench was stifling, time trifling, and the malaise so contagious even the flies stood still. While we welfare mothers sat and dazed, yawning workers idly gazed at empty pages. As our squirming toddlers whined and cried, something inside seemed to have died. Our dignity got blown away by whirring fans. The wall clock ticked and tocked. I watched and waited, then answered, pleaded, explained, complained, repeated the process constantly to be recertified for Medicaid and ADC lacerating deeply my humanity. I was reduced in spirit to a minuscule dot, smaller than a ditto mark on their file folders. A faceless, personless boob who should shoulder the blame for making my life a mess and a moocher nonetheless.

I used to pray not to get a black social worker. You would think they'd be empathetic, but most often they were abrasive and hostile. Living one paycheck from poverty themselves, they daren't show compassion, lest they suffer negative repercussions and end up on the other side of the desk in distress. Keeping their J-O-B became more important than any inclinations they might have had to help me. When someone feels powerless, how corrupting a little power can be, especially when wielded against the person one rung down on the ladder, trying to climb up. People can become very high and mighty when given authority over pencils and paper and they get to sign their names to something. You can't touch them with a ten-foot pole!

That's one of the foibles about black people. Some of us don't like to see others get ahead. Like crabs in a bucket, as soon as they see you trying to climb out of your situation, they reach up and pull you down. I had to learn how to play the game to remain in the system. I told them what they wanted to hear, ignored their sneers, hid my tears, suppressed my fears, and persevered.

The system itself was slower to repent than individuals, locking women into hopeless poverty by not providing a viable way out for its recipients. The woman who tried to use the system to help herself was punished for her efforts. Saving money, attending school, or getting a job were all good cause for terminating benefits.

Still I believed success was gettable, but I'd have to do a lot of work. Mama had instilled in us a work ethic, not to sit back and collect a check. Left in the lurches by youthful rebellion and unable to earn a decent living, I decided to return to school, this time the city university, a working-class institution. When you grow up railing against society, it's natural to want to serve society by performing a social or human service. That was my mission in wanting to become a teacher. Passionate and headstrong about things I believed in, I thought I could influence kids.

Adults have trouble mixing, but little children don't. I suppose that's why I liked it in their world. They play together honestly, and when spats happen, they make up quickly, so there's no lingering pain and bitterness. I'd have been a great candidate for Mr. Roger's Neighborhood, with its fantasy, magic, and puppetry focused on simplicity and kindness. 'Twas the type of place I needed to go to heal.

As my circumstances propelled me toward responsibility, I went along learning how to make ends meet like I'd seen Mama do. Living on welfare, you barely get enough to stay alive. Contrary to popular belief, it was no joy ride! But I'd made a decision about the type of life I wanted to have, which meant abandoning the ranks of the needy, the greedy, and the lazy who chronically live on ADC. I wanted to do something important with my life to try and make a difference.

Reentering school was a first step. Getting up the gumption to just "go on and do it" seemed a monumental task, the process of registration a morass of frustration. I reached into myself and found determination. When you dive headfirst in deep water, you really need to believe in your ability to survive. I didn't have strong confidence but knew I *had* to do something. College would be my door to independence. Black women in my family had a history of achievement that I could look back on, not necessarily educationally, but they were women of substance and strength who overcame by faith. I drew on the support system of a family I knew would be proud of me. A strong mother at home, who I watched hold a bad marriage together, work, and rear her kids, impacted me greatly.

Everything from that point on was a deep-breathing uphill climb and a constant fight to make it. Either Malik was sick or I was. As school progressed, there was the pressure of taking tests, meeting deadlines, getting financial assistance, burning midnight oil to study and write papers, concerns with my GPA, and the madness of the grading process adding to my stress. I had little personal time and no outside support.

I didn't yet have the fortitude I needed to make it alone but thought I had to prove myself. This placed me on my nettle to do my best. I was so fragile, but my crumbly self-image improved as I saw myself building skills and ability in the field of education. With time God added armor onto me, not all at once, but in overlapping scales. By Malik's first birthday, I'd managed to wangle my own little apartment near Mom for security but my responsibility.

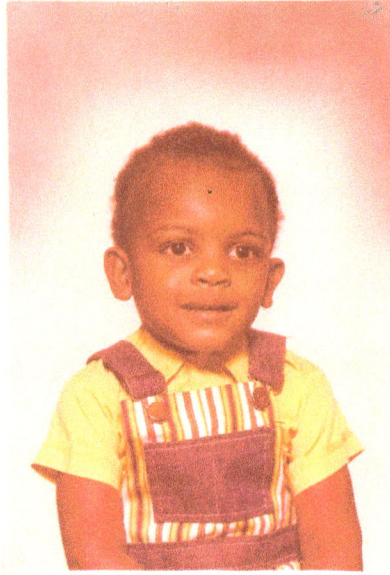

Malik as a toddler.

Each morning before daybreak I had to take Malik downtown to my sister's for babysitting, then make my way to school riding two trains and a bus or walk blocks to a sitter, carrying stacks of books, dragging Malik by the hand. When other young women students were whistling a happy tune without a care in the world, for me it was books and baby night and day.

Once I got past the wonderment of welcoming the precious new life that sprung from my loins, I began to discover single motherhood wasn't easy! I was always on call, always having to show tenderness, always having to provide. I sometimes felt angry and deprived. There were lots of things I couldn't have. I found myself coutured in Salvation Army clothes as the baby's needs always came first. Financial problems hounded me. Trying to do everything on my own depleted my energy. There was no one reaching out to me. Government subsidy was my only help. I felt ashamed I'd let myself get into this predicament.

Life became a constant battle against forces beyond my control. I felt powerless and victimized by my situation. Everything was way out of balance, and I lived under so much condemnation. I longed to break free, but my role as a mother called for dedication to meet the insatiable demands of the child. His father was allowed to shirk his responsibility, but I was being held accountable. I'd taken him to court, and the judge asked him if he had a job, to which his reply was negative. Hammering the gavel, the judge shouted, "Case dismissed!" then put *me* through the third-degree, berating me while letting him go free. Underneath, I felt resentful that I was left "holding the bag." When you are going through ups and downs, it is difficult to see your children as the blessings they really are, until the dark clouds roll away. Seems I'm only focusing on what I gave to him and saying nothing of the oodles of love he gave me any and every time I needed it and the structure, purpose, and direction he brought to my life. Nurturing him taught me to hold gently, caress lovingly, and give totally to someone who needed me.

In the early seventies, impetus toward remedying the inequities of the past racial injustices lost steam. The activism of the sixties died. Even voting seemed a waste of time. Barriers that kept blacks from voting had been removed, but apathy and a sense of hopelessness took its place. Political whims, ebbs, and flows trickled down to total conservatism on the part of the public about civil rights. There was so much lying and deception in the government during the Nixon years all trust in government was lost. Distrust left me disillusioned about my ability to contribute to the political process.

I'd become a true urbanite, coolly uncomfortable, up against the grit, grappling to cross the gridiron, trying to make it. I listened to the voices of whispering spirits guiding me along, the voice of my father saying, "Hold your own!" Mama's voice saying, "Trust God!" and Mr. Lewis's voice saying, "Beware, be wise, and be careful!" It had been a period of defining who I was.

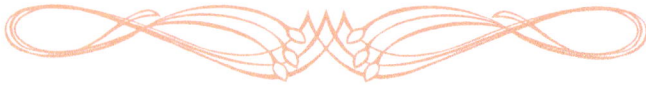

CHAPTER FIFTEEN
On Becoming

IT was the 1970s, age of pop art, pop psychology, paisley shirts, platform shoes, polyester, *Play Boy* and Hugh Hefner, the Tate-LaBianca killings, and Attica uprisings. Things were changing—families, culture, the world. A number of things weren't the way they used to be. But some things, particularly for black Americans, remained the same. In poverty there was continuity. A good many people broke with the shared beliefs of the past and chased the illusion of affluence. For most, it was a torturesome stretch to take a bite out of a big apple, always yanked out of reach, leaving mouths watering and stomachs cringing.

The myth of starting at the bottom and working our way upward wasn't working. We started at the bottom and stayed there like heavy silt and sediment. There was no buoyancy, nothing that took us up. The cycle always pulled downward. Inability to earn a decent wage to support a family was often a problem for black men. As Martin Luther King once said, "Starvation wages can never help a man overcome poverty."

Many of our people were in bondage to fear, ignorance, and low self-esteem. Others so locked in self-centeredness couldn't be concerned about anyone else. Looking to save our own necks and seeking personal gain, we put our well-being above any cause or movement—focused on me, my, mine, and all I can get for myself. Busily going after material wealth, we couldn't get involved in children's programs, community groups, or self-improvement.

As we began to worship autonomy and believed in every man for himself, our community life worsened. Each individual took the view it's somebody else's job to do something about conditions. Apathy kept folks from getting out to vote. Shock and fear loomed at seeing our leaders wiped out and cops getting away with "legitimized murder" of militants. Ordinary people realized it could happen to them. Though blacks spent millions of dollars yearly consuming, we didn't, by in large, support black businesses, and cash wasn't funneled back into our communities. Those who achieved middle-class status most often moved away and did not give their resources back to help their own. Apathy bred inactivity.

Multitudes remained in bondage to the environment, as there was no access to success for a large portion of us. Too many were sucked under by the downward pull of poverty and negative environmental forces. Poverty for white men was a temporary lack of funds or loss of a job. But for black men, it was a constant state of being unable to break free of the cycle or change his estate.

Those who did manage to move up to better jobs or into better housing found getting more didn't solve our problems. We just moved up to a higher class of losing. The opportunities provided weren't enough to help us catch up. We were outpaced by those around us. The terrible legacy of racism we inherited functioned to undermine our self-esteem and self-love. Becoming our own worst enemies, we at once loved, hated, and undermined ourselves by our actions. And society, through the media especially, compounded the poor perception of our group.

Oftentimes whites didn't permit us into neighborhoods until those areas were ailing and on the decline. By the time minorities got a foothold, decay was well underway. Problems were left for us to fix with limited capital or resources. Immediately we would be blamed for coming in and ruining the neighborhood, when the seeds of destruction had long since been sown. We remained, for the most part, cordoned off in well-defined areas, which became highly impacted by too many poor concentrated in one place. Overcrowding led to a build-up of dirt and put stress on city services.

In the cusps of the seventies, we looked forward to the promised social changes civil rights and integration should have brought. Our expectations were too high. White fear and distrust were too deeply entrenched. They kept running, and we kept heading out after them. Ten years after *Brown v. the Board of Education*, schools in Boston and other northern cities still were not integrated. Discouragement became a weight we continually struggled under. A great many people never came to the realization of their abilities and were not empowered to change their lives. Living in bad conditions is very depressing. Substandard housing, decaying neighborhoods easily gets one down, makes you feel helpless. Living the American dream for numerous Americans was just a pipe dream.

Before long, there was a sharp increase in recreational drug use as people sought release and temporary euphoria. Some turned to heroin and cocaine. Methadone centers sprung up across black districts to treat those addicted to heroin. But the substitute was even more addictive, exacerbating the problem. Addicts often visited the welfare center, picked up their checks and food stamps, then traded them for methadone. Some were mothers of small children breaking ground for a new generation who would face an even more deadly epidemic, HIV and AIDS. These women had lacerated faces, tracks on their arms, and many punctures in their spirits.

We all crossed paths at "the office," that wasteland of human degradation: Women who'd had too many lovers and kids. Children who'd had too few hugs or meals. Men who had no jobs and too many drinks, whose egos had suffered many fisticuffs and uppercuts, in that place where we were reminded quite brutally, you are on the bottom, being given something undeserved, and should be *ashamed!* They made us feel like cheats—people unworthy of life and substance—by their tone of voice, body posturing and attitude, lack of eye contact, intimidating and personal questions, investigations into our private lives, and suggestive questions implying we were immoral and beggarly. It was the hub of life in poor areas, where inductees came together in a strange comradery, knowing whether man or woman, black or Hispanic, young or old, we at least had one thing in common. We all belonged to a system that kept us living and dying at the same time.

It was quite a jump to go regularly from the world of the hopeless to the world of the hopeful—the college campus. To believe, in spite of it all, that I was *worthy* when so many things around me were saying I was not. I lingered in purgatory, wondering if I'd ever break free or remain in that state.

During those times, loneliness and depression dropped by so often. In avoidance, I left the house, went out to clubs to be in a celebratory atmosphere, hoping to find a mate who would make drinking the bitters of life a little sweeter. But I felt the other girls had more guy appeal than I. I searched for Mr. Right and practiced on five or six wrong along the way, suffering the pain of broken relationships and many emotional scars, as I got caught up in the craziness of the dating game.

Every Friday and Saturday night, I went zipping around the corner to the Monterey Club, a popular wet spot where they kept rum flowing, reggae music going, and the pickings, especially among Jamaican men, were plenteous. Its crops, I soon discovered, yielded a lot of bruised and damaged fruit—guys who could barely afford the cover charge let alone bring a date and buy her drinks. So I went Dutch—came in alone and went home alone, unless, in my loneliness, I let someone come home with me. There was always some guy who wanted to help me make it through the night. But I knew he'd be *gone* before the morning light. Those types of men were not bitter-enders, didn't stick around for the long haul, and certainly weren't interested in built-in families.

I got involved with promiscuity, thought I had to sleep with one to keep him. You know how it is! You start dropping your guard, lowering standards just to say you have a man in your life. You do things you know you shouldn't do, allow yourself to be used, then offer rationalizations to make justifications. I altered my thoughts, values, and habits to suit the situation, did things that were not me, not what I believed in, and not what I'd been taught.

I found myself clinging to a liquor glass, pretending I was having a ball, trying to forget it all, saying it really didn't matter while inside I felt shattered, unattractive, and disposable. In that world where "beautiful people" came out at night to be seen in the dazzle of disco lights, music pumped passions to a frenzy, and go-gos performed dances in slinky minis, I sat singing,

> Rescue me, take me in your arms,
> Rescue me, I want to feel your charms,
> 'Cause I'm lonely and I'm blue,
> Won't somebody come on and rescue me?

In those vacant, empty moments that seemed a thousand hours in duration, as I waited for my prince to come and we go sailing across the dance floor like at a palace ball, that same tempter started hanging around me who used to hang around with Daddy, keeping him company in his misery, whispering ever so sweetly, "Come on, I'll show you a place to hide, to get away from the smooth-talking guys with all their lies. Everything is gonna be all right. I'll help you make it through the night!" Alcohol kept beckoning to me with its flirtatious tease, promising to put my mind at ease. But I would not be snared by his charms or run into his waiting arms. I would not lie with him on my bed and let him fill my head with lies. I was too wise! Besides, I knew if I responded to his wink, into despair I would sink. At best, he would only accelerate my loneliness. Realizing that was so, I decided to let go.

One day I just didn't return, knowing my special someone was never going to show. Think that's when I stopped believing in fairy princes. My season for fantasy had ended. The therapist told me I needed to "take control" of my life. Taking that control involved decision-making and risk-taking. I felt ready.

Each time you bond with someone romantically and have to let go, you lose a little of yourself and your ability to sustain intimacy. Emotions become entangled. Wounds don't want to heal. I tended to nurse a drink when I was hurting (still have that tendency), but I've substituted intoxicants with coffee. I joined the league of man-less black women who sat and bellyached about things men do, said how I wasn't gonna be no fool. In mutual commiseration we shared stories. It seemed if you didn't have a story to tell, you weren't normal. There's nothing louder or livelier than a cadre of black women cussedly complaining about what some man has done. It's kinda our way of having fun. I asserted independently that I didn't *need* one.

They say in urban centers there are four females for every male. Naturally, problems arose as some women became desperate to attract and keep one of their own—cattiness, backstabbing, man stealing, swapping, viciousness, and envy while smiling in each other's faces. We have yet to learn true sisterhood, but many ban together in a spirit of man hatred and bespatter the names of all mankind.

In the mid '70s, unemployment in New York City for whites was at a high of 9 percent. Inflation was on the rise. Mounting costs forced cutbacks, and chronic money shortages precipitated lay-offs. The country had gone into a recession. For minorities it was more like the Depression with up to 14 percent unemployed. Black women, many of them single heads of household, had to scramble for jobs. With the push of the women's movement, traditionally men's jobs opened to women. However, black women weren't going down to take their husband's seat on the board. They were getting those low-paying jobs that take everything out of you.

After a workday like that, back home they weren't "taking no stuff" off men or their kids. Women started earning their own money, bought new clothes, took themselves out, and asked, "What can a man do for me?" If they didn't have something to offer, they pushed them farther out of their lives. Men were valued primarily for their paychecks. The emotional schism between black men and women became an ever-widening gulf as the feminist movement got underway.

Black women unwittingly colluded with the system to pull the rug out from under our men by devaluating their role in the family, usurping their authority in the home, and taking jobs for which many were suited. Men are emasculated by not being allowed to work. For males, ego is often tied in with job performance. The man who doesn't work becomes a nobody. Some of our men sought ways of becoming "somebody" by doing things illegal to bring in fast, easy money, i.e., crime and drugs, thereby channeling their needs in a destructive direction. Others became vain Adonises, lovers of many women, committed to none, but eager to live off a woman's good graces.

Finding a suitable mate was harder than ever before for a black woman, with the high crime rate and men being killed off or incarcerated. The woman with more education found her dating pool brimming with polliwogs but very scant of fish. Black churches were teeming with women looking for a Christian man. They knew Christ could change a man's reputation and his station.

My desire to make something of my life induced me to work hard at becoming a teacher. It drove me to keep trying and not give up. Doing it for myself as well as Malik made me persist despite obstacles. When I reached my graduate year, I had practically repeated all my course work, when the city university changed its transfer policy and decided to accept my former credits. Therefore, I had 170 credits, when only 124 were required. The extra course work provided valuable enrichment. I graduated from Lehman College cum laude and made the dean's list several semesters. I beamed with the pride of accomplishment, just as my grandparents had when they traded in their horse and wagon for a real automobile.

Mom and Fay took me out for a Chinese dinner, and I was presented with a gold pocket watch inscribed, "Grad 74 To Jean." It became my treasured keepsake, which I have until now, tucked away amid the clutter of many years. The degree, hat, tassel, and wilted corsage are in a file drawer in my garage. Its faded brown petals remind me sadly of the fading hopes of today's generation to do better than their parents, regardless of education. To us an education was a valuable commodity, the key to upward mobility, almost a guarantee of a better life, something that could open doors for you in the white world. We thought it was the answer, but many whites with less earn more than blacks who have more, so it is not the only factor.

America gives and takes away, gives jobs and takes them back according to the times. When well-educated whites begin losing jobs, things are taken back from minorities and the poor. Even white kids now worry about doing better than their parent generation because of tough economic times. Still education is important, and too few minority students are making it across the portals of college institutions for lack of financial assistance. A college degree offers no guarantee, but without it, there is an assurance of difficult straits ahead.

I was the first member of the New York contingent of our clan to finish college. It made me especially proud when Mom followed in my footsteps, went back to school, got an associate degree, gave up her cleaning job, and entered the classroom as an assistant teacher. Mama, understanding hardship very well, cautioned me never to forget from whence I'd come, nor the bridge that brought me over. I never did.

Conditions under, through, and by which we live tell us something about our strengths and resilience as women. The media projects us as people who are failures, not overcomers. Unsung black heroines have been the backbones of families and whole communities throughout American history, bearing upon their warm breasts and strong backs the children of this nation. Yet we often endure a particular kind of degradation. Compared to other women of the world, we're treated like fake pearls having no beauty or value.

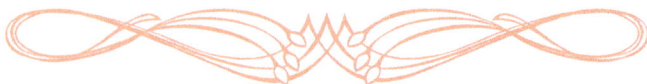

CHAPTER SIXTEEN
Ms. Barrett, TM

THE year I began teaching, President Nixon resigned in disgrace, Gerald Ford took office, and my uncontested divorce through legal aid became finalized. The cost of living was very high and unemployment spiraled. The declining economy and withdrawal of the country's commitment to economic justice left the essentials of a decent life no more available to masses of blacks than had been years before. Moral leadership was lacking. Legislators sought to pass full employment programs to guarantee the right to useful and meaningful jobs to all who were willing and able to work. There was talk of work requirements for welfare recipients undergirded by job development and child care. Also, talk of comprehensive health care programs to give full coverage to all Americans. Those promises are still wafting the winds.

In 1974, there were still many problems nationally—an energy crisis, decaying cities, swelling welfare rolls, and segregated schools in many parts of the country. Whites rallied vehemently against bussing. There were calls for law and order, which meant to us, "Keep them Niggers under control and in their places!" Internationally, the United States domination of the world, both militarily and economically, unraveled. The country was in a no-win situation in Vietnam. Europe and Japan were fast becoming industrial powers. The Soviets were an ominous threat, and the Third World countries gained military might. Nations in the Middle East seized control of oil resources. The stage was being set across the globe for Brown Power, Red Power, Yellow Power, Black Power, and Women's Power. The US was having to stand up and take notice.

By then, most of the hippies had gone back home somewhat disillusioned, carrying a sense of commitment, I believe, to make this a better world. They entered the job market as doctors, lawyers, and service providers, leaping in the same boat along with everyone else out there trying to make a dollar and climb the economic ladder. Everyone joined the rat race. We all wanted to get more and have more. Before long, it became a national obsession. As new products and services became available, it took more and more *things* to be considered average. The gap between the haves and the have-nots grew. The dual societies, as described by the Kerner Commission Report, remained worlds apart. Its recommendations for massive programs to improve conditions in the ghettoes went unheeded.

Mama started getting new things for her home, wall-to-wall carpeting, a large entertainment center, a king-size bed, a modern kitchen with new appliances—every type of gadget and convenience to make family life comfortable. While she trenched in and tried to keep up with the mortgage payments, masses of poor across the nation were still howling and complaining. But society continued to quieten, control, and contain them, making only half-hearted attempts at remediation.

The old generation believed in two worlds, this one struggle and the next one glory. Ours was the first generation that expected to find happiness in this world. For that reason, we felt more despair because we never achieved it.

Soldiers were returning from the rice fields of Southeast Asia to the killing fields of American cities, from the front lines to the unemployment lines, from roles of honor and duty to positions of insignificance and insecurity. It was a position black men knew well.

After Malik's birth, I came to the realization I couldn't change the world. It was too big, violent, and crazy. I still remember the terror-stricken faces of Vietnamese mothers and children fleeing burning villages being napalmed to end war and bring about "lasting peace." Soon strife erupted in other parts of the globe and military intervention again became "necessary." We knew how to put a man on the moon but not how to resolve basic human conflicts. I decided to just try and change the little world around me, somehow to affect the people whose lives I touched, particularly children. I thought if I could change the world for a child, then I'd indeed *change* the world.

In fact, their world mirrored the type of world I wanted to live in. Watching preschoolers at play, one easily sees they have a great deal to teach us about human relations. Kids come together regardless of race, without a lot of words or rules, and get a game going. Too bad the nations of the world, who are always fighting, can't play ball that way. Children are like beautiful flowers in a garden—reflections of God's infinite creativity. Each has his own place in the sun.

As I entered the teaching profession, I continued asking myself those gnawing questions: Who am I? What do I believe? What are my goals? What can I do about the have-nots? How can I turn my moral outrage into personal action? My focus turned from learning to teaching. I wanted to help poor kids coming from where I came, to say I'd walked that road and could lead the way. I made a commitment to *serve* them.

I landed my first position teaching kindergarten at a nursery school near Freeman Street in the South Bronx. My interest was in early childhood education. We have twenty short years to enculturate kids to our language, culture, ethics, and ideals. I felt it best to reach them in the formative years, before bad habits become established.

I went to work in "the gitto," in an area known as Fort Apache, bringing with me the prejudices of an outsider. I assumed the people were less, although I was really not much better off, living hand-to-mouth from day to day. I looked superficially at the neighborhood and easily saw the degradation, poverty, and filth but almost missed the vibrance, energy, and determination the people had to survive against all odds and obstacles. In the ghetto there is a lot of good, some bad, but a lot of *life*.

I started working with kids who tasted what I never had: wanton neglect. My childhood was fairly bucolic, having grown up in simpler times. Sometimes they were able to laugh and smile; other days their hearts sank in despair. They were the helpless, hapless victims of something they knew nothing about or could understand. They only knew they needed love, and it wasn't always there; they needed security and to feel wanted. I ended up trying to create a homelike environment in my classroom. Being more a surrogate mommy, my first priority became to comfort and reassure.

With them, I was able to put forth a stronger posture. My creativity transferred into teaching ability and allowed others to focus on what I could *do* rather than on *me*. This helped manage feelings of inadequacy. Teaching gave me a positive new identity, and I went at it passionately.

By then, kids could not have normal childhoods and no longer just had fun. The world for them had taken a turn for the worse. Their lives were perpetually threatened growing up in unsafe environments. Chaos, violence, drugs, homes filled with turbulence, and rapid change brought no stability. The essentials—food, clothing, and shelter—were not always available. Home training was lacking as the primary caregivers worked. Mothers went out seeking self-actualization and careers, leaving their little ones in my care. And I left mine with others to be there. I prayed someone was doing for him what I tried to do with them.

Children were under a lot of pressure to perform and read early, to get a head start in the race to achieve in the future. They were being hurried, pushed, dragged kicking and screaming from place to place, left in the hands of strangers or precocious teens to fit into adult work schedules. Some got dropped off just so young mothers could go out and have fun.

I thought about the new freedoms that came with women's lib and what it meant for these youngsters. Women were free, liberated, out discovering their potential, competing with men for the throne of dominance, while children became unseen victims, cast-bys, latch-key kids, far down on their parents' list of priorities. Likewise, they were far down on society's too, in a time when we were more concerned with what was happening in space than in the home of the American family.

I remember well a little boy of Hispanic background who always had this broad smile. It seemed strange because of its constancy, even when not appropriate, like when he was hurt, tired, or hungry. I inquired into his family history and was told he lived with his mother and her boyfriend who was easily set off. Whining, crying, or a sad look sent him into a frenzy. It was reported he put cigarettes out on the child's skin and once put his naked bottom on the eye of a stove as punishment. The incessant smile became his defense against cruel and inhuman torture.

Kids who extract life daily amid the glass and rubble of ghetto neighborhoods are born with the same pride and laughter as everyone else, but their surroundings nurture anger and hostility in a society that doesn't support their self-worth. These kids feel love, pain, and compassion. All those emotions swirl around inside, looking for outlets. They need time and physical touch from someone who will respond in kind.

I saw they were not cowards or quitters; rather, it was society that had given up on them. Things we see in our surroundings reflect back things we see in ourselves. When our surroundings are cruel, harsh, litter strewn, and violent, it brings out the worse qualities in us. Likewise, when our surroundings are fostering, wholesome, and supportive, it brings out lovingkindness, tenderness, and hope. The lack was not in the children. They were lively and curious like all kids. Surrounding forces conspired to rob them of their best chances to develop secure, stable lifestyles.

As a teacher, I idolized women who were models of Victorian beauty and grace—who reverenced God and had good morals. I was particularly impressed by well-educated, articulate paragons who came alive in front of a group, sang, told stories, and captured audiences with endless mirth and song—mannequin beauties like Mary Poppins in *The Sound of Music* and Mrs. Anna in the 1956 musical *The King and I*. I wanted to emulate those prissy, prim, amusingly prudish pedagogues who were true devotees to their profession. Like them, I wanted to help youngsters see the world through my eyes.

Working with small children helped develop my resourcefulness because I always had to be thinking of new ways to teach them. Therefore, art became not just an avenue for self-expression but a valuable teaching tool. I made things by hand to stimulate their imaginations, then moved on to concepts in reading and math. These were kids who had never seen a rainbow or smelled the earth after a summer rain. For them, I needed to dip a brush in paint and trace a palette of color across the heavenlies, even bring twinkling stars down where they could touch them. The smog in their lives had been keeping them from view. They couldn't see vistas of what lie ahead.

This was not my maiden voyage in the classroom. I'd had numerous experiences volunteering and substituting all over the Bronx. But it was here that things came together for me. A creative teaching approach was born out of the need to motivate kids whose most faithful parent at home was the TV set to get them to talk, move, express, and share what was on their minds. Crafts, playacting, and storytelling became my forte. I established easy rapport with them and began to speak their language. I'd found my comfort zone. Working with the children of the sub city—the so-called underprivileged—was a very great privilege. In reaching out to them, I found my natural gifts and saw as a teacher I could be useful.

They say if you teach young children, by them you will be taught. I learned to greet each new day with openness and a mind for discovery, to accept new people without bias or prejudice, to look at things in nature with awe and wonderment, to laugh even when faced with adversity, and to take hold of someone's hand as I walked the mean streets of life. Children don't naturally exhibit prejudice. It has to be carefully taught. They must be taught to hate all the people their family hates. A prejudicial attitude begins at home. Therefore, it's in the home that it must be excised.

By this time, bedsheets were pattery and pretty colored, some made for mattresses filled with water. Ladies stopped carrying matching hat and purse and didn't wear a hat at all to church. In fact, ladies had become very unladylike, cussin' and fussin' worse than men. A new age had fully been ushered in. Wig hats were being worn by Mom's generation, 'Fros by ours that had the look of cottony dandelion flowers.

Mom and I retained our love for old things, Mom, because they kept her connected to bygone days along the byways of the Old South, me, because perhaps I sensed that as those byways were being replaced by super highways, something precious was being lost—chasteness, simplicity, and our sense of peace. The way we looked, worked, and thought was shaken up. Our moors, mores, and values had become as hodgepodge as the funky fashions we wore.

Traditional fashions and furnishings were being upstaged by very up-to-date mod styling. A weekly sequel, *The Mod Squad*, on TV featured three young hotshots who were hip, cool, and sexy. Everyone developed a penchant for the new and wanted to be in with the in crowd too. Cool and the Gang sang, "It's your thang. Do what you wanna do! I can't tell you who to sock it to!" There was a tenor of disrespect for God, authority, and traditional values. Looseness and laxity became okay. Distinctions between the sexes were getting blurry as unisex got underway.

Dads no longer stayed close by to chaperone their daughters the way Grandpa did when Mom and her dates tried to steal a kiss while sitting on the old porch swing. Dating relationships commonly involved sex, and living together without marriage hardly caused a stir, though there was some attempt at hiding it to show respect for elders. Girls weren't being chased away from home or forced to marry when they got P-R-E-G. Abortion for many was becoming a viable option; few thought about adoption. It was "the Pepsi generation" play but don't pay. A lot of people played; a lot paid.

At home we rocked to Motown, while Mom and Dad still held on to those down-home blues—Bobby Bland, Jimmy Lee Hooker, Muddy Waters. Seemed like they knew old things you just oughta hold on to 'cause they have value.

Often, I dreamed of going and starting a new life somewhere else, to the South mostly where country cousins fared better than we Northerners. Old board houses were being abandoned for new ranch-styled homes and late-model cars. Jobs were opening, the pace was slower, and crime was lower. What is more important, the South exerted a peculiar hold on my spirit because of the rich memories of childhood days, when I played barefoot in the grass, broke off

Grandma's pretty zinnias and put them in a glass. I nursed them with unusual devotion, believing one day I'd get the notion to pick up and go. Yet I was not ready to chase my dreams and put them on hold.

As a young aspiring teacher, I went at each new day with that key wound level of energy and enthusiasm, so happy to at last have my own classroom and hang out my shingle, "Ms. Barrett, TM" (Teacher/Mom). Time came and went, relationships also. But I took nothing seriously, except my job and kid. Those two roles meant the most to me—became who I *was*. Sometimes the roles conflicted when I had to put Malik's needs aside to do homework, make projects, and study. But they overlapped when I was able to use the same songs, stories, and handmade things to teach him as time permitted. Trying hard to make it in the material world, I concentrated on developing my mind but not my *soul*. And there was still a lot of stuff I didn't know.

I did know that if I wanted to remain in teaching, I'd need a graduate degree. In thinking about environments where art is used as a therapeutic tool, I began taking courses at Columbia University to test my aptitude and see what was out there. I found monies were available through PL 94-142 to train teachers for the disabled. The new law guaranteed a free, appropriate public education to every disabled student in the least restrictive environment. Impetus was toward mainstreaming them in regular classrooms. A new disenfranchised group had become the focus of federal legislation. I won a scholarship for full-time study for an MA in special education of the physically handicapped. I was on my way!

When I entered grad school in 1976 at the age of twenty-seven, a whole new genre of students entered with me. They didn't talk much about politics. Chitchat was career oriented—where they were going, how they would get there, and what they'd buy when they "arrived." The hippies of the '60s prepared to become the yuppies of the '80s. They weren't hungry for a taste of justice or committed to public service. They wanted to get that coveted "piece of paper" so they could get that job, earn that income, buy that house, drive that car, take that vacation, and on and on. It was all about achieving and, in so doing, to be found *worthy*. Everyone let their hair down.

Professors and students were on a first-name basis. The uptightness of higher institutions had become passé.

Fairness and respect were meted out equitably in the program. Still, there was only *one* of me. Others smiled, talked. They were real nice. It was mostly in the lunchroom that you could see the pairing off, people organizing by race, still seeking friendships where they were most comfortable. As I was a loner, I was always alone, with neither black nor white. I would say most whites wished me well and, to the extent they dared, came close and helped as much as possible. I made no lasting friendships. There was no taking home or going out to lunch. They didn't pursue it; I didn't either. We remained respectful but in our mutual corners.

Many today get no further than associating on the job or in business situations. Outside there is distancing and fear of involvement. Boundaries are still drawn around our relationships.

But I got along well. Teachers and students lauded me, told me how proud I should be proud of myself, how my efforts got me that far. Said I was a "credit to my race," not like all the rest, as if it was rare for us to be capable and carry ourselves with comportment. Sometimes I patted myself on the back and felt complimented, but deep down I knew it wasn't true.

Many afternoons I walked across 116th Street, across Broadway to the other side of the track, down off "the hill" to the Harlem I knew, the place that grew me. Down past gray tenements that had the appearance of bombed-out buildings after World War II, looking at the dismal faces of poor kids playing in the gutter. It brought bitterness knowing only a few would walk the hallowed halls of a major university in the future. Again I felt unfairly chosen.

Race is still a controlling factor in the quality of life and opportunities in America. Myths of self-determination and equal opportunity don't hold much validity for kids who don't see college as "doable" and are growing up feeling powerless to make a difference in the overall swing of things. With so much beyond their control affecting their lives like violence and drugs, most don't have the right circumstances or the constitution to make it. They need others to show the way, to believe in them, to encourage and push.

Many feel so despised and rejected they won't even try. Their frustration never gets articulated, except in the resounding blast of an illegal handgun, when a fifteen-year-old starts wanting something he can't have, mugs somebody, and some innocent person dies.

People don't have high expectations of black young men beyond sports, music, or criminality. Some live up to the negative prospect by becoming "diablos," robbing from the haves to feed their needs or greed. Most victims are their own black brothers and sisters. Crime and violence so permeate city life they see few options. No one is organizing to lead them where they need to go. Society hasn't widened the path for more to become successful.

There was only one slot at Teacher's College for a minority student in my program. What happened to the other welfare survivors who perhaps had potential but not the finances to attend college? They were left hopelessly entrapped in their situations. What of those who didn't have the support systems I had, a strong mother, close family ties, special someones along the way to light my path? Decisions about who goes to Columbia and who goes to jail are made outside poor communities. In the future, we will either invest in creating more options or invest in prisons to house more inmates. Someday there'll be no place left to put them.

Maybe the system wants it that way; after all, it keeps a lot of people employed. Doctors have jobs sewing up gunshot victims. Lawyers get cases representing criminals in court. Judges get to hammer their gavels and say "Twenty years!" to guys who are back on the streets in two weeks. Legislators promise to pass tougher gun laws, while politicians vow to "keep the streets safe for all our citizens." A lot of jobs are dependent upon having an abundance of poor people and the criminal element. But can we be content with that?

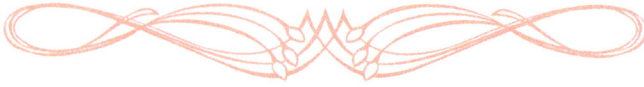

CHAPTER SEVENTEEN
Exceptionality

THAT harried September, I was catapulted headlong into a year of intensive study of the exceptional child. From a medical model, we studied physically disabling conditions and their effects on the human body. From a service model, we discussed the call for educational accessibility and the implications for instructing physically challenged students in regular classrooms. From a legal model, we examined the constructs of Public Law 94-142 (the Education for all Handicapped Children Act of 1975) and its mandate for a free, appropriate, public education, in the least restrictive environment.

But we never heard from disabled people, what they had to say for or about themselves. As always, it was the majority defining a minority's existence, describing what they are like, their needs and problems. Professors told us about their impairments and how to work with them. They taught us to test and assess to see how they measure up, perform in our world, on our terms, within parameters we set. I picked up the notion *they* had all the needs and we were preparing to serve *them*. There was never any suggestion they had anything to teach us or (I dare say) that there is any benefit to being as they are.

Historically public attitudes toward the disabled have been negative. Certain folks call them slow, problem kids, retards, dummies, rejects, pinheads, the brain dead, or "poor, unfortunate *things*." If you say you work with them, they squeeze your hand and add "God bless you!" as if you're such a wonderful human being for what you're doing and deserve a medal. Some think they are funny, repulsive, or pitiful. A few say lock 'em away, out of sight, because they pose a threat as they are not responsible for what they do. (You know, dangerous, unpredictable, and bent on violence or oversexed and can't control their urges.)

Others feel they are a nuisance, in the way, a burden to society, consuming money that could be better spent on more "productive" members of the human race. They are thought to be needy, dependent, and having nothing to give, only able to take. To many families they are an embarrassment, evidence of bad blood in the family line, products of faulty or errant genes. Some think what they have is contagious, like if you shake hands with one of them, it might rub off on you. Still others feel brought down in social stature by association or somehow diminished in their presence. And there are the ones who like to gawk and stare the way we would at the world's tallest man or the enormous fat lady in a circus show. They seem particularly obsessed with oddities, like to point and poke fun, while at the same time being repulsed.

Anything that makes us stand out or marks us differently is seen as bad and becomes a social stigma. Those who are different are ostracized for it. No one wants to be the person with the thick glasses, the stutter when he talks, the funny walk, the crossed eyes, the crutches, the hearing aid, the wheelchair, or the deformed or missing limbs, let alone a severe mental impediment. These things are thought to say something about your lack of wholeness as a person. You may be considered of imperfect stock, a freak of nature, a mistake, degenerate, mentally incompetent, retarded and not nice to look at or be around.

In this country there is little appreciation for uniqueness. It is seen as deviance in a negative sense. Everyone aspires to be that individual with skill, personality, and intellect, who wows the world with both body and brains. Those paralytic, sedentary folk who aren't "contributing members of society" aren't seen as valuable to have around, especially those who can't hold their own, earn their keep, and pay their own way. We carry around images of beauty and virility conditioned by the American gladiators on TV, though few of us really fit in that stellar company. Such qualities as gentleness, creativity, sensitivity, purity, childlikeness, loveableness, simplicity, joyfulness are seen as signs of weakness and vulnerability. There are those who believe the disabled members of our society live in a state of blissful innocence, protected by their own limited feeble minds from the intentional stabs of others and the jabs and frustrations of life. They believe the disabled have it easy, live a pampered existence, while having everything given to and done for them.

Being labeled disabled is thought to be financially beneficial, that lots of perks come along with the position in society: Medicaid, Medicare, food stamps, and social security. It is believed to mean free everything—housing, education, equipment, and transportation services provided by organizations that contribute thousands of dollars and sponsor programs. This is not true in most cases, but what's important is that people *think* so.

My first student teaching assignment with special needs children was at a day program that gave respite to parents while providing stimulation to the kids. In close contact for the first time with a multiply handicapped child, I was reminded of a baby starling I once found that had fallen from its nest. It was so utterly helpless, broken and ugly; I was taken aback. I had been unconsciously marinated in negative attitudes over the years and brought my uncomfortableness into the situation with me. I had to become acclimated to this new subgroup.

Suddenly I was confronted with children who had gnarled torsos with twisted limbs growing from them like strange unearthly appendages, making them appear better suited for the world beneath the sea or out in space than this terrestrial planet. Some had bodies molded into L-shapes by the wheelchairs in which they sat. Others were locked in fetal positions by muscles that had become like rigid vises, from which they could not be freed. Faces were pulled in uncanny grimaces with mouths agape. Saliva trickled at will from their openings. Utterances were more like guttural chirps and gurgles intermixed with gasps and gags, as flow backed up when weakened muscles got too tired to pump. The only visible bodily activities were the athetoid wanderings of fingers and toes that just never seemed to obey, sudden tremors lacing through hurriedly in quivers and quakes, and the little twitches that followed in aftershocks along with behaviors like self-biting, masturbating, and head banging lulled only by rhythmic rocking back and forth.

I remember clearly what their bodies looked like. But I also remember their faces, how their eyes twinkled with the light of hope, and their lips most often parted in engaging smiles when they had every reason to be sad. It was a striking contrast. I began thinking, surely they must know something I don't know about the "well-being of life." They were not overcome by concerns as I was, and I don't think it was because of diminished capacity. Since none spoke, it is hard to say what went through their minds, yet in spite of it all, many seemed to be at peace.

I didn't like the feelings they garnered up in me toward God as I questioned how He could so cruelly afflict such innocents as these, mar them for life and cut them off from communicating. Why place them in these earthly temples so like prisons from which there was no escape? For what crimes were they being punished?

I was moved with compassion and touched by them in ways no one else had before. As I began to hold and work with them, my fears slowly melted away. I locked into their humanity, felt compelled to give more and more of myself. I had to mobilize all my strength and match it with my training in order to be of assistance. Strangely, I found enablement by working with disabled children, sharing their joys and fears. As I went along, something deep inside was being satiated. I found myself bouncing through the door each day, not because of what I was doing for them, but because of what they were doing for me.

These were kids who didn't improve overnight. There were no one-shot deals. I learned there something about faithfulness, making long-term commitments, and celebrating tiny accomplishments when they happened. Each one of those kids deserved a drum roll, a salute, and a red badge of courage in facing life. They were tender yet tough little people. I felt called to work with the disadvantaged, the unfortunate, "the least of these God's children." But I would have to grow into it like anything else.

My second placement down on Twenty-Third Street gave a startling glimpse of how we ascribe worth or don't ascribe worth to the lives of others depending on where we carve their notch on our measuring stick. I was placed in a class of eight to ten severely retarded children with cerebral palsy, working with a young blond teacher and her assistant. Students in the group had a range of responsiveness from mild to none at all, except to food.

The staff regularly conducted fire drills, and every classroom had to have a plan for evacuating the children in the event of an emergency. The teacher promptly pointed to a chart on the wall bearing each child's name entitled "The Triage Chart." Triage refers to the act of assigning priorities for the sake of expediency when only limited help is available. It was used during the war on battlefields, when medics had to make a choice of giving medical treatment to casualties most likely to survive. It is used also on our urban battlefronts, in city emergency rooms by doctors who try to treat the critically ill and wounded first, then get to others as they can. It is a crude concept based on using scarce resources where they can do the most good, or in the latter case, where life depends on it.

The teacher's plan of whom to administer help to first was based on the qualitative value she placed on each of their lives dependent upon the severity of their disability and level of function. The highest functioning were to be taken out first, then the rest in descending order. Obviously, she valued those closer to normal more than the very low functioning. What's more, she displayed the chart unabashedly, as if this was perfectly okay!

It became clear, it was not only the general public that has contemptible attitudes toward the disabled but those who worked in the field also. Unfortunately, they are the ones who can do the most harm because of their proximity and direct involvement. At that time, service in general was meted out to the ones thought most likely to "survive" in the mainstream, another application of triage.

I believe all people have equal and infinite value no matter how seemingly insignificant or impaired. We have lost something of the sanctity of life today. In our *thing*-oriented society, we treat people like goods, judge them by whether they are useful, convenient, and serviceable and what *image* they project. Like commodities, we pick our favorite type, style, shape, and color and which attributes we esteem best, denying God's right—in His wisdom—to do things we don't understand, even in creating those with severe limitations and placing them in our world. I still don't know why He does it, but I haven't met a person yet who has been in a close relationship with someone with a disability and not had their lives altered in a meaningful way.

As a nation, we still don't have our priorities straight. We'd passed the twenty-fifth anniversary of the Apollo II moonwalk and just got around to passing comprehensive civil rights legislation (ADA) for the disabled and developing a public policy. Evidently, in 1969 we thought it more important to enable three men to take an adventure walk on the moon than to remove the barriers in society that prevented millions of individuals with disabilities from venturing out of their homes to go to the bank, a place of business, a school, a restaurant, a job if desired—to have full enjoyment of society's goods and services. Some Americans have made it to outer space, while others are still trying to make it around the corner independently.

As I expanded, Malik did too. He was bouncy, round, cute, and *different*, slower than other kids his age. I noticed the slowness but did not want to acknowledge it, preferred to think I was just an easily frightened first-time mother with exaggerated fears. In time, Malik sprouted from a roly-poly toddler to a rather leguminous-looking preschooler with happy eyes and two beaver-like front teeth. He remained clumsy, fearful, and didn't grasp things quickly.

As a single parent, I curtailed my social life and bore the ups 'n' downs of first-time parenthood alone, with all my unanswered questions. I oriented myself around him, sacrificed continually for his benefit, and tried to make him feel special and build confidence. My circuits were often overloaded. I spent every minute I could doing the things parents and kids are supposed to while working around my teaching responsibilities. A significant part of my identity had become "Malik's mom." The role was so engrossing it weighed heavily upon all my choices. I carried an extra burden because of his perceived slowness, overdoing to compensate for lack. I wanted to do all I could to ensure his success. I had such feelings of liability that if I couldn't be there in every way without aberration, I thought I was failing.

A part of my graduate training involved working in the Teacher's College Child Study Center, helping with administration of psychometric tests, scoring, and writing evaluations. I gained knowledge of how to pinpoint a special needs learner. Learning problems can be so devious because they cloak themselves in the normal foibles and follies of early childhood. However, my suspicions were aroused, so I decided to have Malik tested. To my chagrin, my suspicions were confirmed. He had a learning disability to a degree that would require special schooling.

Suddenly, terms that had been applied only to *them* were now being applied to *my* son. It made a world of difference. No longer was it an anonymous kid being wheeled into the testing room by his distraught mother. Now it was me in the hot seat and my child under the glare of the spotlight. I couldn't just sit and talk dispassionately about stats, stanines, and test results. My insides were thrown into a tumult, guts wrenched back and forth, head pounded, and heart fluttered like the notes of a piccolo. I had to struggle to keep my eyes from overflowing with tears. The evaluator's recount of her findings was barely audible above the blare of my own inner voice crying out, "Why my little boy? And why me?"

It was easier when it was somebody else's problem and I just wrote a report, gave a little input, and suggested what *they* should do. When I had to take the problem home and live with it myself, answers weren't so clear-cut. I couldn't be strictly professional because he was my child. My emotions were too entangled; there was too much pain. I was too scared. My internal alarm system rang at 1,000 decibels. So loud I could not hear the voice of any assurance everything was going to be all right. She said there was help out there for him. I wouldn't have to do this alone. The words, like paper planes, sailed past me. The seeming enormity of the problem dwarfed what little resources I had for dealing with it.

I tried to buttress myself as always, said I would carry the load, be strong. My timid eyes scanned her face, imploring, "Are you sure?" It's one of those moments that got frozen in time, remains like an ice block in the far reaches of my mind.

It was a scary and unfamiliar world I was suddenly thrust into. I knew some, but as they say, "A little knowledge can be dangerous." I had no support. There was no group to go to help fend off my fears, no "how-to" books to tell me what to do. I was more the expert than most of the people I met. Even doctors had little awareness of LD kids beyond symptoms of hyperactivity, in which case, they prescribed Ritalin to put them in a stupor and control them. Whom do you turn to when you are the "expert"? I found myself trying to educate my family and friends. Since it was a hidden disability, people wondered if it wasn't in my head instead of his.

I was floored by the realization my suspicions were true and not just the product of my imaginings. The boogie man was out of the closet. There was no more denying. I was terrorized and overwhelmed by all the decisions I would have to make and the responsibility for planning for his education. When I dropped him off at the babysitter, I didn't know what kind of care he'd be getting. Where would I go from there, knowing there was so little I could afford?

I didn't know what to do, what was right or wrong. Maybe he was misdiagnosed! I felt tormented inside. What would be his future? I tried to accept him and live happily ever after, but it didn't work that way. My heart lamented. I went in and out of potholes of despair, from anger, to feeling bad, to losing hope, to trying again. I don't believe there are words to adequately express the guilt and agony I felt. I poured out all the blame on myself. Was it the attempted suicide? Prenatal neglect? Trauma at birth? I didn't know. I just felt it was all my fault. The unction of guilt anointed me from head to toe. I took up the task to make up for what I had done.

We used to tell this joke about Jewish people at home. It's said when they lullaby their babies to sleep at night, they sing, "Go to sleep, little doctor! Go to sleep, little lawyer!" having a profession in view from the day they're born. I suppose that's every parent's dream, but as a black mother, I just prayed he would grow up to be a decent, responsible family man who was employed and stable. With that, I would have been satisfied.

No one wants to accept their child has a problem. Dealing with it became so time-consuming and captivating of my attention. Guilt kicked in and gobbled me up like a hungry hound, clinched me in its teeth, held me, and wouldn't let go. I couldn't break free of the worry and frustration. Frequently, I wanted to escape, then more guilt came in cycles that went round and around. I had no way to vent the strong emotions that I had and at the same time felt those emotions weren't legitimate. This was *my* burden; I was supposed to carry it!

I found myself lashing out at people that I shouldn't, especially those closest to me. I felt so helpless. My inner resources were often taxed to the limit. I'd been through a lot already. This was just one more straw thrown on the heap. I wondered if God really knew how much I could bear. I wanted to rail upward, but I had to accept the situation, like it or not. I took so much responsibility on my shoulders for making sure his future would be consistent with what my hopes were for him. I believed the child had been entrusted to me by God and I had to bear his affliction. I "carried my cross" willingly, but not without many moments of agony and sleepless nights feeling at times forsaken. Yet I know He was always there in the darkness, holding my hand.

Having a child with a disability is a life-changing experience because of all the things you feel and must do, all the special concerns and worries you have about him, all the arrangements you must make for his care and education, all the extras you give personally that tax your strength and drain you emotionally, the feelings there are no allies in your struggle, that you are alone. Your spirit grieves and groans for the little boy you envisioned when you carried him in your womb. You still love and accept this one, but your heart is in bitter anguish for what you've lost. You live in the midst of distress and self-analysis. Life gets harder.

But there were also the rewards I got each time he made it over some little hurdle, achieved some goal or small victory, like when he finally learned to ride a bike after endless hours wheeling him up and down the street, holding the handlebars, yelling, "Pedal! Pedal!"

What a day of rejoicing for me and for him! Those moments were like a battery charge and helped me to keep going—gave me an energy boost.

Troubling circumstances in our lives often send us calling upon the Lord, especially with regard to our children. This poem was written during that period:

> If upon my cup great burden were brought to bear,
> I the suffering trough,
> Would extend my hand to touch His hair,
> And kiss His garment cloth.

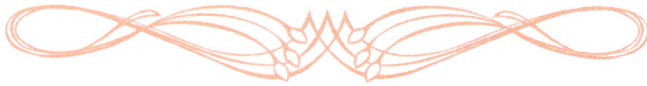

CHAPTER EIGHTEEN
New Horizons

THE school year's momentum moved quickly toward graduation day. Once more I donned ceremonial robes, crossed the stage, MA in hand. Soon I was in the market for a new job. A position was offered as an educational evaluator at a hospital for the physically disabled upstate. It would require that I relocate to staff quarters on the grounds and leave Malik behind. This left me on the horns of a dilemma. Life gets complicated when it's time to go away. I had strong feelings that he needed me. Out of necessity, I left Malik—immature and unready—with his grandma, clutching his bear and dragging a wagon along. It was terribly hard, yet I was urged along by my desire to make a better life. Meanwhile, I shuttle bused back and forth to see him.

Living in the city matures you. You become jaded and a bit cynical. Nothing surprises you. Once you've breathed everybody's breath and smelled their sweat, it all becomes overwhelmingly foul. It's like eating an overly seasoned meal. While you're taking it in, it tastes very pleasing, but once it goes down, it stirs up a fiery mess in your inward parts. You want to puke the whole thing back up and take in a light salad. Upstate was a salad bowl—crisp, fresh, green, with bits of color and a light sprinkling of flavor. Whereas suburban life is healthful, the urban regimen is rich in carcinogens that bring cancer to the soul.

Once settled in, I began to experience how cloistered institutional life can be. Monotony lulls one into feeling secure. The outer world is not like that, because of those untimed, unexpected dealings and doings that create excitement. At lunchtime workers sat around telling dirty jokes to splice the boredom or bragging about the new toys they had acquired—a car, a boat, a new set of fishing rods. Staff consisted of an average crew of professionals owning homes in the area, who pulled up every day like clockwork, put in time, took up space, and covered up for their ineptness with high-sounding words and mock efficiency. Like dead wood, many were decaying in those state jobs but couldn't be fired.

The patients provided them livelihoods, while their own lives were cutoff, lacking in all the things only a family unit could give: loving attention, support and encouragement, a feeling of acceptance and belonging. On visiting days I watched a trickle of kin come and go. Only a few took the ride upstate every once in a while to see little so and so, then headed back to complicated lives out in the real world, leaving the children sheltered, clothed, and fed but very much alone.

Through varying experiences, I'd developed talents but lacked audacity to use them. Folks saw me as more capable than I saw myself. Despite holding two degrees, I still did not feel "qualified." I was overly concerned with others' opinions of me, feared scrutiny, and always tried to be Ms. Nicey-Nicey, even when I didn't feel that way inwardly. I wasn't comfortable with anger—mine or anyone else's. I stood alone but wanted to be accepted. I suffered stage fright, was pretty uptight and nervous, yet I played it cool—held it all together. Inner conflict beleaguered me due to feelings of inferiority. Whenever we feel either better or less than others, it's hard to operate in balance.

As a people, we develop so many fissures and underground caverns in our collective personality that our confidence becomes disturbed. There are so many undercurrents to our experience. It's as if we pick up radar signals telling us to stay black and stay back, that we can't succeed and we are not to exceed boundaries. I worried so much about how I would be received or perceived, always carrying with me the burden of my race. I feared the group wasn't going to accept Ms. Black New York City offering suggestions on what to do and wouldn't take me seriously. I felt they wanted me to show no real intellect and not challenge their remarks and decisions. So for the most part, I did just that. Why? Because it felt safer. When I did let what I knew show through, it seemed to make others uncomfortable. Before long, I was out of a job. Of course, no one told me "You're fired!" It was that my services were no longer necessary as they had to rethink the position.

Being a minority on a job is a constant balancing act. On the one hand, I wanted to be a team player. On the other, I wanted to be true to my cultural identity and had sensitivity in certain areas. Most of all, I wanted to be true to my own proclivities and not be what everyone else expected of me.

I am reminded of a luncheon the staff planned to celebrate cultural diversity, which boiled down to placing everyone in boxes. I guess they typecast me as a typical Negro, so they asked me to bring in a dish of pig's feet and collard greens. I didn't eat that and hadn't the faintest idea how to cook it because I shied away from pork. I was a lot more familiar with bagels and cream cheese, but I couldn't tell them that. Therefore, in a spirit of cooperation, I consented.

I rushed to the phone to call a friend to get her recipe. And in my haste I scribbled among the ingredients a cup of vinegar for the pig's feet instead of a cap and a spoon of baking soda for the greens instead of a speck. Well, I went out, did my shopping, and faithfully cooked up my "soul food," adding a little more of each to give it pizzazz. It didn't come out too badly, except the pig's feet had a kick that could take the roof off a house and the greens were about the best purgative I'd ever come across. I should have bottled it!

Placed in an attractive dish, it was at the center of the table the following day. Everyone milled around sampling this or that. Someone took the lid off, and it was as if everyone was immediately etherized by the fumes. Yet they kept plastic smiles on their faces and behaved as politely as possible out of respect for my "culture."

On another occasion, I was invited to dinner by coworkers getting together over lasagna, which at first was really appreciated, as I was feeling quite isolated. I had eaten my fill and was enjoying the atmosphere when one person shouted, "Why don't we ask Jean to clean the dishes and take out the trash?" I responded, "Oh certainly!" before stopping to realize why he'd chosen me. Some whites assumed we should be maids and valets. In those years they were not so inclined to call you Nigger but still had a tendency to treat you like one.

We are a piebald nation, spotted in two colors though our cultures very much overlap. We are not as dissimilar as people like to think. Incomes place many of us in separate brackets; however, a lot of our experiences, values, and beliefs are similar. Instead of typing Americans and focusing on disparities, we need to accentuate what is the same—the commonalities of our experiences cross-culturally. To acknowledge racial differences is good if it helps to promote understanding, but to play on it is not. It's time to stop seeing everything in terms of black and white. It's really a very colorful planet we live on. And our country is taking on lovely hues of yellow and brown with many newcomers coming to town. The world is at our doorstep, knocking to be let in.

I'd gone upstate to escape the smogged-out city, with its car exhaust and smorgasbord of woes. In the dusk of evening, I used to stroll out, find a pretty spot, sit looking at the rolling hills while drinking in the freshness of the air. But before long, squiggly things slithered from under the moss-laden rocks, and I heard ugly whisperings in the crackling brush. Rumor had it that patients were having sex with staff and relations with each other, hopping in and out of beds at night. Staff members played vicious little games of hardball to keep their jobs or to advance to higher positions. There was an older white man sliding notes under my door, propositioning me for paid sex, a married man wanting to take me off in the woods and park, and a doctor who wanted to have secret rendezvous in his room while on call on those l-o-n-g weekends.

I thought things didn't happen in those picture-perfect towns with houses nestled in the trees like down in the city. Was I wrong! Slowly I realized there were no more Mayberrys, conservative backwater towns, untainted by the immorality of the age. I was no longer so idealistic. I was losing my innocence; America had already lost hers.

I did complain to the administration about the guy harassing me with notes but received a mere "We'll take care of it. He's been working here a long time, and we wouldn't want him to lose his job!" It was quickly and quietly swept under the rug. Funny how they were so discreet and protective of *him*, not me.

You never know why things happen. I believe the Lord allowed that brief interlude up there just so I could meet Annie, a black teenager with paraplegia, insensate from her waist down. She was diagnosed also as severely emotionally disturbed and prone to self-mutilation of her lower extremities with sharp objects. When she came into the hospital, they put her in an isolated room, in a high walled bed much like a cage, and kept everything out of reach so she couldn't hurt herself. As she had no visitors, one nurse brought an old phonograph and records to entertain her. Hearing of the case one evening when I was in low spirits, I wandered the halls and ended up in her room, not knowing what to expect from this "insane patient."

When I entered the room, she seemed quite comfortable with me. As she was nonverbal, she merely smiled and made sounds while pointing to her stereo. I got the message, turned it on, selected a record, and played it. She immediately began to gyrate her torso, seeming to imitate dancers she had seen on TV. I smiled, popped my fingers, and goaded her on. Then she pointed at my feet, and I understood she wanted me to do the footwork. She took my hand, worked her upper body, while I shuffled my feet. Before I knew it, all sadness slipped away. We were both giggling and having a ball.

I learned a great life lesson in the room that night, from an unlikely teacher. That pitiful young girl, robbed of her freedom to move about, cut off from social contact, unable to communicate, and very limited in her mental capacity, was still able to make the best of her world and even bring joy into it. She used what she had, I supplied what was lacking, and together we were a team. In our bond there was strength. Isn't that the gist of human interaction? People coming together, filling in for each other's needs, bearing one another's burdens? I thank Annie for a powerful message and for the healing she brought to my tendency to pout and complain.

Minority group members trying to maneuver the employment world often lack the resources, connections, and network of contacts to move easily from job to job. We don't, for the most part, have well-placed friends or family who can help us get our foot in the door, belong to professional clubs or organizations, and often depend on minority hiring projects or turn to newspaper ads or agencies, which don't work well for us. Therefore, we usually come in at the bottom and, in many cases, stay there.

I felt the impulse to take off, heading who knows where, to travel that mystical journey across the country along Route 66, to explore, be free, and find *me*. But it would just have been an odyssey into the heartlands of hate where I'd be pointed at and called ugly names. It's likely no one would have wanted me as their neighbor, save my own, nor would willingly share the labor fields so I could eat. Guess that's why our folks horded in the major cities.

I was hearkened back to my roost by a postcard from the Board of Education of the City of New York, a job notice for teacher of common branch subjects based on an exam I'd taken years before. God provides; He's always right on time!

The black community remained distinct from all others—the sights, the sounds, the stir, the movements, the voices, the laughter, the comings and goings, the richness and beauty of its people. On my return to the old neighborhood, I found the underpinnings of our commune slipping away and the climate of the city getting more jungle-like every day. The block was being inundated with new faces—move-ups from the South Bronx and foreigners (Jamaicans, but not of the hardworking sort I had grown up with). These were hooligans that sat on stoops or hung around street corners selling nickel bags of pot to kids, members of a posse who carried guns, blasted music, and hurdled expletives into the air. Those menacing immigrants brought a new sense of fear and lack of cohesiveness to the area. I winced at seeing the newcomers, just as Italians had when they saw us coming years before.

There was another new arrival: White Girl, little rocks called by many street names (crack, smack, horse, etc.). Men in cars came from far and wide to court her graces. She, like a brazen harlot, for a few dollars gladly hopped in, and they sped away to get "beamed up." For the first time, I witnessed open drug sales…I was shocked!

My natural emotion was one of sadness for what was being lost in the quality of life for city dwellers as the quiet destruction of our sanctuary unfolded. Everyone began hiding behind closed doors and putting bars over their windows. People stopped sitting out enjoying the open air on folding chairs, leaving bikes on sidewalks or flower pots on their porches. Personal property had to be locked up or chained down. Residents were now walking, looking back over their shoulders. Survival on the streets was becoming more and more a roulette game. You never knew when bad luck would call your name. The neighborhood was no longer an extension of our well-kept homes. Long-established families talked of moving away. Kung Fu movies were coming out in theaters. Kids drop kicked and chopped each other up as play. The mood turned really violent.

Decline and demoralization was evident in marauding bands of toughs roving the avenue, swearing, fighting, and stealing from stores. Lunchtime merchants were forced to lock their doors. These were but harbingers of the trend toward senseless violence that was to come.

There was a foulness in the air; ill winds were brewing. Personal security was pushed in the corner like an old corn broom. I used to carry shopping bags full of corn down on the bus from upstate, wanting to bring some of the bounty of that place to share with my family. It amounted to too little too late. Nothing could sandbag the raging flood headed our way.

Peace and love went the way of bell-bottom pants and platform shoes. They got packed away like yesterday's clothes. We only take them out now for pleasant memories. They are no longer a part of our present reality as fear of violence permeates our consciousness and families have fallen into disarray. Bell bottoms and platforms came back in the nineties, stylized, fashion accessorized, and costing a fortune. I wish we could do something to bring back peace and love. I'd like to see that back in vogue. In 1994, they held a second Woodstock for hippies, who have grown older and fatter but still haven't found a way to make this a safer world. Many of their kids went to try and relive the experience, to find out what it was really all about. They probably went to see if it was all a fraud, if there ever was any such thing as peace and love, or for that matter, ever will be. It will be hard to convince them.

I'd still like to escape to a bygone era. Perhaps that's why I've taken to *The Lawrence Welk Show* with its accordion players, jaunty polkas, beautiful Irish tenors, and Brazilian sambas. It's a pleasant junket back to a simpler time. I especially enjoy the old love songs with timeless appeal…still like rides on tinkling carousels and swirling cones of ice cream, reminiscences of how things used to be. In this age of women fighting to be like men, men changing into women, AIDS, I want to go back to the good ol' days! Sometimes I wonder if they were real or as fanciful as the painted wooden pony I giddyapped on as I kicked at his sides with my heels.

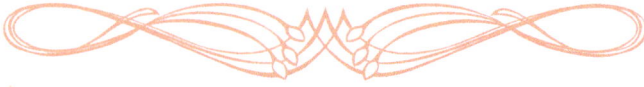

CHAPTER NINETEEN
A Higher Education

BACK to the push and busy of New York City life shoved and hurried me along. I had no time for inward reflection or meditation. My most frequent emotions were fear and trepidation. Returning, after time away, made me more aware of the cultural shift. The city had become a big sordid mess, and I was getting caught up in its craziness. My dating relationships were so fleeting and unsure, and I struggled with job failure. There I was, looking to connect and find intimacy in a world gone zany and wild.

I sought new answers for the goings-on around me. I'd come into my own in a sense, but deep down I was lonely, searching, and disillusioned. I'd worked on developing my mind but neglected my spirit. Though somewhat intelligent, I still needed help with *life*. The answers were not in my books or with my learned associates who were as messed up as I was. Secular theories confounded me. This one said this; that one said that. I wanted absolute truth. I decided to go back to church for grounding in the fundamentals of Christianity. This time, I listened as never before. I needed someone more experienced to guide me, to come alongside and shore me up, to make me not feel so weak. Who better than an all-knowing and all-seeing God?

On the horns of the '80s, we had rapidly advanced to the age of consumerism, a time of muchness and success for many, a period of wanting and not having for most. Science had given us powerful medications and quick-fix solutions. People no longer believed in suffering through things, trying to make them work, and asking the Lord to see you through. Now it was the fast way out, changing partners, divorce, suicide, and the guy on the corner saying, "I want it, you've got it. I'm gonna take it away from you by any means necessary!" (Violence, rip-offs, deception, you name it.)

That little song we sang back when I went to Sunday school, "Jesus loves me, this I know," had been rewritten by the new generation to go, "I love myself, yes I do. It's all about me, later for you!" In the past, people believed the Bible was a light unto their paths and a lamp unto their feet. The New Agers looked to how-to-books, Dr. Spock, talk shows, situation comedies, soaps, parenting and marriage manuals, and sex gurus. We had knowledge to know how to dissect life under a microscope down to its molecular structure. But I searched for wisdom to know how to put things in my life together.

One Sunday the minister gave an altar call with the words of Jesus, "Come unto me all ye who labor and are heavy laden and I will give you rest." I decided to accept the Lord's offer of forgiveness. The message promised solutions for my problems, healing of my hurts, and strength to break free of bad habits and sins that were wrong. I made that long walk down the aisle to make a public confession of faith and took on a new identity as a child of God. I remember having a sweatshirt printed with the words "Yes, Jesus Loves Me." Now that faith that was in Fannie Bell, then Ernestine, had come alive in me.

When I came to the Lord, I remembered my grandmother, how strength was always in the lines of her face and warmth in her smile—how she was clothed in dignity and showed tender compassion to all. I loved her genuine, simplistic ways. We need more folks around like her these days.

Things began to change in my life. I took up the mantle of advancing Christ's agenda to the world. God had given me the privilege of getting an education. I wanted to use it to shape young lives. The church became a place to learn how to teach and reach kids and change the route of their lives. The teaching/learning process helped me grow in faith. It gave my idealism form and solidity, made me more substantive. I was no longer standing alone; the Lord was in the battle with me. I believed Jesus would help me find direction. I received lots of support and encouragement from my church family. For many of us, the church has served as a springboard for our talents.

It also helped assuage my feelings about race. I learned all men have value in the eyes of God for we were created in His image. The issue became no longer someone else's estimation of me, but faith in God and acceptance of His love for me as His child. That feeling of *worthlessness* and self-rejection began to subside, as did anger toward other racial groups. I came to understand the problem of racism proceeds out of an evil heart, not inherent superiority. In the words of a song,

> In the beloved He sees me,
> In the beloved accepted and free!

I went through a transformation, began viewing things differently, and became concerned with what was right from a divine standpoint. I wanted God's influence on my mind. Things didn't all of a sudden become perfect as I'd hoped, but I gained a new perspective on life and had a friend in a high place.

Christ's presence has been a garland woven throughout my experiences, tying them all together. Unlike a Christmas tree that's thrown out annually, I grew year after year and spiraled upward. I weathered many unkind New York winters and found strength for every new circumstance. His wonderful provisions abounded in me and produced fruits of patience. Therefore, as I continue picking up my experiences and hanging them like ornaments on a tree, it is with great awe I place that shining star on top whose ambient glow gave everything flow and a luster of richness. It's the reason I've stored them away so carefully in the trunk box of my mind. I can take them out from time to time, blow the dust off, and display them like precious heirlooms.

I began working to preserve kids' rights to have a wholesome childhood. What happened to it is a true American enigma. It exists only in our memories of days past. Gone are the old shows I grew up on. Imperfect though they were, they modeled socially acceptable behavior. TV land is no longer a safe place for kids' minds to wander and idle, as it has become increasingly violent and sensual. If they step off Sesame Street or turn a corner from Mr. Roger's neighborhood, they are likely to encounter Dirty Doggie, Super Stud, Mighty Mouth, Seedie Bird, Sexeralla, or the Thriller Killer. It's called "reality TV," but it's the kind of reality that awakens fears, provides no answers, and doesn't say what is right or wrong.

With further social decline, kids couldn't just be sent out to play. The old couldn't go out and sit. Couples couldn't take a stroll in the park after dark. Against this backdrop, I entered the rough and tumble of the public school system, teaching third grade in the East Bronx, working with kids who knew all the four-letter words but couldn't read a three-letter word, who used the F-word as a verb, adjective, and adverb. My horizon was not vivid with hope.

When I started, I was so overwhelmed, determined, and scared. Given my room key, it was do or die. By that time, crack had cracked a lot of poor families up. There were many one-parent and some with none. Though a predominantly white school in a nice area, it was undergoing a population shift. There were lots of changes and instability as many cultures came together.

Some parents didn't speak English, which made it difficult for them to get involved. Others were kids themselves, barely out of high school, now saddled with parenting responsibilities. This placed a number of students at risk before they ever had a chance to get going.

I recall vividly standing in front of that patchwork of cleanly scrubbed faces for the first time, how nervous I was yet excited. I felt if we could work things out under one roof in that classroom, maybe they could work things out in the world. I can run through the first school play we put on in assembly as if it were yesterday. Its theme? The Pilgrims and the Indians pulling together to survive the harsh winter and sharing the harvest in fall. I can still hear the words to the song we sang ringing in my ears, "Let there be peace on earth and let it begin with me!" I had the unfailing belief that hand in hand we could end ethnic fighting. A glance across the global stage could easily convince one I was wrong.

I remember hurtfully the white parents, how they came into my room and asked for the teacher assuming I was just an aide, and blushed with embarrassment when I said, "I am she"; how at lunchtime a coworker drove me to see the neighborhood, and when we passed through Edgewater Park, a small area of boathouses near the water, the people surrounded the car, pointed, and laughed, calling, "Nigger, Nigger!" Hard to believe this took place in New York City, but it did.

When I visited the East Tremont area fourteen years later, nothing much had changed. There were still enclaves of whites who were hostile to blacks like the business owner who told me to get the "F" away from there when I showed up to buy furnishings. Strange how racial problems are not cured with time. They only get set like an ugly smudge or stain. Racism in America is similar to a nagging backache; we just work around it. We try to carp and complain it away, but it has perpetuity.

Once on staff, I finally began to see my colleagues as equals. But my insides knew I would never be, especially not in their eyes, for I would always be the black teacher with emphasis on *black*. There was this notion that blacks who were educated should go and help their own people. We were not thought to be good enough to teach whites. They devalued our worth. My hiring signaled to me they had a bottom class with tough minority kids and wanted someone who could "handle them."

In northern cities, whites were believed to be liberal and unbiased. But the dynamics of racism got played out in covert rather than overt ways. As African Americans, we learn to identify prejudice by how it *feels* to us, although it is not always expressed in words and often doesn't have a tangible form that can be pointed at. Like love, it's invisible but manifests itself in gestures, posturing, eye movements, attitudes, slights of speech, and manner that telegraph messages without ever a spoken word. The message is, "I'm suspicious of you. You don't belong here. You don't measure up. You make me uncomfortable. You're a threat to me. You might do something or steal something or step out of place in some way, or you're here to take over." I've heard blacks say they don't like the way others look at them, makes them feel strange. But I don't like the way some won't look at me or make eye contact, as if to look would mean they'd have to sanction me and acknowledge my personhood.

We learned to hear what was not said regarding race through code words that signaled what the real issues were, i.e., opposition to busing, or the construction of low-income housing in white areas was a code for opposition to integration. Law and order was perceived as white protection and black suppression. Tough on crime seemed to mean tough on us, and welfare reform meant, "We are tired of *you people* getting something for nothing!"

Society itself perpetuates an atmosphere of distrust of people of color before we ever do anything. For example, a black man enters a store. The owner fears he is a robber coming to steal and watches him like a hawk. He buys a new car with hard-earned cash, only to be pulled over by officers checking if it's stolen, or he walks in a white neighborhood and the police hassle him because "he doesn't belong around there" and must be looking for trouble.

The reality of race in America is that it is still an issue. That's what makes the black experience so painful. While we continually try to maneuver through the entrails of the system, other groups have found ways to be absorbed. An impermeable membrane holds us back. The system's normal osmotic tendencies haven't worked for us.

Overtime I learned to "fit in" with whites, adopted the same tastes and clothing styles, and had that accent like someone from upstate New York. I practiced proper diction and politeness of speech and relished sophistication—didn't like jiveyness, that so-called black way of behaving (rolling necks, hands on hips, the slap me five, and the honey child, or as they say today, "girlfriend"). I'd become the quintessential black professional, educated, bilingual (spoke English and Ebonics). Though a native of the city, I dressed like Ms. Sally Sue from West Kalamazoo—prim, ladyish, loved dainty embroidery, pearls, and lace. My outerwear reflected my internals—soft and gentle. Others might say I liked to act white. I say that was just me. I am more than my racial identity. But black is the only thing some people ever see.

By the end of the school year there were a few success stories in my group which brought praise and congrats. I liked that. More important, I won the confidence and respect of those who doubted me, which shows attitudes can be broken down by direct contact and interaction when both sides make an investment in the outcome. Control of a group and keeping interest I learned by trial and error. Some of the kids were holy terrors, but with time the experience got better.

Once I developed a reputation for being able to handle trouble-makers, all were dumped in my room, so I figured, if I was going to work with "those kids," I might as well transfer to special education classes with fewer on roster. Jobs in public school are work intensive and stress intensive. Purely teaching was sometimes the smallest part of what we did as issues of control, management, planning, reports, paperwork, and testing weighed so heavily on our responsibilities.

By then, God had been expelled from school. They didn't want Him hanging around the kids. Words like *authority*, *decency*, and *morality* had become old hat. There was little respect for the position of parents, policemen, teachers, and the like. Obedience to rules was sometimes scoffed at. Discipline was a major problem. Keeping them in a seat, maintaining some semblance of order, and surviving until 3:00 p.m. was basically my job.

This was a reflection of changes in the home. Children were no longer raised by the book. They weren't expected to mind any-more. Everything had become negotiable. I'm your friend; you're my friend. I listen to you; you listen to me. No one wanted to submit. It was a recipe for chaos!

I was always trying to hold it all in check and remain focused while rebounding from problems with my love life, family, or son. In kindergarten, Malik's reading and math difficulties started right away. Where some kids flung right along, he didn't. He was poorly coordinated, couldn't sit still and focus. His mind frequently wan-dered, and he was starting to stand out from the others socially as well.

Seeing what was happening in the public schools, I was afraid he would be like putty in the hands of tough kids. I began looking for a private school with specialized training to provide a safety net. Since I couldn't pay, I'd ask the Board of Education for funding. This meant fighting the board's new policy of inclusion of special kids in regular classes.

The Committee on the Handicapped would have to decide. Not knowing how to advocate, I feared a bureaucratic mess and was baffled by the appeals process. I knew they'd seek the least expensive option, and the burden of proof was on me to show special need. I studied my old school notes, wanting to be able to explain the difference between the letter of the law (children are to be educated in the least restrictive environment) and the spirit of the law to give parents and kids greater choice. I believed Malik would fare better in a special setting.

Warned not to appear too eager, it was a delicate game of trying to walk through a mind field and not set off any explosives. I was afraid I'd blow the whole thing. In the grips of intense agony and frustration, I felt my performance would determine his future. I didn't feel adequate to make my case. I went in sweaty, heart in hand, bearing test reports and pleading with a mother's ardor for help. Somehow the Lord pulled me through. He was given funding.

An anvil had been lifted from my shoulders, but only temporarily, for I had to trek back through that door year after year to prove his continued need. I almost prayed he wouldn't make any progress just so his improvement couldn't be used to justify terminating funds. It's a shame the system places parents in that kind of bind.

He was placed in a lovely cocoon environment, the Gateway School, with a sensitive, highly skilled staff who understood his problems and had the resources to help. The school was a demonstration model for working with LD kids, then under the direction of Elizabeth Freidus, an outstanding educator in the field. Located in a prestigious area, Madison Avenue in the '50s, the students were generally well off. It pleased me to be a poor mother from the Bronx and have my child in attendance there; it gave me peace of mind to focus more on my work. When the yellow school bus pulled up at the door each morning, it lit my day. I couldn't have been happier, not only for Malik, but for the opportunity to learn along the way.

With a new license to teach HC-30 class, I was transferred from the East to the South Bronx for what I thought would be an art teacher cluster position. It turned out they wanted a coordinator for a large unit of classes for the emotionally handicapped consisting of 90 percent tough, streetwise older boys.

On entering the building, suddenly I was overpowered by a towering mural of famous black Americans, a monument to consciousness and pride. The halls teemed with movement and living color. In the air a romp and beatbox cadence crescendoed to a raucous din. In short, it was a madhouse!

The principal, hip in appearance, wore Afrocentric dress, yet conceit in her countenance said, "Call me Your Royal Highness." Her staff was a garden variety of characters, including party people, rabble-rousers, Hispanics, bulldog-looking women you better not mess with, fast-buck makers selling earrings and hot things, fast-talking sugar daddies and "high-class blacks" pulling up in caddies, mercenaries there to "enculturate the heathens, to bring them out of darkness, into the marvelous light, "great white father" or mother types, outsiders slumming to get a paycheck, whose cars encircled the school like Conestoga wagons so they could get in, earn the money, and get out easily without any community involvement, and a remnant of fine, dedicated workers of all races who labored valiantly to bring out the best in the students, struggling daily against this culture of poverty.

The special wing was being controlled with an iron fist by teachers with a baseball bat mentality because, "You know how you have to be with those kids!" The boys in the unit couldn't compete on an intellectual level with main body students. Prone toward music and sports, most wanted to grow up to be a DJ, a musician, or a basketball star. They didn't see books and success in school as a viable way out of poverty and showed little motivation. Behaviors they picked up on the street (i.e., boasting, taunting, false bravado, energetic play, and aggressiveness) belied success in the classroom, where sitting quietly and working long hours was required.

The message had filtered down to them that if you're black, you can't be no brainiac, that they must be opposites (white kids—studious nerds; blacks—jive talkin' homeboys who carry no books). Lacking in positive role models, many never saw a leader or saw the wrong type of leaders in new heroes—gang members, drug dealers, and pimps. A "*man*" on the street was someone who could fight, curse, fornicate, and never cry. It was not safe to let show your vulnerability.

These students were growing up feeling like losers, not winners. It's hard to see the qualities of a winner in yourself growing up in a negative environment. With the focus on control rather than teaching and learning in the classrooms, their fears were heightened of themselves and each other. There was always some sort of threat looming over them from tougher kids or adults.

God planted raw material in all of us, but somehow when you have never been approached as a winner, you internalize failure, even opt for it because you're afraid to succeed; it's too foreign to your experience. The kids did need firm discipline and work required of them, but what they needed most was to see "I believe in you!" in someone's eyes and hear it in their voice. They had missed out on a lot of molding during the formative years when bad habits get established. Often latchkey kids, left in the hands of older siblings or hanging out on street corners, there wasn't much encouragement or security. Some had no one to look up to and didn't see much to feel positive about around them. These kids were literally backed in a corner by society and didn't feel like they were worth much. Most lacked the wherewithal to "just say no" to street life.

In early grades, they usually did okay, but by third grade, they were labeled troublemakers as those behaviors that worked well on the street collided with what was expected in the classroom and was often misread by white teachers. Written off, they were shipped to EH class and inducted into special education. White kids hardly ever ended up there, even those with behavior problems as it was felt they'd be preyed upon by tough black kids. The system made other arrangements for them. Thus, EH became a dumping ground for black and Hispanic youth whom regular class teachers couldn't handle.

The same mentality operated in some prisons where whites were separated from blacks for their own "protection" and put in more favorable conditions even though they were all criminals.

With our kids, I believe teachers from minority backgrounds have an edge. They demonstrate education can be attained even though the system often works unfavorably and have themselves as proof. I feel they are less likely to throw their hands up and say, "Well, what are you going to do?" given the preponderant factors warring against them. Making a personal investment is linked to knowing the children's future is our future. Not to suggest black teachers should only teach black kids and whites teach white, for any dedicated, sensitive teacher can help a needy child of any race, if willing to go the distance. With the absence of black male role models on the lower grades, a valuable modeling opportunity is lost.

I felt incapable, not the woman for the job. The circumstances looked too overwhelming. I was not a controlling, regulating, highly structured person—couldn't see how to make *me* work there. Extremely doubtful of my leadership capacity, my insecurities came strongly into play. My attitude was, "I'm not as good as I'd like to be. There are others who are more capable than I am. I am afraid of failing—afraid I can't follow through." Self-doubt was such a weighty and controlling factor. I asked myself, "What if I can't handle it?" I resisted success, told myself, "I can't do this!" I went through a crisis of confidence.

Assuming leadership only figuratively, I never put myself on the spot to be tested before the crowd, never went out on the limb. I stayed in my comfort zone, hidden in the front office, avoiding difficult staff members who relished confrontation. I didn't wish to stand out or go toe-to-toe with anyone over their methods. I had creative ideas for the program but never blurted them out because I was afraid to defend my position and approach. I always felt, "Let somebody else be the one to take them on." I didn't want the stress of proving myself. I just didn't have the courage to step out there, believe, and take risks. I felt like a failure and continually focused on what I thought I was lacking, which continually robbed me of my esteem. My image of myself kept me out of what I was supposed to do.

But the Lord rallied the staff around me, shored me up, and I made it through the year. Obviously, they saw leadership in me though I was resistant. They seemed at ease with my low-key manner and preferred having me over someone more demanding. No one likes the crack of a whip! Things went remarkably well, frighteningly smooth. I knew I wasn't in control, yet it was being controlled, which I attribute to Christ.

Before long, I came to the conclusion I was just not meant to be a team leader or player. I wanted to work one on one with students and not have to communicate with and depend on others frequently to carry out my job. I preferred the safety and security of my own classroom and direct contact with kids in a world I would create and orchestrate. I wanted to work with younger kids before they became hardened, so to speak, where my artsy-crafty approach would be a plus. I was more inspired to attend to the needs of youngsters whose lives had the potential of being nasty and short, if they got stuck in the mire of city streets. Giving kids dreams and teaching them to persist would be my goal.

I loved the tenacity of poor kids and the die-hardness they exhibited while struggling to grow up in often hostile home environments with the added burden of emotional and learning disabilities. Life was an uphill fight, yet they were high-spirited and full of laughter. When those kids put on an assembly program, they really put their hearts into it. It meant so much as they rarely got a chance to take centerstage and show what they could do. Though few were likely to survive the perils and predators of the environment, most had drive and will to make it.

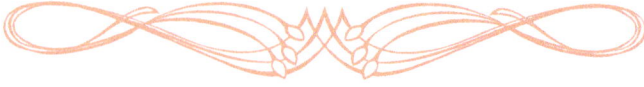

CHAPTER TWENTY
Driven to Give My All

AS we embarked on a new decade, a frightening chapter of change and challenge was in motion. Fear stalked the streets. Anger seethed in steamy housing projects crawling with roaches and pushers. At the same time, disparity between white and black income levels grew. The atmosphere turned more threatening and unsafe as we sank into self-annihilation—brothers killing brothers. No one was saying "Whitey" anymore; it was black-on-black crime. Lack of job opportunities, easy access to weapons, and crack cocaine undermined the black family in ways slavery never could. Young black men with idle time fell under a new yoke. In bondage to drugs, they were willing to rob their mothers or a neighbor's house or snatch an old woman's purse to get money.

Some did this, but not *all*. Most struggled along, taking whatever job they could, out there trying to make it with little acknowledgment and no one to trumpet their accomplishments. Those committing the crimes got the bulk of media attention. Nightly newscasters recanted a sad litany of those arrested for robbery, rape, mayhem, and murder. The faces flashing across the screen were most often black. They didn't have to do that because we all knew the color of the face of our fears.

As I write this entry, it is with deep sadness I listen to news reports of an attack on Mrs. Rosa Parks, the mother of the civil rights movement, mugged in her home by a man who broke in, beat her in the face, and demanded money. It is a shameful irony that a woman who is a living symbol of our pride and dignity should be a victim of senseless violence by black criminals breaking down her door at age eighty-one. The face of our oppressors has changed, but the battle for dignity wages on.

Kids of Generation X seem to have no message. They see nothing worth dying for and revere, honor, respect, or worship nothing but themselves and material goods. This is largely our fault as parents because we were so busy out trying to give our kids all the things we never had; we failed to give them what we did have: old-fashioned values like hard work, self-discipline, respect for others' property and authority figures, also a healthy sense of family and community bound together by our traditions.

We, the baby boomers, let religious training that emphasized doing what was right in God's eyes and taught us self-control go down the drain. We let our kids go unchurched and replaced giving them spiritual food with trying to feed their yearnings for more and more *things*—the hottest fashions, leather sneakers, bikes, gold, video games with push buttons, flashing lights, and music that tinkled like a nickelodeon. Something in their allure captured their childish fancy like a piping calliope, and they could never get enough!

Moving into a new era, parents and kids had so little in common—not music or shared activities, nothing. We were so near yet so far apart. Kids were rappin', scratchin', breakdancin', rankin', dissin', cussin', and swaggerin', while their parents were busy going after money and economic power. When I saw how difficult it was becoming to relate and communicate, I thought back to the days when we took turns doing the swing with Mom and Dad in the middle of the living room floor, playing 45s on the old Victrola. How Daddy had these smooth moves and put a little hop in his steps to make us laugh. We were so faithful to our family institution and its traditions.

Kids started seeing their parents in passing as they ran aerobically in and out of each other's lives. Parents were not living with their kids, being there for them, and loving them sacrificially so that they were willing to give up a lot of things for their sakes. Although as a nation we were great worshipers of youth, we didn't love our children by making policies and decisions in our careers and personal lives that were in their best interests.

They also had no strong moral, ethical giants to look up to, no powerful examples of self-discipline and leadership, no men like Dr. Martin Luther King to feel great reverence for, no people who stood up for their ideals like the Freedom Riders at great personal risk to themselves, no grandmas living in the homes to teach them godly wisdom. All our American heroes and icons had come crashing to the floor like glass idols. People asked what character and integrity had to do with leadership, yet we saw its absence undermining and debilitating our nation. The falling away and breakdown of integrity led to a lack of moral codes and a lowering of standards. Many became unprincipled and irresponsible.

I used to take Malik to see Saturday matinees during the Christmas holidays, remembering back to when we as kids went to the movies, bought buttered popcorn, and stayed all day watching Walt Disney, space monsters, or shoot-'em-up flicks. But the veil of innocence had been lifted off the entertainment world, and moviegoers were being exposed to wanton sex, vulgarity, raw violence, and high-powered weapons. It was shocking! Before Hollywood passed down traditional values, but they too dropped their standards. It was bad enough for poor kids that conditions of deprivation were affecting their choices, but now you had the powerful influence of Hollywood and TV carrying them downhill as well.

What was I to do to protect my child and raise him clean and decent? We spent a lot of time at the zoo or Central Park sitting and talking. Staying close and teaching values was all I knew. Somehow it seemed not enough because, as my father used to say, "Once the horse has escaped from the barn, it's hard to go get him and put him back in there!"

Music no longer brought generations together. Break dancing was for kids only. The older crowd couldn't execute its wild acrobatics. The message of beatbox held no meaning to adults. Likewise, clothing styles identified kids in and everyone else out of their group. Most people my age avoided the club scene fearing things would get out of control and there would be shooting as perception of danger and violence grew. I basically stayed close to kith and kin for safety. Old friends had gone their separate ways, and interest in going out fizzled. Letting my hair down meant sitting in the living room, spinning oldies, crooning like an alley cat, as I started looking back.

Although I had a career and two degrees, there were few social outlets for meeting eligible males. Outside activities centered around my church where I discovered I didn't need a "significant other" to feel validated and to be a good mother. I took on the roles of usher and Sunday school teacher. My participation mushroomed, as well as my sense of my own capabilities.

I began to clip along at a steady pace, headed into the rush of my career, striving to be hardworking, dedicated, and dependable like a member of the Eye Witness News Team. In society in general, however, commitment and loyalty had taken a back seat to selfishness and self-preservation. Intensity was out. Everyone was laid back and casual, while at home marriages and families boiled over with conflict and abuse. Burning embers were becoming a lava flow.

As a real New Yorker, I learned to listen for a light note and find a chuckle amid the cacophony of urban calamity. I looked for a ray of hope shining like a copper penny among the rubble of broken lives. I smelled the sweat, tasted the grit, yet dreamed of a country place where the air was fresh and sweet and blades of grass tickled my feet.

Out in the workaday world, I was into paying bills, planning quick meals, barely keeping my head above water, walking the fine line between just making it and not doing so well. I lived on the edge of a precipice, always with the realization that one slip and I was over the side, back down into the pit of poverty. Earning a teacher's salary, I'd gone from the public roll to lower-middle-class life.

Driven to give my all as a career woman, I was torn between responsibilities to my job and home. I tried not to shove the spiritual aside and let things get out of balance. Often I felt worn out trying to be Mega Mom. I had no timeouts to unwind; it was straight from work to my kid. There was no one to team with to get things done. I had no time to shift gears, rejuvenate, rest, or rebuild. Society said women were supposed to be able to "do it all," but I didn't have endless supplies of energy. The constant output took its toll.

When you have a child and work, *you* become the casualty. There is very little time to take care of your needs, pamper yourself, or give your body attention. You don't have quiet time to be alone, revamp, and revitalize your will. You can't pursue personal goals and interests. You make extreme sacrifices for the sake of your child and abuse yourself for others. I often wondered how I would meet everyone's needs when mine weren't being met.

Typical of me, instead of slowing down, I tended to overcommit, took on more and more things to do, unable to say no or realize I couldn't burn the candle on both ends. It's easy to get caught up in busyness when you believe yesterday is gone, today will pass, only what's done for Jesus Christ will last. That becomes the reason to wear a stack of hats. Like the peddler in the children's story "Caps for Sale," I wished I could get someone to take a few off my head.

I went about coutured in thrift-shop chic and Salvation Army rags. My patchy apartment was done up with bric-a-brac and this 'n' thats of early Goodwill styling. My fashion sense changed from what looked good on to wash-'n'-wear things that I didn't need to iron. Baked beans and wieners we ate plenty, and many days I was down to the penny, living in terror checks would bounce or a goose egg would appear on my savings account. I ate humble pie and had to like it.

Suddenly all those things Mama used to say that were so nagging when I lived at home—"Turn off the lights!" "Don't waste food!" "Use bones to cook!" "Buy on sale!"—took on new meaning. I clung to her every precious word. Sayings that taught me little economies, like, "Waste not, want not!" "Make do with what you've got!" "What's still good, don't throw it away!" "Don't gab, blab, and run up the phone bill!" All the funny truisms that were so rich in wisdom: "A hard head makes a soft behind!" "Every tub has to stand on its own bottom!" "Put up or shut up!" "Don't fight the hand that feeds you or burn the bridge that brought you over!"

I clad myself in midiskirts so my ratty slips wouldn't show, wore pants to hide my flea-bitten stockings, and steered clear of open dressing areas so no one would get to stare at my piecy underwear.

Q-tip got every nip out of my tube of lipstick. I bathed with cheap white soap and bought drugstore cosmetics like dusting powder by Chateau. Vaseline greased my hair, Jergens lotion smoothed my rough edges, and Chantilly made sure I didn't smell like anybody else in my secondhand clothes. Castaways and make-dos were the best I could do. Dollar Days I was on the spot and shopped a lot at Odd Lot. When my deodorant and toothpaste ran out, it was baking soda under my flaps and in my trap. Inevitably being put through these paces made me draw up sap from my roots.

I kept flapping my arms, kicking my feet, trying to stay afloat. My goal was not necessarily to move ahead but to keep what I had, put food on the table, and keep the landlord off my back. With money left over, Malik and I went to Micky D's for a little treat, a Happy Meal or something sweet. I'd been taught you have to go through what you have to go through, stand up like "a real man," and take it. Except, I wasn't a man and needed someone to take my hand. I heard the voice of the Lord like a whisper saying, "Don't worry, I'm here! I'll help you carry the load." He was teaching me how much I could love by having to put aside my needs for my son's.

I liked going in places like the Salvation Army and Goodwill. It was humbling. I loved the people I met inside: the alcoholics who, because of drinking, had lost control but were now making a comeback; the sweet old ladies lumbering with overstuffed garbage bags, having raised five kids, put them through college, now alone finding companionship there; the broken-spirited women whom brutish men had beaten, recovering their pride, finding themselves enabled by coming in, putting dresses on racks, and checking tickets; the foreigners who didn't speak a word of English but who always knew which items were 50 percent off and how to count their change. It was a place where real people shopped—people who lived from day to day and didn't know what tomorrow would bring, who had no cushioning between themselves and life's bitter onslaughts. They were warm and accepting. God had begun His sifting, sanding, sculpting, chipping work in their lives. And they were finding courage to go on.

When you live in a place with many creature comforts like "the burbs," you can become snobbish, self-centered, and enwalled in your own world. But when you reside where poor people are, there is life and spirit, even in the midst of a struggle. There are times you laugh heartily, times you reach out and help each other, times you feel your humanity with your fellow man as when a snowstorm hits and mass transit breaks down. New York brings out your guts, but it also tenderizes and sensitizes you to what's really important—to touch another life.

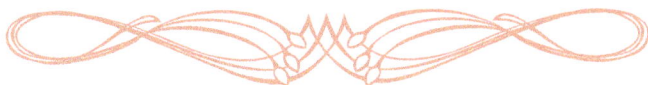

CHAPTER TWENTY-ONE
At War with Hopelessness

BY the nineteen eighties, many city dwellers though bogged in inertia were experiencing vertigo, a feeling that we were whirling out of control. This was a by-product of our overspeeding, overstimulating, overwhelming urban lifestyles.

In Africa, activities of daily living and rearing of children were a communal experience. Each person in the village shared responsibility for the welfare of the group. They believed in the harmony of spirituality and everyday living. They saw the need for faith and community. To them, people meant more than things. Relationships were the keys to an abundant life, and it was important to get along. God reigned sovereignly; He, they depended on. That wisdom, we had lost.

Early forms of Afro-American music were about loving, losing, and going through hard times, but they were filled with hope and reconciliation and never suggested shoot the next person who "disses you" or gets in your face. Neither did they employ nasty lyrics and vulgarity or perform lewd stage acts. New performers capitalized on the negative aspects of our experience. I can imagine, if my grandmother saw some of the latest pop videos, she'd shake her head and say, "Oh Lawd have mussy!" Even the old slave songs never talked of hate or violence, but faith, hope, and love in spite of the cruel system of chattel slavery they endured. The black experience has beauty, vitality, and love, but others often don't realize it because the media tends to leave the good things out when talking about black life. We've shown creative force and durability throughout history undergirded with love, not hate.

The changing labor force of the eighties dashed the hopes of many as the 1950–60s industrial base collapsed. Changes in the economic environment left black men with fewer opportunities, except selling drugs, as new technology and computers took over semiskilled and unskilled jobs. Several large companies either folded or moved to foreign soil where the labor force was cheaper. Our men have always had a difficult time finding decent jobs to support their families, so that wasn't new. More significant was the collapse of a dependent relationship on the Lord. A generation was coming up that was unchurched and lacked the sense of right and wrong Christianity taught. A new root of frustration and bitterness took hold. The sense of hopelessness became so much more pervasive.

You had a lot of young black men wanting the same things everyone else wanted: nice clothes, cars, money, jewelry, without the means to access them legitimately, yet believing they deserved them. Some were not willing to go start at the bottom on one of those low-paying menial jobs, figuring they had been in this country long enough and were tired of playing second fiddle to all the new arrivals. They felt they had to "do what they had to do" to get over. Unfortunately, the drug trade was an equal-opportunity employer and didn't require education and experience like the job market, only that they be willing to risk life and limb for the prospect of pocketing $200–$300 a day. As foot soldiers for the drug trade, these men proved to be crafty, resourceful, resilient, hard workers who put in seven-day weeks and eighteen-hour days. Only death could stop them. What a waste of human potential! Neighborhood activists are now calling these men back to responsibility.

My father believed strongly in work and did so until his retirement. Why is it you never hear about the package handlers, dock workers, maintenance men, parts assemblers, factory workers, and cooks who dredge through snow and rain, bearing up under all sorts of indignities to bring home minimum wage and put it on the dresser?

We always hear about black men who don't work. What about the ones who do? There are many of them!

Society continued to promulgate myths that had been around since slavery that determined how black males were viewed (violent, criminal, babymakers who didn't want to work). Their media image was often musical, athletic, funny, entertaining, yet somewhat pathological. The outworkings of this have had a ripple effect from generation to generation. I believed the best way to turn the tide and break the pattern was through early intervention.

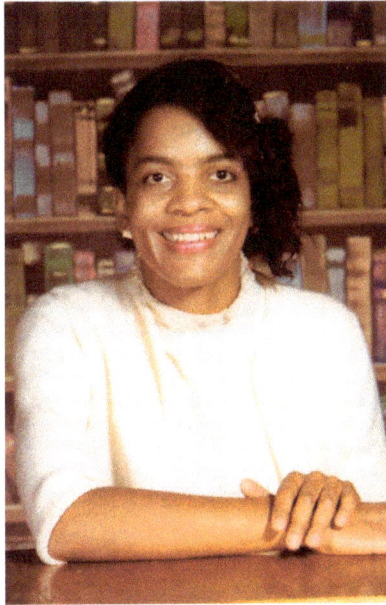

Me as a teacher in Riverdale.

In the year that followed, I was transferred to Riverdale and given a special ed class of rambunctious boys with plenty of zest and zeal. There I would be put to the test and have to make my philosophies real.

The school itself was a good example of how bias gets carried out in an educational setting. It was located in an area of the Bronx where status and money were not strangers to the households. Incomes and test scores were high by borough-wide comparison. The surrounding community consisted of yuppies and well-established families of predominantly Jewish or Irish descent. Japanese students, children of foreign dignitaries and businessman, made up 10–20 percent of the student body, while the number of black and Hispanic kids was less than 3 percent. Needless to say, the school was a showcase for the district.

The special ed wing, isolated on the second floor, presented a vastly different picture. The students from predominantly low-income minority families were bussed in from the West Bronx area near Broadway. They had a hodgepodge of learning problems and scored poorly on tests. In spite of the fact one primary goal of special education is mainstreaming, these students were "ghettoized" in the school. They entered the building through a separate entrance, ate a separate lunch, played in a separate schoolyard, and only came in contact with the main body as they passed quickly in line through the halls. If they were on grade and ready to go back into regular classes, they had to return to a school in "their neighborhood."

The principal's explanation for this was that the students were so different in appearance, clothing, and family backgrounds they wouldn't fit in with the regular kids and would be much happier with others like themselves. To spare them the pain and embarrassment of being thrown in with kids with whom they could not compete or compare, this policy was made for *their* benefit. A prejudicial attitude is revealed in his well-intended benevolence. It should be noted that the Japanese students, some recent arrivals from Japan and culturally very different, were fully integrated because, as he put it, he was "sure they would do well and pick up quickly."

Unfair as this arrangement was, it did provide the kids with an educational setting in nicer surroundings with probably better books and equipment than their homeschool might have had. But it limited the amount of involvement poor parents could have in the program because of distance. For me it was like being a hyphen between two worlds. As the only black teacher on staff, I faced similarly low expectations and stood in the gap. I knew I'd have to prove my competence as well as my students'.

A stately canopy of trees dropped a royal carpet of leaves to welcome my young mascots that crisp September, while fidgety gray squirrels performed like circus aerialists collecting their fall delights. A wily raccoon dressed in winter woollies bedded down on a branch outside our window, providing the perfect opportunity to study seasonal change. Even a dark, fuzzy caterpillar wearing an expensive-looking coat inched out to greet. Nature was quite accommodating that year. The boys burst through the door, antsy, exuberant, filled with leftover summer wildness.

I jumped in and started pitching. Realizing they had to be instinctive and sensory oriented to survive on city streets, I set out to provide a rich visual and auditory environment as well as hands-on experiences to stimulate their appetite for learning academics. Placing things around that were interesting helped set the learning stage and captured their natural curiosity. This became a springboard to reading and writing activities that gave structure and order to our day. Before long we had such a menagerie of animals, fish, and plants our room was more like a zoo-arium than a classroom.

You have to be able to read to succeed in today's times. A child who can't read internalizes frustration and failure early in life, which leads to discipline and behavior problems. Boys who read poorly suffer great pain and embarrassment, feel dumb, and are inclined to act out. However, if you can give a kid a system for attacking words, deciphering them and not guessing, many bad habits already developed can be remedied. A rich intellectual life can be opened up through reading. The world becomes so much bigger. Those who don't read don't know another world is out there. Reading can present an orderly world to a child who is surrounded with disorder.

Reading, writing, and language arts go hand in hand. Society does not complain about rap music until artists start talking about cop killing, but look at the job teachers have teaching minority kids standard English, when the linguistic model braying through their headsets is so unenriching. The detrimental effect is seen years later when those students go for job interviews and can't communicate well. It works to their undoing.

Whites said the key to success for the disadvantaged was education when, in fact, what some hated most was an educated black person, particularly males, preferring those who were entertaining, jivey, and fit the stereotypes that made them feel comfortable. They had expectation for black youth to do well in music and athletics, but not math and science. When a high percentage of students in a school were minority, funding to teach these subjects well was usually low. Consequently, many didn't acquire the skills to compete in the changing job market.

As for those who did succeed, our group was so cut off from knowing who they were, what they'd accomplished, and how they made their attainments; it is as if they were no longer ours. They became lost to us, out of reach. We so easily lost connection with our achievers because the media kept our success stories secret while bombarding us with images of our failure. This hurt the broader society also because not heralding the positives caused negative attitudes to persist. A lot has been kept from us about our contributions throughout history. The record has to be set straight.

Knowledge is powerful. There is a need for African Americans to make reading an integral part of our home life. Half the children of the world are unable to pick up a book and read it. We who live in a land of abundance should make use of our informational resources.

I believed the lack of leadership and positive role models in the schools was linked to the lack of followship by the kids. Teachers were failing because society put the worse to teach the worse. Teachers who couldn't cut it anywhere else were often hired to teach poor, deficient, or disabled students. The best were given to the gifted and talented. Actually, it should have been the other way around. The slower kids really needed a very clever and skilled teacher to motivate them and maximize their learning potential. Brighter kids picked up without too much help.

In the classroom, I was like the little old lady who lived in a shoe, ripping, racing, running behind, trying to serve, control, and mold, making things, putting on plays, having lots going on simultaneously. This required planning, preparation, and burning midnight oil. I tried to strike a balance between control and freedom knowing there was a need for both. Latchkey kids spend little quality time with parents reading, sharing, doing things, and going places. I became their surrogate mother, as concerned with who didn't have breakfast and whose hair wasn't combed or whose clothes weren't tidy, as I was with teaching the three *R*s.

From the crack of dawn they were on the bus—sometimes hungry, sick, unprepared, or dealing with family issues that made them insecure and fearful like domestic violence, drug abuse, or alcoholism. They tended to be clingy, yearning for encouragement and support, and always wanted someone to listen. Sometimes they drained so much from me because they were so emotionally needy.

I found teaching had little to do with the methods classes I took in college. It really had to do with encapsulating information into a form they could swallow, digest, and want to come back for more. If it never gets down the throat, it never becomes useful to the body. My students were controlled, not by a club, but through an environment that put knowledge within reach bringing reading and math to life in everyday experiences that were familiar to them. They were given freedom to move, to pick and choose, to be social while learning in partnership with friends, to explore their natural gifts by providing outlets for self-expression in creative rather than destructive ways.

The parents and the system already having failed the kids, I asked myself if I should get in there, play savior, and try to work miracles overnight, or should I roll with the punches, earn my money, and go home? So many older, more experienced teachers had been there for years and done nothing. Why should I make waves? I was just a young whippersnapper. I questioned what my responsibility was to the kids, myself, the staff, and my school. Should I stand together with other professionals in a wall of silence? Tenured teachers couldn't be fired. They just got transferred from school to school, some carrying bad habits with them. Many of the really bad ones had been in the system for years.

I lived with frustration day and night, mulling over ideas and problems, asking myself if I should stick my neck out and become the sacrificial lamb. It called into question what I really believed in. Fear told me my beliefs were just shields to keep me from accepting the real world. Those inner voices can be the hardest to silence. I wrestled with issues both ethical and moral. I was confronted with the harsh realities of life like hunger and child abuse each time I saw whelps on a kid's body, stood close enough to hear stomachs roll, or looked in a small face and saw the worn countenance of someone whose life was in turmoil when there should have been mirth and lightheartedness. Today there are very tough issues to deal with, like cyberbullying, teen suicide, and school shootings. I basically went along with the program because I too had a child to feed and lived from paycheck to paycheck, but I tried not to compromise my values.

The same old feeling kept haunting me that I couldn't make a difference. I had to continually remind myself that I was a teacher and my job was to teach, not to preach or try to take on the bigger issues singlehandedly. I tried to close the door, shut the world out and just do my job well. I figured even if I didn't impact the system, if I touched the life of one child, then I did something worthwhile. Public school education is more about the board, the union, and the staff than it is about the kids. Maybe that's what made me compatible with them. I felt weak and vulnerable, and so did they. We bonded together for strength. They needed me and I them, which created a link.

I began to develop intuitiveness and instinctiveness for teaching through many trials and failures. How to do it is not in the books. It's something you pull out of yourself day by day. Neither is it glamorous work. But it's real and earnest and can be quite rewarding when you see a light bulb go off in a student's head and know you've gotten through. It's the type of job you often have to put your guts on the table for class examination because along with instruction, the kids want to know what's deep inside of you, what makes you tick, and if you really care. That tug-of-war between you and the student is the basis of the teaching dynamic. As they say in the Century 21 ads, "People don't care how much you know until they know how much you care."

The 1980s brought movies into homes and increased viewing considerably. This cut studying and homework down to nil and whittled away family time for communicating and playing games. Eyes were glued to the tube. Along came the computer chip, which some say was the greatest invention since the paperback book. Video games began exciting kids visually but didn't challenge them intellectually. They just had to push a button and become mesmerized by sights, sounds, and music. Who would suffer through the ropes of reading when such entertainment was available, providing an easy leap to the fanciful and magical? For a teacher, this was tough competition. It forced us to take out bells and whistles and pull out all the stops.

Making headway required commitment to give hours to planning, working with parents, pulling kids together as a team, challenging them to go beyond themselves, having heart-to-heart talks, rallying their energy, letting them know I believed they could succeed, bringing success down to their level, listening to problems at home, visiting homes to intercede, engaging in weekend activities, constantly redoubling my efforts. It was like pulling teeth.

Teaching is seizing teachable moments and making the best of them. My best moments as a teacher were unplanned, unpolished, and unprogrammed. They just happened as the kids and I joined in discovering new things. I can't take credit for any success I may have had. I will say God used whatever gifts I had to help them. There were many dips and moments of discouragement, but the Lord was my stay.

Today we have a whole generation of kids who are in jeopardy of being lost because they lack a fundamental personal morality on which to build their lives and need to be rescued. Communities must assume leadership in throwing out a lifeline to our kids and not depend on the usual societal interventions. We can't let teaching become just a job while schools turn into bloody battlefields with gangs recruiting for members.

Kids today wish things were decent and easy like in the 1950s, when everyone knew the rules even if they didn't obey them. They live in fear of violence and worry if they will even live to see tomorrow. That makes things like tests seem unimportant. Some have sex as early as nine, begin dating, get pregnant, have babies and abortions, contract STDs or HIV, and have gone through so much that by the age of twenty, they feel they are ready to die, feel like there is nothing left to do. They yearn for the peace and innocence of the America we once knew. We don't have an enemy anymore or an ideology to hate, like communism except violent extremism. It's time to turn our eyes inward, see what's happened to our soul, our spirituality, to examine what is causing our strife and ask ourselves what kind of legacy we are passing on to them.

The Spanish kids honored me by calling me simply "Maestra." It made me feel I was a real teacher in their eyes. I tended to press the kids hard sometimes, but with loving chastisement, not arrogance, contempt, or belittlement. I tried to go beyond cultural barriers by learning as much Spanish as I could pick up and conveying respect for roots.

For many minority kids, school is a hostile place where they are convinced of failure rather than success. Their unique problems, ways of approaching things, speech, and manner are often misread and not understood by whites. The learning they get in school seems unrelated to their world. Society has so many labels for people: disabled, culturally disadvantaged, economically deprived. I don't think we have as much challenge overcoming our own limitations as we have breaking out of the boxes we are placed in and getting to do what we *can* do. Not having the confidence of people is a tremendous holdback.

I used to allow students to get together in my room and let their hair down to street music in order to build a spirit of comradery like the slaves did when they assembled in clandestine hideaways to plan a trip over yonder to freedom land. Back in those times, slaves could only rock, clap, or stomp their feet because they weren't permitted drums to beat. Music has long been a vehicle for expressing deep-seated need. The boys needed a place to belong, a sense of family, to feel bonds of friendship and oneness in an atmosphere that was nonthreatening and safe. Adults think kids today want sex, condoms, stimulants, and all sorts of liberties. But what they really want is a safe, orderly world that makes sense, that they feel connected to, accepted by, and worthwhile in. They like to do simple things with people who think they matter and make them feel capable.

I found it hard to sit in the staff room and listen to other teachers talk whose realities were so different from mine. They'd say, "If only we could get them to realize they could improve their lives, if they would just study and learn and conform and...and...and..." Trouble is, there is always something more we have to do to become acceptable. In the end, we never get the M&M or whatever the prize is because we never quite measure up, remain in a mode of continually having to prove and reprove ourselves. That is the lot of many in this country.

It was hard also to go into the classroom daily and give kids a reason to try, when reason, logic, and everything around said it was hopeless and they were not going to get anywhere, that they were stuck on the bottom. Some kids lie down and dream wonderful dreams of great conquests. Others you actually have to teach how to dream, then help make it a reality. When you're standing on the shore looking out at the channel separating you from those on the other side, it takes great confidence and faith to believe you can make it across, especially when you have no boat or navigator and the gulf is ever widening.

Sometimes I wonder if the whole system isn't really just a farce. You see the kids appear in September all shiny faced and new, wearing clothes their parents sweated to buy, and watch them leave in June flinging books into the air. In between there are those months of pulling, tugging, and doing the best you can. What's so sad is you can almost predict where the kids with limited academic skills will wind up unless they make significant progress, perhaps filling the jails or on the welfare roll. I felt like just a pawn in the game.

That's why hope is so important, because when everything around you is conspiring to pull you down, you really need to be able to, as the slaves did, fix your eyes on that bright and shiny star and trust it to guide the way.

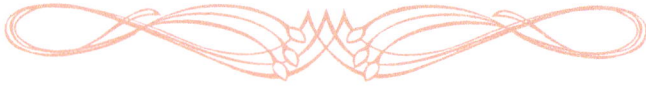

CHAPTER TWENTY-TWO
One Son, then Two

THE student who affected me most was a twelve-year-old Dominican boy named Danny. I guess you might say it was love at first bite. He was one of those naughty kids who could charm the pants off you with an elfin smile that made everything he did seem forgivable. Other teachers spoke of him with utmost venom, but to me he was just a wayward youth needing love. His dark eyes were crossed just enough to make me feel sorry for him, but his behavior was sufficient to throw any classroom into a tumult. He came from a group home in the area. His mother had a house full of other children and couldn't contend with his romp and riot. He had been passed around from teacher to teacher, and many calls went out to his counselor saying he was wreaking havoc in the school.

The Sunday school department at my church developed an outreach ministry to draw kids. We held Friday night socials to bring teens and preteens through our doors. I thought Danny would be a perfect candidate as I was sure a wholesome family environment would do him good. I began inviting him on weekends and taking him and Malik to the program. The principal and guidance counselor were to some extent aware of the special relationship we were building but advised against it for fear personal involvement, in his case, would backfire. Indeed it almost did.

There were episodes at the school with Danny involving theft, vandalism, and rock throwing. On one occasion a small child was hit and had to be taken to the hospital. Defiantly, he took up a pail of water and doused me with it, but that didn't drown my enthusiasm for helping him. For months, he was invited on weekends and included in activities of my family life. I imagined if things worked out, I possibly could take him in as a foster child. Unfortunately, as Danny sailed into his teen years, he initiated more acts of rebellion, always testing rules and challenging authority. I recall one incident when Danny allowed me to walk several feet ahead, then ran up behind and yanked my pocketbook from my arm in a sort of "game." I should have known something was amiss.

A few weeks later, I received word from his mother he had been arrested, charged with purse snatching and robbery at gunpoint. She asked me to go to court and see about him. The social worker indicated Danny could be released if an adult were willing to accept responsibility. I consented, and he was freed in my custody. We left taking the train to his mom's in Queens. In the madness of the rush-hour crowds, Danny disappeared. So did my hopes of rescuing him from the cycle.

I set out in a search, pounding the pavement in a Latino section of Queens, asking questions of residents who weren't too eager to divulge anything even if they knew. Every day after work, I searched, feeling I was to blame. I went in and out of haunts I thought he might frequent, to no avail. Weeks later, detectives who were obviously better at tracking people down than I located and rearrested him, ending one of the most frightening sagas of my teaching career.

Although things didn't work out exactly as I envisioned, God used the situation as a catalyst for change. Danny's mom, seeing the effort made to help, became convinced her son was worth saving and began participating more fully in planning for his care. Also it let me know there was room in my heart for another child. I thought to have a big brother would be good for Malik. Adopting an older child seemed a reasonable alternative.

Little did I know the Lord already had just the right son waiting in the wings. In fact, he had been coming along on many excursions with Danny as they were good friends. As my relationship with Danny waned, Hector continued coming and seemed right for our family. I knew he was the one. I made the commitment that if given the opportunity, I'd faithfully assume the role of mother. Sure enough, when I approached the counselors, I was told he was freed for adoption and they would consider it. I felt the way a woman feels when she learns she's pregnant—scared, nerves ajangle, but overjoyed!

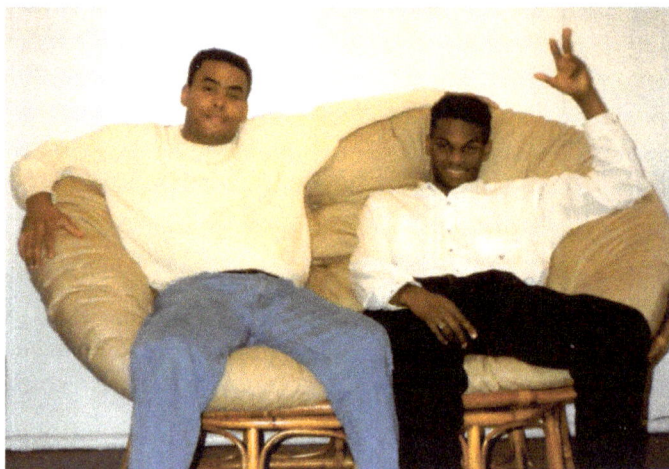

My sons Malik and Hector.

Of course, there'd be a year of foster care to try it out, akin to nine months of the birthing process, with accompanying birth pangs and frustration. Reams of paperwork, evaluations, and social worker visits were required to meet stringent codes as well as an extensive background check. For me, it was like laboring to bring a child into the world. After a year of intense scrutiny, I finally "birthed" a 125 lb. handsome brown-skinned Hispanic son. Hector went through considerable birth trauma. Malik too, when he no longer had his mama to himself. Also it meant finding a bigger apartment so each could have a room and sharing whatever we had three ways.

We faced continuous economic problems and stress. But the Lord filled in the gaps plus provided extra income through the state. Just when we needed it, a three-bedroom unit was offered by one of the ministers of our church. The junior high across from us admitted him so that I'd be close by. And our gym teacher gave him a job helping with after-school athletics to keep busy. Other staff kind of "adopted" him too, supplying needed encouragement. A blend of resources and support was created right around us so that all went well.

Our home became a harmonious mix of cultural traditions richly overlaid with language, foods, and music. Our landlords were Nigerian and our friends from the Caribbean. The pleasing blend created an aroma of a fresh potpourri, which spiced the air with the sway and rhythms of the Third World. As we gradually began to merge, I learned to cook cross-culturally and practiced making foreign words part of my vocabulary. Close interaction brought stronger awareness I did have cultural identity as an African American. This contradicted the erroneous impression I had growing up that we were sort of acultural.

My hands were full with the class, the church, and my two sons. Growing responsibility made me feel like I was on a treadmill moving rapidly and I didn't know how to regulate the flow. Everything was "andale, andale, go, go, go." My life seemed to have no Off button. I was burning myself out but couldn't stop. As women, we grow up learning how to serve others but often fail to realize we must serve ourselves by doing things to unwind.

There was the weekly gruel and grind to get my check then stretch and s-t-r-e-t-c-h. Most of the time I only had tokens to go to work, but no lunch money. So I'd buy coffee and fill my stomach with air while walking across the bridge to go peering in windows of little shops at things I wanted but couldn't afford. I especially favored the display of old-fashioned toys—a rocking horse, miniature cars, overstuffed teddies, a train set, baseball cards, and soldiers made of tin—reminders of the warm days of my youth. That generation of playthings was being replaced by the new—neon pens, stickers, trinket boxes, goop, all nonsensical confetti that fed the desire to have objects of little use. Prices for this fiddle-faddle were astronomical, but they were guaranteed to wile an unsuspecting child.

I had no car or credit cards and couldn't afford a vacation, a weekend excursion, or a shopping spree. I seldom took a trip to the house of beauty, while other women were spending $100 a pop on cosmetology. It made little difference, I'm sure, for those things don't change the heart and soul. It's only external prettiness.

People were becoming very concerned with how they looked on the outside, not on the inside, and gave little time to spiritual matters. Everyone was obsessed with physical well-being and wanted to look slim and trim. We were all so active. Our whole generation and society had become so active and attractive.

At home I had no microwave to nuke my food. I zoomed in the door, started boiling, chopping, and fixing while picking up room to room. On weekends I let dust fly with the broom. We ate lots of chicken a la everything during those streak o' lean years. I actually don't know how I did it, but the Lord made a way out of no way. Christ Himself is a hardy staple.

Soon I started having mini breakdowns—sick a few days, then back in the saddle feeling debilitated, exhausted, suffering voice strain and fatigue. The combination of bad weather, yelling, and stress made my throat a mess. My battery was constantly winding down and needing to be energized. Being able to go to worship, pray, and reflect refreshed me for the daily battle.

Eighty's women traded their high-heeled pumps for jogging sneakers and puffy down coats to brave the slip and slide of brutal New York winters, looking like colorful airbags zipping past the bleak cityscape. After thirteen years, I traded in my short Afro for "the wet look" at age thirty-one. A miracle of modern science gave black women sticky spiral curls with just a squirt from a yellow spray bottle. Advanced technology made practically anything you wanted for your home or person available, but not equally accessible. A common sight was our men queuing up by the thousands in blizzard weather to pick up job applications in all major cities. Most blacks still lived with that "I don't have, can't have, but would like to have mentality," which held poor people in bondage.

Yet we had a federal administration that showed little pity. Political winds changed when the Republicans took office.

Commitment to remedying social problems like inadequate housing died. Many poor were forced to live on the streets. At the same time political leaders used the rising crime statistics to fan the fires of fear and further polarize the races.

In the 1980s, the first cases of the fatal disease AIDS began to surface along with the suggestion it started with blacks in Africa having sex with monkeys and affected minority group members disproportionately because of their "highly promiscuous lifestyles." People were told their tax dollars were going to support folks who didn't deserve it as they brought this condition on themselves. Suddenly the dating game took on deadly consequences. The death toll among our ranks began to mount. Again the black community was identified as a harborage for evil.

Prices rose at the gas pump because of a Middle East oil shortage. More layoffs and job freezes ensued. White middle- and upper-class workers started pounding the pavement looking for work too. People who are insecure about their own job's future are not concerned and giving. This led to a lack of interest in social programs to help the poor. Shelters filled with homeless persons with no options. Hemlines yo-yoed up and down along with the stock market. Everyone felt the crunch and squeeze.

The face of the family had changed since my parents' time, when most kids had two parents in the home. A large number of black women, my age or younger, had no husbands, lived with boyfriends, or had children by different fathers. This was looked upon as okay. Kids growing up under these new arrangements experienced extreme turmoil trying to work out complicated relationships with transient household members. Growing up with a not-so-perfect father is preferable to no dad at all, or having people bouncing in and out and you don't even know what to call them. The infrastructure of our roads and bridges was crumbling. Likewise, the infrastructure of the family was crumbling. Kids sought security and family support outside that normally nurturant body.

Right wasn't the same anymore either. People no longer used God as a standard. Churches, schools, and policemen no longer worked in tandem to reinforce one view of right and wrong. We had relativism, humanism, and situational ethics. In other words, what seemed right to you, that's what you did. That "anything goes" mentality severely impacted poor areas of town where all of society's ills were compressed and intensified. It led to further disintegration of the black community. The ugly blemish of kids killing kids erupted on our visage and bedeviled efforts to throw off the stigma of being violence prone.

So much of what I took for granted would always be there like morality, decency, and accountability disappeared in the air like a puff of smoke. A down and dirty attitude that survived on cynically trashing everyone and everything took hold. It embraced that which was debase, fed on the pain and hurt of others, and mocked anything that purported to have dignity, honesty, or virtue. The farther we moved toward that end, the more I realized the old way was the way to go.

New faces appeared in the media. New stars burst across the stellar heavens of Hollywood—new rich and famous who were younger but lacked real glamor, cult idols of rock, pop, film, and fashion. Their excessive lifestyles centered around numerous relationships, public private lives, spats, divorce, undignified speech and manner, letting punches fly, and airing dirty laundry before the world. Hollywood, the media, and social scientists continued stretching the limits of acceptable behavior, writing new definitions that threatened our most cherished institutions—marriage and family. The concept of a family being a father, mother, and a couple of kids became obsolete.

My mother used to like Ray Charles's soulful rendition of the song "America, America, God shed His grace on thee, and crown thy good with brotherhood from sea to shining sea." However, the nation's bright light had begun to dim. It was not being defeated from without, but from within by growing violence and moral decay. Though still the richest nation in the world, people were very spiritually lacking, empty, and searching for answers to insurmountable problems. A civil war of values was well underway. The silent majority had been driven into the closet for fear of ostracization if they expressed views that were no longer "politically correct." American homes and consciousness were under siege by people and a media that did not hold traditional values. There was a severe shortage of moral leaders in politics. The sociopolitical climate was in transition.

We had advanced from Negro History Week to Black History Month. Comedians joked they deliberately gave us February because it is the shortest month of the year. In our school, you would never have known of its existence anyway, as little attention was paid. Whites tended to regard black holidays and issues as not their concern and saw no benefit in participating. I remember asking a mixed group of students who Dr. Martin Luther King was, and one white kid raised his hand and said, "Yeah, he was the king of *you people*, right?"

Nevertheless, I came to fit in very well there, had found my niche. With time, more minority teachers got hired and reading materials depicting children with chocolate-colored faces began appearing in various places. But on the whole, we had little input in designing curriculum and selecting the literature students read.

Kids had come a long way from "Eeny, meeny, miny moe" back in my Dick and Jane days. They were now learning to interact with inanimate objects on a computer but desperately needed to learn to solve problems with each other. Gangs and weapons were becoming evident in the schools. Seemed like the only peaceful place left was in computer cyberspace. They were being told life was like making choices from a Chinese menu—take one from group A, two from B. But no guidelines were given for making good selections. Some chose to take a human life in a robbery, to settle a score, or just because someone looked at them funny. This left mouths agape with horror at juvenile murders.

We had gone from Jocko back in the fifties to a new host of radio jocks who replaced music to get you in the groove with rumbling, angry music that clobbered you over the head. These "rappers" were not just baying at the moon and seemed to encourage gun violence and disrespect for authority and women. My sons were hip-hopping right along with the rest, causing great consternation. I wondered how long I could keep them under the shadow of my wing and safe from the tide of misplaced anger sweeping the streets.

Gangs operate like a magnetic sphere, drawing boys in by offering a sense of power to those who feel powerless. How would I teach mine to be assets rather than liabilities? Would I learn to be attentive to their special needs, realizing as a black female even I am treated differently? I felt Hector might have a better chance because of his Hispanic surname. Society seemed to prefer people be anything, except just plain black. Malik used to say, "Mommy, you look at me as if I'm *bad*!" Who knows how my exaggerated fears of those teen years were being manifested.

The more loose and amoral things got, the more society held parents responsible for what their children did. My parents could let us go free. But I had to pray each time mine walked out of the door that they'd make it back safely. Inside I practically sat with my finger on the remote button, trying to weed out the new programs coming on TV. Hollywood decided if we wouldn't go to the theater to see trash, they would send it right into our homes (no favor to me). Sometimes there was no warning material would be objectionable. What I thought was offensive, somebody in Hollywood land deemed it okay. Parenting had taken on an all-new stress-laden dimension from making sure the food they ate wasn't laced with sugar to making certain what they fed on in other ways built good character. I tried to provide a home life quiet and stable, while they clamored for Atari, Nintendo, a VCR, and cable. Malik especially was a video game junky.

The increasing rage of young black men could be seen in changing Hollywood depictions of them from bowing and shuffling to sulking and sullen, to angry and defiant. We heard their bray and brawl in the streets and the public outcry for cops to lock 'em up and throw away the keys, while the government lay as if asleep, heedless to their needs. We listened to the statistics on crime and death in the urban centers and watched cities like LA go up in flames in the flash of a moment's rampaging anguish. People asked, "What's it all about?" scratching their heads in utter bewilderment. But I knew!

It was about power, respect, and access to what everybody else wanted and not believing they could get it; about being tired, bored, and frustrated with being ignored, locked out of the system by a society that wouldn't admit them. It was about the myths, the lies, and the promises never kept that if we marched, voted, got an education, looked a certain way, lived in a particular neighborhood, and held a professional job, things would get better when in reality nothing removed the drawback of being black in America.

It was also about wanting things without having to work and getting things fast, no waiting; about making having them so important that you'd kill; about believing you could get something for nothing, believing I deserve to have what I want to have; about seeing sports stars on TV who "had it all" and wanting the same in order to feel like you're *somebody*; about bad influences from the media that fed us on a constant diet of violence and murder; about being stupefied, made immune so that "offing a person" seemed as innocent as killing a bad guy in a video game; about glorifying violence as a way to solve conflict, like in a Clint Eastwood movie where he says, "Go on, make my day!"; about having no fathers in the home to set limits and maintain control; about permissiveness and lack of codes for conduct; about letting money supersede values and brotherly love.

The rancor in the streets came from a root of bitterness about the lack of access to success for so many in spite of four centuries' efforts. We'd gone from a proclamation to emancipation, to demonstrations, to legislation, to integration, to education, through many administrations and then incarceration as the solution to what to do about the black man. Stored-up wrath erupted in seemingly senseless violence. Indeed, many of those young men, if asked, wouldn't be able to articulate their pain and anger. They just walked around feeling so much rage and didn't know whom to direct it at, frequently lashing out at the innocent. Their own black brothers and sisters were often targeted. Like in any family, we hurt the ones closest to us most. When looking at this violence, we must try and understand its root.

There was a whole other side to this story fed by selfish desire to gain attention, money, and power, even at the expense of corrupting a legitimate cause to fulfill self-serving needs. Public performances, records, tapes, and videos were ways of attracting a following and an audience who worshiped and adored them. Hollywood and TV popularized the attitude of the bad boy, the brat, and the rebel. In films, the handsome expletive-shouting young punkster who took on the world often got the girl. Street clothing and speech were top sellers. Rap paraphernalia and cassettes earned millions around the world. Its expressions antiquated standard English. The surrounding hype was used to push everything from hamburgers to soda pop.

Those rebels not in the limelight as stars and artists survived on fear and intimidation, taking over neighborhoods, setting up headquarters in abandoned buildings on every block where the city failed to take action and allowed urban decay and the downturn of communities. We heard the thud and rumble of their stereo boxes as they went galloping through the darkness in expensive cars bought with drug money. They held court under cover of night with a kingly entourage of followers who did their bidding for just a few shillings and the opportunity to be associated with their fame. They became sexual conquistadores—diablos, with no noble cause save to gorge themselves at everyone's expense.

I loved kids—mine, the ones at church, those in school. Each time they came barreling through the door with little superhero lunch boxes, I was reminded of the lack of real heroes in their lives. Instead, music and sports figures, notorious for drugs, womanizing, and brushes with the law, were placed on pedestals. Blacks made tremendous strides in the fields of sports and entertainment, earning money and recognition. However, some left behind the obligation to, like Hank Aaron and Jackie Robinson, be our heroes asserting their lives were their own and they owed no responsibility to the black community to be role models for kids. Many sank into lifestyles that were less than inspiring. Drug arrests and jailings were highly publicized. Still, they drove big flashy cars and carried high profiles. Some even wore diamonds in their teeth! This sent a powerfully wrong message of what it was to succeed. Their lives were as gilded as the heavy gold chains dangling from their necks, while underneath lay only spiritual emptiness.

Blacks had gained access to the national pastime baseball, a game about winning and losing with much social significance to all Americans. Yet its new stars didn't emphasize character, good sportsmanship, discipline, or teamwork—skills kids desperately needed to learn. They taught go for money, fame, frills, thrills, and media attention, even if negative. Never mind fair play or watching hard work pay off. Their acts stain the memory of our cultural history as a people who strived for excellence in sports to open doors. Our aspirations got mired in their disgrace and failure to hold up a standard. A player like Willie Mays was respected not only for who he was but what he stood for.

Back in the fifties, boys played stick ball, handball, scuzzies, or shoot 'em up with cap pistols. By the eighties they were having real shootouts with real guns and bullets. In place of Saturday matinees, they watched friends gunned down on street corners, caught in the crossfire of rival gangs or used as human shields. Violence for amusement led to a loss of the sanctity of human life. A terrible inheritance we left Generation X—a society abounding in violence, cops in the schools, weakened families, and a world with no clear rules.

When I was little, older people had humility, feared the Lord, and respected themselves and others. God was right, the Bible was "the Good Book," the minister was prominent, and Jesus was the way, the truth, and the light. Even if everyone didn't adhere, they all accepted the sovereignty of God, the moral absolutes, and His codes for human conduct. Latter-day blacks, in an attempt to assert a strong new sense of identity, rejected "the white man's religion," which the slave master gave us for bad but accomplished our good.

To the contemporary culture, God had become an anonymous higher power subject to individual interpretation. Your guess was as good as mine about who He was and how to worship Him. We were told to live and let live, to tolerate all points of view, but believe in nothing except our own personal fulfilment. There was no right or wrong, only *opinions*. How you *felt* and what you *had* were more important than what you believed. In the new times, nurturing your spiritual self seemed unimportant, and expressing views that were not "PC" could subject you to persecution at home, on the job, and in schools.

Religious beliefs were not to be expressed in public. Christians were viewed as either fanatics, hypocrites, or weak-minded followers who lacked education or reason. The teachings of the Gospel were repressed by the media, while other points of view were given prominence. The notion of freedom of religion was being interpreted as a guarantee of freedom from religion by our lawmakers. A pronounced effort was seen to keep mention of God, prayer, Christian beliefs or symbols out of public life. As we embraced materialism, we began to reject spiritualism, defying our need for God. Grandma's generation had true dependence on the Lord as the only source who could supply all their needs. We didn't need Him 'cause we had plastic to give us access to the finer things. The more sated we became, the less we thought of Him.

Simultaneously, the old Protestant ethic that valued hard work, starting at the bottom, and working your way up seemed to fade. Those with few technical skills and limited education started at the bottom and stayed there. The notion of choosing and remaining in a job for a lifetime or a man being known by the quality of his work fizzed out. Modern technology and computerization brought rapid turnover, increased mobility, and devalued the individual worker. Everyone wanted to go straight to the top by having the right connections, knowing the right people and learning how to play the game. CEOs, fresh out of diapers, were heading major corporations.

A devastating cultural shift was taking place right before my eyes, and I was left wondering how to respond to it. When I looked at the general picture, it all appeared like an abstract painting, just one big mess. Everything had become so complex. I had the feeling of being swept along by something so much bigger than I was, something impossible to stop or do anything about. I couldn't see how my paltry efforts could restore God, family, and community. Still, as a schoolmarm, I was in there pitching every day, doing my own little thing in a seemingly futile way.

When Grandma visited us in the city years ago, she'd stay just one week, then say she *had* to get back to her simple life down in the country. I wasn't yet old but felt my peace being stolen away as we went speeding into the nineties. My sense was that we were headed for desolation as a nation. Black people, who came forth with great strength and blessing from God, after breaking off the shackles of segregation and ignorance in the '60s, had fallen under a reproach, having lost that which was greater than ourselves guiding us out of bondage.

Many of our youth had no sense of identity or rootedness. The struggles of the past meant nothing, only the momentary pleasures of the present when they got some *thing*, whether by force, robbery, selling of drugs, or killing, that made them feel validated. Their crimes were becoming more vicious and merciless as restraints were removed from their consciences. I decided whatever happened, Christ and I would have to face it together, as I watched a disturbing new chapter unfold.

The gross national product was up a thousand percent. Likewise, violence, crime, and illegitimate births were multiplying. These weren't easy times for me either, for although I was a working professional, I wrestled with old fears of being rejected, not fitting in, not being valued for my contribution, or of trusting and opening up then getting betrayed. I stood out like the dark lines on fancy wall paper. Some days I relished being different for dark lines are an important accent, but other times I wanted to blend in with the background, preferring the safety of anonymity. Besides, my white coworkers expressed themselves verbally so much better than I did, which made me feel intimidated.

Inwardly I resented them, feeling I went through the same ropes as they had to get my education, yet they appeared to have everything, while my life was a constant struggle. To me they were like princesses, heirs to privilege with every advantage at hand, and I was the poor hoi-polloi having to scrimp, scrape, and suffer. It hurt knowing at the end of the day we were heading off to two very different worlds. They'd hop in their nice cars and speed off to fine homes in Westchester, New Jersey, or to a condo right there in Riverdale, while I lugged a satchel full of books and my classroom pets on city buses with cursing, fighting school kids for a two-hour journey across town to a neighborhood crumbling down. I had to get beyond my condemning ideas and realize we each had to meet the other halfway and sometimes go all the way in order to break down barriers.

I went from an underprivileged student to a disadvantaged teacher who couldn't afford the accouterments of middle-class life, being saddled with student loans to pay back and two kids to keep track of. Homework, schoolwork, and church work weighed heavily upon me, and I had very little money. Boy, do I remember those long walks pulling my shopping cart to Pathmark to try to get a bargain on food, the nervous stares at the cash register, and after making it through, quick breezes into Toys-R-Us in response to my son's pleadings. Recall holidays, sons waiting for Kris Kringle, with not a jingle in my pockets. And those wrenching yuletide morns praying they'd feel glee when they saw what Ma put under the tree. Just when I thought I would break under the load, the Lord made provisions in an unexpected way, and I didn't have to burn green candles or scent my house with money-blessing spray!

I'd been working as a temporary sub, being called back yearly, earning minimal salary but doing the work of a tenured teacher. I didn't get the salary I should have because I wasn't a permanent hire. The system did that quite often to minority teachers, reaping the benefits of our labors, holding over the threat of easy dismissal, and paying only a minimum of what we were really worth, saving lots of money in the process. I had my degrees and had taken tests, but my name hadn't come up yet for appointment. The union rep found this to be an error. The fact that I should've been paid a higher wage all those years worked out well for us. I received a lump sum and decided to put it down on a home for the boys and me. Yippee! This poor woman was on top of the world. Finally, I was gonna have something to call my own!

I wanted to move to a good neighborhood, which usually meant white. I felt like running off to a quaint little town, lock the door behind, and throw away the key so no one could follow me, particularly not my people. Really, I wanted black people there, but the "right kind of blacks," folks with good values who were community minded.

We were all affected by hearing too much of our tragedies and not enough of our triumphs in the media. Whites said they didn't fear black women but feared our male children. We feared one another because the majority of us were law-abiding citizens who were frequently victims rather than perpetrators of crime. We remained limited in our choice of places to live, not by legal restriction, but by social coercion—stares and suspicious looks, being followed around in stores, uncomfortably cold behavior, nonaccepting attitudes, rudeness, or being totally ignored.

Another impediment was my dependence on public transportation. Like many working poor, I had no vehicle and needed to ride the bus to work. Suburban areas often turn down rapid transit as a way of keeping "undesirables" out. Distance and travel became inhibitory factors.

I discovered prices for housing in white areas were often lower than ours, contrary to popular belief. However, finding someone to rent to us or getting a bank to secure a loan for a home outside a designated target area was no easy task. It was twice as hard for a minority person to get a mortgage from a bank. They simply didn't believe in our success. A major stumbling block was they looked for a history of stability and security, which many didn't have, or relatives to put up cash for collateral. Despite a large down payment, I had to turn to a small loan company and pay high interest rates, which burdened me with a hefty monthly payment.

Some African Americans actually prefer living in black communities, deeming it more healthful for their children in developing a strong group identity. As a mark of cultural pride and for the freedom to live in a manner most comfortable, they hold on to that which is familiar. Many other ethnic minorities do the same—live where they find products and services conducive to their needs such as foods, fashions, hair care, and entertainment. We also exercise greater political strength when concentrated in large numbers.

The main issue for me was to find a place where my sons and I would feel safe, be accepted, and have friends. Everyone wants to fit in. Black teens often were harassed in white areas by cops or gangs of white youth protecting "their turf." I feared having to defend my home and children from abuse, as sometimes others show little respect for black home ownership. Our safety as well as our security was at stake. I considered buying into Co-op City, an integrated development where whites didn't seem to run when they saw us coming. I liked the idea of a mutually respectful relationship that wasn't forced as I didn't wish to cram myself down anyone's throat. But I was told although residents lived together, whites felt *they* ought to run things.

How I wish I didn't have to go around with an awareness that I am a black American living in a white society, having to worry where I can go, fit in, and be accepted, and who'll give me a chance. Wish I could be just like everybody else and have society's vote of confidence, until I give people reason to think otherwise. There are those now saying American society is unmeltable, that we will always be a multicultural society fractured by poor race relations, but I am hoping to see the day we become a nation of gorgeous hues as we come together. It will take a communication revolution to break down barriers.

One notion that grew out of the civil rights era was that we all had to be side by side in order for high standards to be maintained as in schools. I didn't agree. I wanted to believe in our ability to establish and take care of our own. Many blacks were talking about taking back our communities and had stopped pushing for integration. I decided to approach things from that perspective, stay where I had roots and felt commitment to make conditions better. My North Bronx neighborhood meant something to me, for it embodied my history and cradled my family. So I walked right around the corner and spotted a little house that once was the garage of the people next door but had been remodeled. Though a tiny salt box, it was big enough for us.

I purchased it, moved in, but immediately began having problems with my new neighbors. One of the few Italian families left in that vicinity, their attitude was one of "We may be poor, but we are still white!" The mother particularly showed her dislike, told her children not to play with mine, blocked my driveway all the time with her car, and stuffed dirty rags into the fence, creating an ongoing nuisance. I thought she was implying things looking run-down for us was okay. I saw no resort but to go to court to get respect for boundaries.

There was a hopeful ray; her son came on over to play anyway. She'd be outside calling while he'd be in there hiding, and I'd have to chase him home. She would have freaked if she had known! Our sons were great friends in spite of her and me not speaking. With time, we followed their lead and started communicating. Soon we realized we were much the same, just two single moms doing the best we could to see our kids grow up good. The Bible says, "A little child shall lead them."

We got down to a lot of last chickens during those red beans and rice years. Living on a teacher's salary, we couldn't afford a lot of things but pulled our belts tightly and managed. Eventually, I was able to make additions, plant landscaping, and buy new furnishings. God supplied a witty older woman close by to mentor me in all the little things I needed to know to grow as a home owner. His ever-present grace was always sufficient.

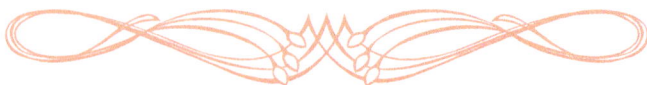

CHAPTER TWENTY-THREE
The Pinnacle

I had gone through a period of rebellion and separation—of marriage and childbearing, of returning, repenting, refocusing, rebuilding, then seeking and attaining. Now, it was establishment and accomplishment. Many new years had become old years past and thirty-five balls dropped on Forty-Second Street. Times Square had become the bedroom of the homeless, the porn halls, the prostitutes, the gays and sleaze. Crime, injustice, and family disintegration were all around. There were changes, changes, so many changes!

We'd evolved into a throwaway society based on consuming. We lived to take in and feed the self. It was a time of junk food and junk bonds. Satisfaction always had to be immediate, solutions fast. The buzzwords of the eighties were *self-help*, *discovery*, *determination*, and *fulfilment*. We believed we were masters of our fate and captains of our souls, that we were in control and could create our own security. We were no longer talking about moonwalks but moon colonies. Test tube babies had become a reality. We had more knowledge, technology, and information, but less wisdom. In our striving to acquire wealth and prestige, we didn't always notice what was happening to, around, or in us.

It was a scientific era. We'd advanced from the discovery of electricity to genetic engineering and were trying to crack the code to life itself. Scientists were supposedly closing in on diseases that plagued man for centuries developing new medicines and procedures for practically anything that ailed you. Man was attempting to manipulate genes, trying to play God, threatening to eliminate all individuality and difference because according to man's wisdom, some of us are highly desirable, while others we'd be better off without. By the twenty-first century, we hoped to be able to influence the human blueprint, and indeed we'd opened the door by managing to clone sheep. However, God's creative process remained a mystery, as did His reasons for making us different—some black, some white, some Oriental, some "normal," and some exceptional.

Changes in how we got goods and services were evident. An information superhighway was being formed by computer networks. Telephones, satellites, and fax machines were making the world smaller. We began talking about the world as our neighborhood, world economies, and global communities. Black America had Oprah, OJ, the Mikes (Jordan, Jackson, and Tyson), the Cosbys, Aretha and Tina, Maya and Alice Walker, as well as a host of political figures. Yet most were still traveling dirt back roads, looking for an access road. We continued to have difficult human conflicts to conquer as a nation called to world leadership.

New York City turned into a Barnum & Bailey Circus and every motley clown put on a show, except their characterizations were sad rather than funny. The center attraction was Mayor Koch, acting as ringmaster, cracking his whip trying to keep the animals under control. And there I was, a juggler, attempting to toss the balls of life, balance the ups and downs, keep them all in sync. The pace was fast moving, nonstop, no time limits. Watches with alarms kept us all on track. My life was pressure packed, stressed out. As I went after prosperity, I struggled to hold on to my sanity. Life was driving me into overload because of my extreme sense of responsibility for everyone else's.

I went on playing "messiah," always overextending myself. At church I was an usher, Sunday school teacher, summer camp director, and food bank organizer. At home, I was chief cook and bottle washer, while at school teaching and taking computer training. "Success" was demanding more each day, and I was stretching to cover all the bases. But we were supposed to learn to deal with many factors going on simultaneously and take risks, so said the popular rhetoric.

Around me there were many broken and hurting people. I was enmeshed in their lives, being motivated by pain. I felt deeply concerned about my parents. My father's drinking worsened, in spite of constant prayer and beseeching God. Their communication declined. They became like two remote islands separated by a broad and torrent sea, with me trying to swim from shore to shore. Yet they remained under the same roof. My sister's marriage had ended, and brother Sonny was searching. Everyone had problems, and I was always stepping in to solve them. I'd become accustomed to the rescuer role.

When you live that way, it is easy to become fragmented. I placed a little of myself here, a little there. It became a battle to hold it all together—meeting the boss's expectations, carrying on the role of teacher-mom and my obligations to my church family, being a provider and home manager, getting repairs done, being the family guardian and protector, trying to have a social life and me time, being the spiritual leader of my home, and taking courses for advancement. I constantly felt drained and strained.

I set myself up as an old mule, a beast of burden, bearing all the responsibility with no one to help carry the load. I didn't know how to work, play, eat, rest, and sing a little and didn't require enough of others.

I wanted a man in my life but was unwilling to just grab anyone. Black women had so few choices of good men, and there were many cads out there looking for someone to use and abuse, for a place to flop, deal drugs, and go in and out freely. They desired no commitment and had very little to offer, except free cocaine or babies. I couldn't see letting myself become that type of victim.

Time kept edging onward; the boys got older. Before long, Hector was off to a special high school to study baking and Malik transferred to another private setting. They were becoming more socially active outside our home. I did my best to stay abreast of what was going on. I saw teens dangling off the backs of city buses, scrawling graffiti on walls, and riding atop subway cars in a need for strange kicks and thrills by doing destructive things. Even the "good kids" didn't want to be wholesome and squeaky clean. I asked myself, what would all this mean?

We were headed toward a new decade, in the era of new technologies, the information age. White kids' families began sending them abroad to study and gain international experience in preparation for performance on the world stage. Minority kids rarely got a chance to get out of their inner-city neighborhoods, not even to see other parts of this country, let alone another. And there were still places they couldn't go and feel welcomed. As potential future employees, they were becoming as obsolete as burgeoning file cabinets were for storing information or as black rotary desk phones were for dialing. Urban schools needed more machinery to make kids adequate for a job market that would require highly specialized skills in the use of computers.

I was asked to help bring new technology to my special ed classroom by participating in a computer-based project to help kids read. It involved equipping the room with three PCs to be used as writing tools the way chalk and blackboard or pencil and paper were used in the past. A method of putting ideas down was taught using phonetic spelling. The children could compose stories, edit, then print storybooks to be read aloud. The accompanying software provided auditory and picture clues to help develop their skill, reducing some of the frustration the students felt in not being able to spell well. Once written, the children would be eager to read stories to others, paying off in rewards of self-confidence in having achieved. Parents in turn offered praise and undivided attention, providing encouragement to do more. Fear of failure removed, success was then undergirded by positive reinforcement.

This was wonderful for me, as I had a number of boys who seemed particularly drawn to the computer screen and were masters at action video games. They had natural affinity for 3D and were fascinated by machines. It easily captured their interest. The results were phenomenal! Within a short time, each student could "boot up" the computer, type in their text, and print it out at will. What a thrill it was to see their smiling faces at having conquered the machine, which even I was afraid of because it was so brainy and made me feel dumb. All this newfangled technology was much more frightening to my generation than theirs. Buttons to press, diskettes, lights, sounds whirring around inside, those tabletop monsters were as threatening as an attacking gorilla. Thought I'd never get it together!

When the computer training opportunity came up, the principal selected me and a white alternate. I didn't know if it was to have equal racial representation or an assumption I might fail and she'd be there to pick up the slack. I certainly didn't feel capable of becoming a computer hack. There was no monetary compensation, and perhaps they just needed someone who wouldn't run from a lot of extra work. Well anyway, I was sent; I went and did quite well. Much better than I ever expected of myself.

Before long, my classroom became the demonstration model for that project in the Bronx. Educators came to see our workshop in progress and learn how to set it up. Student teachers were assigned to be my apprentices. An instructional video was made of the students at work and their books displayed at the head office. I received verbal accolades, gifts of appreciation from parents, and congrats from other staff. In the halls they whispered, "Here comes Ms. Barrett!" whenever I approached. I started taking myself seriously, though embarrassed by all the attention. An article appeared in an educational publication about our success. The only downside was that article bore the picture of a blond-haired teacher standing over a student working at a computer station. Apparently, someone felt that to make the program appear sound and workable, the teacher in charge needed to be white.

Nevertheless, I started having the feeling of having "arrived." Being in the limelight, even for a short time, can give you a jolt of confidence. Little did I know this would be my swan song, for right around the corner lurked something unexpected and I was unprepared to deal with. Just when I'd reached a high point in my career, the bottom dropped out and I was caught off guard!

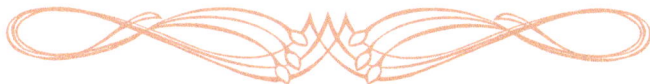

CHAPTER TWENTY-FOUR
The Crucible

IT happens often in life that moments of great triumph are juxtaposed with events of defeat, downfall, and sadness. We all fear sickness and death and never imagine it coming into our lives, particularly at a young age. Inevitably, we all must face a bend in the road. It is God who changes our times and epochs. All of a sudden, my little world broke down.

It began quite innocuously with a bad bout with laryngitis, physical exhaustion, and fatigue, which seemed to occur with greater frequency as the years accelerated. I blamed it on the severe New York winters traipsing the streets in snow and rain not well covered. In any case, it would soon be Christmas break, and I more than needed time off. I stayed out a full two weeks, unable to speak, throat so sore swallowing my own saliva was a chore. I did the usual—bed rest, lozenges, hot tea, popping pills—but their effect was nil. This happened many times in the past, and I'd always had difficulty projecting my voice. Years before at a college seminar on speech disorders, I was duly warned to get it checked, but I said what the heck. Those portentous words now return to haunt.

My two-week hiatus ran into the holiday recess, giving me two additional weeks to pamper myself, which made me physically better, but my speech remained barely audible above a squeak or whisper. I appeared in school after New Year's, determined to ride it out, give the kids busy work a few more days, until I snapped out of it. The problem is, I didn't snap.

It appeared to be trying to return, but it was scraggly and draggy like an old hag. I felt demon possessed. Each time I opened my mouth and strange awful sounds came out, I asked myself who was that talking. I couldn't believe it was actually me and started wondering if some supernatural hocus-pocus hadn't really taken place, if there was an evil spirit speaking from within. I sounded like a 45 rpm played on slow speed. Of course, no one could figure out what on earth I was saying, and the kids were all quite alarmed. One little darling raised her hand and asked if I were turning into the wicked witch. That comment sent me packing to an ENT hospital to see a specialist. After a pharyngological exam, I was told they saw a chink in my vocal cords and that I needed voice rest. How long? Perhaps not long.

I headed straight back to school. Were they crazy? I couldn't take time off! The program couldn't go on without *me*. I was responsible! The whole show would collapse if I wasn't there to do what I had to do. There was no time to take care of myself. Besides, I needed my paycheck.

I tried to improvise by using speech amplification devices, thinking if I could just get by with a microphone for a while and not stress my vocal cords, they'd come back to themselves. Each day I went in flapping my hands, playing charades to get the kids to understand, trying to keep control. Things were worsening. It was obvious I couldn't continue much longer, in fairness to the kids for they were not learning.

After several trips back to clinic, I was advised if I wanted to regain my speech, I'd have to give up teaching and go on complete voice rest. Vocal stress had taken its toll, and I'd need a change of professions. On February 2, I'd planned to go in and tell the kids whether the groundhog had seen its shadow foretelling six more weeks of winter—a pleasant bit of senseless nonsense on a bitter cold frosty day. Instead, I had to go in and announce that I was going away, retiring for health reasons. A shadow now loomed over me and was making me afraid.

There comes a time in life we all must do hard things. Life is not fair. It brings a progression of tough choices. The choice to stop work and seek help for my voice problem was one of the most difficult I ever had to make. I asked myself, "Am I doing the right thing? Making the right decision?" It took every ounce of courage I could muster up. God! I would miss the kids so much! I had a tremendous battle with guilt feeling I was abandoning them and shirking my duties. Never before had I put my needs before others, but I knew I had to let go, walk away. There was no getting around it. The job had already cost me more than I should be asked to give.

It was a bitter irony that just when I thought I'd found my nest, had gotten comfortable, lined it with down and feathers, and was settling in for many more winters, I had to take the wings of faith and fly off into a dark foreboding sky, headed who knows where. Unlike birds who seem to be guided by internal sensors, I had no idea where I was going or how I would survive. Most of all I feared this "demon" that had taken over my body and needed to be exorcized.

The principal was quite understanding, knowing how I'd agonized before coming to that decision. He phoned a request in for a disability pension, which would provide me with one-third of my pay. At least I'd walk away with something. The mechanics and processing, however, would take months. Meanwhile, I'd have to find a way to make it. Thank God, I'd get a sizeable tax return in April to help me over the hurdle! But what then? When work life is finished, we think it's the end because we feel no longer useful and know retirement is usually followed by death.

In the span of a day, I went from the pinnacle of my career to joblessness and possibly soon homelessness, if I didn't get income fast. I couldn't let show how devastated I was, so I tried to face it stoically like my father, keep the door shut on my emotions and not divulge my intense fear. I was in denial. I remember spending the day hiding in my classroom, coworkers likewise hiding in theirs, no one knowing what to say. It's easier to avoid talking about pain, especially when you can't speak, but I knew my liquid eyes would give me away. At dismissal I went out into the hall with a big smile and a gentle nod (my way of saying, "See you tomorrow!"), knowing it was a lie, fighting to hold back the flood of tears welling up inside.

I bit my bottom lip and said, "I can handle this!" because even women were expected to be "real men" and not flinch when hurting. Yet I was trembling in my shoes and wanted to collapse in someone's arms for reassurance. I just couldn't punch that clock and walk out the front door, so I collected my things and slipped out a side exit, unable to say goodbye. I was picked up on the corner by my son Hector, holding a box full of memories and my turtle, Benjy. He pretended not to see that I was crushed and just let quiet reign still in the purring automobile the long way home. Sons can be kind sometimes. It's good to have them!

Once in the house, it wasn't too bad. You know how you tell yourself you're going to enjoy this, do all the things you always wanted to do—lay in bed, watch TV, enjoy the garden. Retirement is the life! You know, watching other people heading to work from your window. That only lasted about two weeks before I wanted to get busy again.

When moving into unchartered waters, the fear is intense, and so is the uncertainty. You don't know where to go or what to do. My occupation, finances, and whole identity were at stake. Life became confusion mixed with frustration, multiplied by anxiety. I was like a flickering star shining in the night whose light suddenly went out. Quietly I fell from view. No one saw me within the four walls of my room. That position that meant so much was gone. Ms. Barrett? Why, she was gone too. There seemed no doubt I was through!

I felt devastated, paralyzed by my situation. All my life I'd tried to be a person who could. Nothing prepared me to accept that I couldn't, and there was no view beyond my immediate circumstances. I asked myself, What am I going to do? Why did this happen to me? I was perplexed, didn't know where God was leading.

It's difficult to walk away emotionally from what you do. You always think you can put the past behind, but some mornings it's right there staring you in the face. Some things I couldn't forget, especially those precious moments with the kids when we enjoyed a special relationship and I saw love sparkle like sunny twinkles in their eyes. When I made a breakthrough and knew they understood, it felt good. I missed the vibrancy of the teaching dynamic.

What happens when the things you hope in disappear? You hope in your job, become disabled, you lose your job. You hope in your bank account, become disabled, the bank account dwindles to nothing. You hope in friends, become disabled, friends are first to go. You hope in health and strength. Chronic illness takes that away. My only real hope was in the Lord to meet all my needs. I began asking in view of my loss, "Who am I?"

Am I what I have? My things? Savings? My furniture? The house? Am I what I do? My job? My position?

Am I what I have achieved? My goals? My degrees? My licenses?

When you develop a disability, all these become threatened. You must reevaluate and redefine your life, value new things, see yourself in a new way, change the focus from externals to internals.

I plunged rashly into a new identity crisis. It was so painful not being able to make myself understood. I had lost *me*, not only as a teacher, but personally. How we express ourselves is a very important aspect of our self-concept and identity. Words are revelations of the people who speak them. They make things knowable about us. What would I do without them? How would I reveal myself? I had an MA in education. Now I would earn an MS in self-doubt. I would go through a practicum in the other side of disability—what it means to live with it. My mind would have to be remodeled to a new way of thinking about myself and a new way of living.

When you're traveling down a dark and unfamiliar path, there are lots of questions. You don't know where the edges of the cliffs are. You must trust God to go ahead and open the door. We conquer not by leaps and bounds but by just continuing day by day as we put our trust in Christ, finding strength to take another step. Life doesn't get easier; it gets harder. You can't just go sit in a corner and become disabled. All of life's responsibilities go on as well as the pressures and problems of everyday living, particularly within families. The disability becomes an added burden tacked onto everything else. Its impact made me feel like I was going insane!

But I've always been a compliant person, even with my disability. I wasn't so inclined to rail upward at God and say, "Why did you do this to me?" Guess I'd learned enough about Him to understand His sovereignty. I knew if He allowed it to happen, I'd not be left alone to deal with it. I was also somewhat of a challenging person in the sense that I said, "Well, let me go and just see what I can do about it." (You know, take care of business.) I set out to go to speech therapy, do my vocal exercises, and wade through it, hoping voila! It would get better. Even Christians pray for quick solutions. When tough times come, we all want to get it over as fast as possible.

When you are young, strong, and well, you get the idea you have the world in your pocket, that you are invincible. It isn't until something happens that you realize your fragility and your mortality. You turn to God and want to know He will be there for you. I felt like a child lost in the night. Behind every shadow lies fear. I curled up, tried to comfort myself, and prayed to be rescued, that Mommy and Daddy would come soon and save me. I wanted my heavenly Father to "let this cup pass from me" so I could go on and do what I had to do. One of the hardest things is knowing you can't do anything for yourself and those around you, whom you've always turned to for comfort, can't do a thing for you either. You must bear your grief alone.

I found myself like the child in this song:

> Whenever I feel afraid,
> I hold my head erect,
> And whistle a happy tune so no one will suspect,
> I'm afraid.
> Though shivering in my shoes,
> I strike a careless pose
> Sing fa la la la,
> So no one ever knows I'm afraid.

I was in need of a comforter but was called on to live out this experience. It wasn't going to just go away as I had hoped.

When you develop a disability, you feel like you have walked down a dead-end street, that you're out of action and ready for the garbage heap. You feel ashamed you have this weakness. You feel incompetent and vulnerable. You feel deformed and different.

It's impossible to describe how it is to be able to think CAT, but when you open your mouth, it comes out gibberish. It's like having a computer virus in your brain! My impulse was to take my hand and bang my head a few times really hard because the message wasn't coming through. I couldn't figure out why. That little word looked so easy. I knew what I intended to say, but no one knew what I meant. "Normal" people don't think about talking. They just speak effortlessly. Folks looked at me like I was crazy. Their curled expressions suggested something was seriously wrong with me, though they wouldn't come right out and say it. Deep breathing and relaxation techniques didn't help. My brain was not transmitting the messages correctly. Doctors said maybe something was wrong with my nerve endings (the myelin sheath). I continued therapy sessions weeks and months for "dysphonia," paid partly by my mom and sis. The financial burden was considerable—fifty dollars a visit, five days a week. It's beautiful how family can pull together to help when a crisis occurs. Every day I took the train downtown to my speech lesson with a glimmer of hope that my voice would be restored soon and I'd be back in the running.

Each day I awakened, the first thing I did lying there was to try and speak one word. It seemed I lived for that moment when I'd open my eyes and mouth simultaneously to see if my voice came back. When it hadn't, there was no apparent reason to get out of bed, like what was the use of living in this condition? As time passed it got harder and harder to find cause to go on. I waited twenty-four hours for just one moment to wake up and try. And when I couldn't, the other twenty-three hours and fifty-nine minutes hardly seemed worthwhile.

The speech therapist was a real gem. She made our sessions lighthearted and fun, I suppose knowing the weight the experience carried with it. Practice lists of silly words and jingles were drawn up to say. The first contained two syllable words like *mama* and *papa*, but what came out was blah blah. Another list was prepared, but this time of monosyllables like *cat, fat, hat,* and I flubbed that. She cut it to just a consonant and a vowel, *ma, pa, da,* but I didn't get very far. Instead of improving, I was progressively declining and feeling more and more frustrated. All the while, she kept smiling and telling me how good I was doing, wanting to keep my spirits high. We went on down to single-letter sounds like *c, b, d, f, l,* and I said ugh, ugh, ugh, ugh!

I remember the day of reckoning, the day I knew it was *gone,* I mean totally gone. I went in for my usual lesson, and the therapist had an assistant working with her. Of course, being a student, she was gung-ho on proving herself and her ability to teach speech. She took me aside with my word lists, and we started from the top. With each try her face was like, "But that's so easy. Surely you can say that!" I kept struggling and trying, but all that came out were awful grunts and ugly guttural sounds. I couldn't even purse my lips in the shape of letters without their trembling and wandering all over my face. I was losing muscle control in my labial area.

In frustration, she threw up her hands and said, "Well, let's hear you say *um hum* or *uh uhhh* like for yes or no!" I pushed and squeezed the muscles of my chest and stomach together to try to at least do that but could only make a high-pitched noise or grunts and groans like an animal. I pounced my head down on the table and sobbed bitterly. I knew at that moment it was gone and there was no sense holding on to hope. It was like a rope had slipped through my fingers. Suddenly I was falling down into a deep and bottomless pit and nothing could stop it. I had gone all the way to the bottom emotionally and would have to learn how to crawl back out of this well of pity or I would drown.

With the loss of speech came the feeling I was no longer *normal* and I was now of lower estate. I began to grieve deeply for the me I used to be. I reminded myself of the apelike creature called Chewie in the *Stars Wars* movie. At least I had one soul mate! I felt I needed to walk with my head hung down and eyes cast down. I felt like there was something terribly wrong with me, but I didn't know what. I found out what real hopelessness feels like. The Lord would have to show me how to navigate this trial, not by giving me a road map to get out of it, but by guiding me through it. Even though the way was dark and I was afraid, I knew I could trust Him. He had given me a promise, "If you make your bed in hell, I will be there!" I would not make any progress until I could say, "Nevertheless, not my will but thine be done."

How do we handle change that cannot change? I felt so helpless and overwhelmed by all I had to do in spite of my disability to live on, to put food on the table, pay bills, and take care of my sons. I wondered how I would ever make it this way.

I'll never forget riding home on the subway one day, coming back from therapy, sitting, nodding, about to fall asleep, when all of a sudden, a Hispanic teenager across from me jumped up and yanked my gold chain from my neck. In a split second, he popped through the closing doors and ran down the platform, leaving me so stunned I was unable to react and, even worse, unable to call for help or explain what had happened. That moment, I realized how absolutely vulnerable I was. Other passengers gathering around called the transit cop while I just sat in total helplessness, wanting to vent outrage at such an act which robbed me of a token of love given to me on my birthday.

Sometimes the things we think are secure pass away. It can be a job, a car, a home, a loved one, even ourselves, and it rips up our heart and soul. That's the way I felt, like I had actually died. Inside I listened to my own sad requiem. When things we've struggled and fought so hard for are gone, we feel distressed by the emptiness left behind. I couldn't get *me* off my mind, sat missing myself and what I used to be like all the time. I went through a period of lamentation, of deep, deep loss. I grieved the loss of my esteem as a teacher, the loss of choices because of the disability, the loss of daily interaction with family and friends—all those not so obvious hidden losses that came along with it.

So much had changed—the times, my look, our family, my body, circumstances. All this would take great adjustment. I would have to work my way through the loss so that I wouldn't sit and grow filled with bitterness at being cut off so suddenly from what I loved to do and loved ones around me. I had to find a new purpose and direction for my life.

The only model I had of a mute was the endearing rogue in the film *Gigio* played sympathetically by Jackie Gleason, who lived in the streets and brothels of France, stole for a living, and became the town buffoon. The tenderhearted rascal fell in love with the town prostitute and her child and treated them kindly. He was both mocked and loved by the villagers who were amused by his mime and jocundity.

There was also a mute Swede who came to my home on a work team with black men to repair my sidewalk, whom they affectionately referred to as Dummy. It struck me how he had to abandon his own race to find work and acceptance. I thought about animals like a doe or rabbit, which are silent. I didn't mind being like one of them, but where would I find a place to belong? Was I now a dummy?

I felt forgotten, stripped of everything that made me, *me*. I felt invisible and insignificant like a ghost that didn't really matter. In the old TV sequel *Topper*, only certain people could see or hear him. In my case, everyone could see me, but no one could communicate with me even though I was right in their midst. I couldn't convey anything unless I wrote it down on paper. My sister had visual problems and couldn't read my notes. My younger son didn't read well either because of his learning disability. The older one was away at college and couldn't call to talk. Mom, each time, had to go and find her glasses, and Dad was sort of incoherent when drinking. It was hard on me and them as well.

I suppose the most devastating moment was one day when the telephone rang and an anxious operator asked to speak with Hector's parent. She was calling from the emergency room at Rhode Island Hospital. He had been in a car accident, and they were trying to reach his next of kin. I didn't know if he was alive or dead and couldn't ask. I wanted to say, "Yes, this is me. I am his mother!" But all that came out were meaningless moans and groans. It was heart-rending knowing he needed me and I couldn't respond. I pulled on a coat, rode down to Penn Station, made my way up there, writing notes all along to ask directions. I found him in traction scuffed up pretty badly but okay. I was the one all shaken up! Guess that experience taught me I could still do what I had to.

With the loss of speech, every situation that required good communication became impaired. Panic easily set in. I couldn't get the help I needed and was not able to tell people what was wrong. Outwardly I had no obvious malady. Others may have wanted to help but didn't understand me.

I got sick just in time to run into the notion of a sick person as a health consumer. Those with no job and little insurance had very little clout. I'd quit speech deciding to go for a battery of neurological tests. At first I went to one of those mills for the working poor where you go in, take a number, and sit for what seems like an eternity waiting to be called. Everywhere I went, staff informed doctors I was formerly a teacher, as if that somehow redeemed me from being in my present state and perhaps entitled me to a little consideration in the meting out of service. It didn't much help.

·Those places hire a lot of foreign doctors who don't speak English too well. I'm not mocking anyone's national origin, but speaking strictly in terms of communication. I couldn't say their names, nor they mine, couldn't get any understanding with my scribbled notes. Some foreigners harbor negative attitudes toward members of the Afro-American community, thinking that we are a bunch of sniveling, groveling freeloaders because of what they've heard before arrival here. One Arabic doctor told me, "What do you want me to do, reach my hand in my pocket and take out money and give it to you?" which was a painful insult in response to my noting I was going through financial hardship and worried about the expense of treatment. Tests performed were inconclusive, and there were long delays between appointments. They kept making requests for more tests and sent me to a different doctor each time I came in, putting me in a spin. These guys were nothing like the image of kindly Dr. Welby, who comforted the sick with words of wit while healing hurts, body, mind, and spirit.

Each visit I held my breath thinking someone would say or do something to get down to the root. White-coat intellectuals with stethoscopes hung around their necks are viewed by most Americans as minor gods with all the answers locked up in their heads. I kept looking for the quick fix that would drive my troubles away, ease the pain. But they didn't know, nor did I, its source.

We are all underneath a load or a heavy burden sometimes, all in trouble in one way or the other. As a young girl I wrestled with certain things. When I got older, something new came along. Life is a constant fight to stand and withstand. All it takes is one special problem to cross us up and medical problems pack a heavy wallop! All of a sudden, nothing in my life was simple.

Prolonged illness can throw a family into bankruptcy and bring great stress and financial turmoil. I didn't want to become a financial liability to my family. They had love to give and concern, but no money. I was fast sinking into a morass of bills and didn't wish to drag them through the mud with me. I wanted to be able to go to a teaching hospital with a good reputation instead of a small clinic but needed money for payment. As I had no other insurance coverage, that sent me with open hands to the government entitlement programs—welfare, Medicaid, food stamps—seeking temporary assistance until Social Security kicked in, making me eligible for Medicare.

I'll never get over man's inhumanity to man, how dispassionate some can be to another person's dilemma. When you go to those places, you are not treated like a delicate piece of glass even though your life is in turmoil. People don't handle you gently, don't view you as fragile or precious. They are more apt to rough you up, some deliberately and others because the system itself mandates it. They look upon you with icy stares, so unmoved by your situation. Nothing you say matters. Maybe they've heard it all before, or perhaps they just don't care! Since you are looking for something free, they're not going to make it easy on you. You'll definitely have to pay in dignity. Where some think to show compassion, the mood of the day, which is rage toward those who get something for nothing, deems it unacceptable.

When you develop a disability suddenly, you must depend on the compassion of strangers when nine out of ten have none. A person who needs to depend is anathema in today's culture. I felt like saying, "Hey! I played by the rules, dropped public assistance, got an education, worked, and paid my dues to society. Under the circumstances, I should be able to ask for temporary aid." They didn't think so, leaving me no place to go. It was always, I should be covered under some other agency, not theirs. The Social Security Administration took more than a year to process my claim and provided nothing in between. They also would not just accept my case without a long, drawn-out, complicated rigmarole.

To think I tried to do something with my life, now was back begging. Had prided myself in self-sufficiency, but had returned to dependency. There is an incredible indignity in having to ask for support from the state. You can't have a car, home, savings—nothing. All your assets must be less than the government's guidelines. The Welfare Department wanted total control of my life in exchange for benefits, wanted to pick and pry into every detail of my existence. I had to lay myself bare before them, answer demeaning questions, and accept their humiliation. I presented every one of my important documents for their inspection. All at once my liberty was at risk.

Workers took full control of my time, expected me to sit hours on end, while they took coffee breaks, did lunch, and shuffled papers across their desks, toying with me, enjoying having me at their mercy as life is often merciless to them as low-paid city employees. Regardless to my being traumatized by emotional upheaval, they sat cruelly playing games.

It is this same wicked system that has been so destructive to the black family unit, separating husbands and wives in order for mothers to collect a check. In the present day, with government officials talking about making people bite the bullet, God help those who are in need!

Agency staff appeared callous or impassive, lackadaisically blurting instructions to me when I could hardly hear what they were saying above the rumble of my own angry stomach panging for food. They spoke with complete abandon or total hostility, as if I were a criminal because misfortune had befallen me, being empowered by a little desk job to make my life miserable. As instruments of the system, they quickly asserted they were "just doing their jobs" but became enthralled with the power to control. The city used them like it did us. We were all pawns in the game. Only the power brokers won, while those straw gods got to feel puffed up by stepping on the backs of the people they served.

There was so little compassion for those with limitations. Few were sympathetic to our needs. Most felt if I should be out there working, so should you! You have a disability? Tough! Work around it! Other people had problems and still worked. They sat reciting every code in the book and refused to bend the rules or make exceptions. Mine was no special case. In fact, who was I anyway that they should even blink an eye and give me consideration? To do that would require a heart and a conscience, and both were in short supply at the time.

As many social workers were minority group members, to me this was another form of black-on-black crime with the underlying system pulling the strings. When we saw our own in jobs, we had a tendency to feel a linkage and familiarity with the person, believing they would understand what we were going through. How easily we forget once we are on the other side of the desk! Some drain every ounce of pride out of you, sit there watching you beg with cold-hearted indifference and act as if the money is coming out of their pockets. I realize they have an obligation to act responsibly and must give an account, but when she got up and pranced around with that facial expression like Maid Marion waiting for the peons to bow, it galled me. Others just glued their eyes to their computer screens, I guess because it was easier than looking at the faces of real human beings who were hurting. The popular attitude was, "You're all liars trying to get over on the system!" Sadly, the professional cheats knew exactly what to say and how to skirt the rules. The legitimately needy find it hard to get assistance.

I sat bleary eyed like a zombie in dirty reception areas filled with women puffing on cigarettes, babies whining, their diapers wet—the stench of humanity in my nose. Being ignored made me feel like a nonperson, just ornamentation against a dull background—vomit-green walls, plastic chairs, an exit sign inviting me to leave, if I dared. Who cared? There was nothing but cold stares. Though my insides raged, I'd reached a stage of desperate patience, waited them out, knowing I was as unimportant in their eyes as the little black flies flitting aimlessly around the room, sickened by the gloom. My life became so entangled in red tape and paperwork. I longed to break free and retrieve my dignity. But I was powerless to deal with this system. There wasn't anyone along to help with communication. I wrote reams of notes, which they impatiently tossed aside. At a time when I needed someone to wrap arms around me, no one was there, not family, friends, or even church members. I mulled despairingly, wondering how much it would cost in self-respect to get the government's help. Many times I wanted to bolt, but where was there to go? I was stuck in an unkind system devoid of compassion.

Finally they told me I would have to get rid of my house or let them put a lien on it to get benefits. I was deathly afraid, not knowing how long I could hold on to it, yet dead set on keeping it. The worker said, well, I should have had emergency money to tide me over. Never mind how fast money dissipates when you stop work! I felt like telling her, "Don't try to make me crawl and beg because I'm not going to do it!" They really put me through it! And to put icing on the cake, when they tallied my total benefit, it would have been ten dollars in food stamps, no Medicaid or welfare, after the nightmare of sitting there.

Receiving nothing, I was in a catch-22, not in a position to help myself, but not destitute enough to qualify for public aid. A lot of people find themselves in that awful middle place these days. I got help from a heavenly agency though, and we survived. Over the next long months money always came in to meet our needs. The Lord supplied!

I clung tenaciously to the words of an old gospel song:

> Father I stretch my hands to thee, no other help
> I know,
> If thou withdraw thine help from me o' wither
> shall I go?

I'd exhausted the avenues my PPO offered and was unable to get Medicaid. The only option left was the city hospital, Bellevue, where the insane, the criminal, the infirmed, and the confined mingled in a mind-boggling menagerie of service providers. Doctors worked daily with those experiencing the crushing realities of hard times, treating their distress by compartment, category, and urgency of need.

When I entered, I was immediately overwhelmed by people streaming back and forth, everybody going somewhere, either need-ing a service or performing one. Weirdos, beggars, and such marched shoulder to shoulder with attendants pushing beds, addicts or old people with tremulous legs. The desk clerk told me to take a number and grab a chair. It turned into an all-day affair, which didn't seem fair, but there were many other poor souls waiting, so why squawk? While time-wearied patients caught forty winks, I, being unnerved, closely watched the carnival of fools passing through.

When finally my number got called, I answered a trillion ques-tions for an intake person who had one minute to spend with me because there were five hundred more on line behind. So what did she do? Sent me to a social worker who dealt with "special problems." When you develop a disability, you are no longer a person, but an issue to be taken up or a problem to be solved. It has to be decided by someone else what to do with you.

Thank God for a social worker for the deaf, who received, com-forted, and ran interference for me in that house of madness. How much I needed someone who understood how hard it was not being able to communicate. She signed me up for neurology, although they kept saying send me to psychiatry, which seemed to make more sense. They were befuddled by the fact that I was mute yet could hear. One asked if I drank or used drugs to try to explain my incoherent babble. To that I took offense. Eventually they gave me my ID card number 9 zillion, a hundred and something million.

Every day I returned for appointment after appointment, in department after department, for test after test. I was treated like a guinea pig, to be tapped, pinched, poked, pulled, stuck, measured, and assessed, i.e., "Walk this line! Touch your nose! Wiggle your toes! Look straight ahead, while I look into your eyes!" I felt like they were peering into my soul, looking for dark secrets. Suddenly strangers were invading my body, putting me to the test—tests I didn't know if I needed to pass or fail to be "confirmed." Some doctors carry on a great deal of secrecy, treat patients with casual arrogance and disdain. They know everything, you nothing, and they keep everything a mystery, disclosing only bits and pieces.

I became someone to be analyzed, scrutinized, contemplated, and demonstrated, I guess as an example of what a mute is. With all their evaluations, however, they came up with no answers, except perhaps my problem was "stress related." I was an enigma, a freak, for whom there was no apparent explanation, and they would have to keep searching. Doctors, with their clinical detachment, treated me like a problem that just happened to be encased in a body rather than a person facing a frightening condition. For example, I was placed in an open area during a test, lying uncovered, naked from the waist down, legs agape with a catheter inserted, while male doctors and staff traipsed through. My protestations in moans and groans failed to protect my dignity. No one thought of my humanity.

Big conferences were held in rooms filled with white coats, all eyes glued on me as I performed various tasks to demonstrate who knows what. Like a good girl, I tried to comply—do this, do that, say this, say that. There were only quizzical looks and stares—it never seemed to get anywhere. I kept trying to read their faces to get an inkling of what they were thinking, for their medicalese was as indeciphrable as the jibber-jabber I spoke. Vital statistics were put up on the board, my case constantly in review. I felt like an amoeba in a test tube. They looked at the results of my multitude of tests—the CAT scans, MRIs, spinal taps, and God knows what else. I came away with a sense they weren't convinced I was what I was, but what was I?

Doctors began whispering the letters to a dreadful disease (Lou Gehrig's) known as ALS, which begins by weakening the muscles of the throat and ends with the patient asphyxiating on their own saliva. I was given a muscle test involving having needles poked in my entire body, including my face and tongue. I sat like a human pincushion while the electrodes clicked and ticked and squiggly lines danced across a screen. Afterward I began waking up in night sweats, imagining myself choking or being on a respirator in my dreams. Concluding nothing with that test, doctors began saying maybe my problem was the result of stress that I had turned inward, that I had converted "psychological pain into a physical manifestation." Try to lie down on that one at night and see where it gets you! It made no sense at all, only increased my frustration and made me angry.

They seemed to be suggesting I was looking for a convenient way to escape work by feigning illness. Therefore, I couldn't have the privilege of feeling through no fault of my own this malady had beset me, and I was going to courageously deal with it. Instead I had to ask myself, "Are you some kind of a fruitcake that needs to go check in at a funny farm?" It made me feel, out of cowardice or inability to cope, I had devised this subterfuge to escape work and save face. I wrestled with holding myself responsible for my loss. I wanted to reach back and kick myself in the rear for bringing this on. It created such extreme anger toward my own mind, which they said might have deceived me and cooked up this charade. If it were true, I sure didn't know anything about it!

Everything they alluded to, I ran to a medical book to look up. That can be one of the most frightening experiences in the world because each one you read sounds just like what you have, and they are all horrible and fatal! I perused page after page, carefully noting the symptoms and prognosis and began imagining myself stretched out in a long pine box. I started telling myself and my loved ones goodbye in my mind, tried to distance myself from them physically so that I might be able to let go and cross over to meet my maker. Imagining can be horribly destructive and debilitating to your spirit because you always think the worse. With only a layman's knowledge, you can't begin to put things together and make sense of what they are saying. When it's your brain they are talking about, it's even more alarming, not like having the flu or something. Since it's your control box, if something goes wrong with that, you figure, brother, I'm outta here!

It's more painful and stressful not knowing than knowing. If you know you have this particular disease that will take this course and last this long, and this is how it is treated, it's much easier than knowing you have something serious, but you don't know what it is and don't understand why these things are happening. Yet they've totally disrupted your life. It's hard to remain sane and deal with it.

I'd come to Bellevue because I needed something fixed. Guess I expected to find Ben Casey. When a person came into his hospital with a neurological problem, he took one look, ran a few tests, and 1, 2, 3, knew the answer, then administered the proper procedure, and *wham! Bam!* They were all better before the show went off. No lingering effects, lasting problems, or unanswered questions. But that's TV! Doctors always feel women are hysterical, their ailments imaginary, brought on by excessive need for attention or, as Freud suggested, sexual conflict. If it can't be explained by testing, then it's not real or it's your will that's causing it. The New Age view of illness is that sickness results from a weak or unhealthy mind. I developed an intense fear that I was indeed losing mine, since they weren't able to give me a physiological reason for my problem. I sank so deep into despair with each medical report and doctors raising more questions than answers—all seeming to suggest I was making this up.

Social agencies had said to me, "Prove to us the severity of your circumstances!" Now doctors seemed to be saying, "Prove to us you have a physical problem!" Both seemed to believe I was a fraud. All I knew was that my economic situation and my inability to speak were very real to me.

I got so tired of going to doctors and bracing for the worse, all the tension, fear, and trembling, only to come away with no answers or with answers that were unacceptable to me. I just didn't want to go anymore. I couldn't take the rise and fall of hope. Doctors seemed to be vacillating between two opinions, either that I had this god-awful disease guaranteed to take me out in the worse way or that I had simply checked out mentally because I couldn't stand the pain of my existence. Either way, it was something I didn't want to confront.

I felt like an ugly grub who had crawled into a cocoon to escape the pain of this world, someone who needed to hide and be ashamed of myself. The other option, ALS, conjured up such horrid images of torturous death my mind wouldn't allow me to accept that one as possibly true. What was I to do? I found myself stuck in a holding pattern, not knowing which way to turn or what was wrong. If I could just find it, then I would accept it and move on.

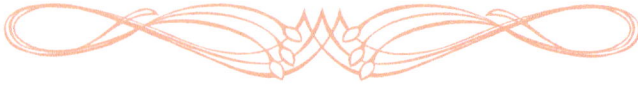

CHAPTER TWENTY-FIVE
Healing Days

AS human beings we are always looking for who is at fault. Self-doubt told me maybe I had concocted an easy way out, although my natural mind said, "Jean, you have never been a person who looks for an escape route, so how can that be true?" When my problem lingered and I didn't know the cause, I tended to walk, act, look, feel, and think down. There was no end in sight, no glimmer of hope on the horizon. I didn't know what to do with myself. I built up a lot of anger and a low opinion of doctors, thinking they were all idiots. I got so fed up I felt like throwing in the towel. I didn't know how to function without the part I was missing.

I feared the loss of love and esteem of family and friends, the lack of control over my body, and the shroud of uncertainty hanging over my future. Most of all, I feared the silence itself, because I was scared of losing connection. Yet through it, the Lord would begin to give me a greater sense of His reality and love.

Most people are more afraid of disability than death. Everyone wants to stay well until their time comes and just die. Disability takes loved ones away or necessitates interaction in new ways. It creates a great deal of distance. Disability faced me with the specter of eminent death; there was only a question of when, which made me think about putting my house in order. But I was not ready to accept its finality and not willing to bid my *self* adieu. I just kept holding on for dear life. My grief for my speech was still too new.

I started really cherishing the little keepsakes I'd collected over the school years given by students as symbols of their affection. Sometimes I called each one by name as I scanned the celluloid frames of my picture album and invited them to join me in the quietness of my room. How I laughed as funny things they said and did came roaring back to me! Holding on to precious memories allowed me to revisit a time when I felt adequate and relive pleasant experiences. I cherished cards and letters I'd long since stashed in a drawer—little niceties sent in times past to say thanks that showed someone appreciated me. They meant so much more now than before and made me feel worthwhile.

It was hard to like myself when I no longer knew who I was, to realize there were people who cared about me when I couldn't feel their care, being blinded by my own emotions. It was difficult coming to terms with it, to develop internal peace that if I remained the way I was, I'd be okay and able to make it. A new me needed time to emerge. Reading scripture helped get me through that lonely trying time.

Inability to communicate what I was experiencing, the doubt, the terror, the hopelessness, the pity, wanting to be rescued were obvious problems of my communication impairment. In an emergency I couldn't respond or couldn't tell others what was wrong. In a confrontation, I couldn't assert myself or present my case. In everyday situations, the people who loved me started getting very frustrated because they couldn't understand me. I began to lose linkage with others.

Everyone else was talking; I was doing all the listening. My side never got expressed. I was never *heard*. There was no give and take, natural interchange, or back and forth flow of ideas. I had been reduced to savage grunts and groans. After a time listening to people became like listening to voices on the radio. I could tune in or out. But I couldn't interact in conversation, so it became hard to stay focused. My insides began speaking too loudly. I lived in a very emotional state, trying to come to grips with the actuality of it. Sometimes I got depressed and hit rock bottom like *kerplonk!*

I was still in a state of shock about the suddenness of the onset of the event and having my life interrupted. My loyalty was to my old experiences, to who I used to be. So many decisions needed to be made in order to go on with my responsibilities.

Suddenly everyone "normal" elevated themselves above me. They all *knew* what I was going through, yet no one understood. Each one became an expert on what I ought to do, but no one could get in touch with my *pain*. Sometimes I just withdrew to try to cope with discouragement. People believed if they hypnotized me, I would speak, or if they scared me badly enough or if I went to church, they looked for some spectacular miracle to just make me suddenly talk. They missed the miracle of God's continual grace that was providing and allowing me to carry on in spite of it.

Each person's life touches so many lives. When we are no longer around, it leaves an empty and awful hole. But when you are still around, yet not around, that hole is even more painful, the gap even wider because the family and friends can see and touch you, but you're a mere shell of who you used to be. There was tremendous stress as we all struggled through the process of adjustment.

My parents agonized over my condition, remembering when I was the teacher in the family they were so proud of. They couldn't accept the new person I'd become either. They wanted me back like I used to be and tended to deny my present state. They'd ask questions and wait for my reply like always. Mom sacrificed and paid for a specialist with an office on Fifth Avenue. She would have paid any price to get me back to myself. She even offered me a pair of her prettiest gold earrings if only I'd speak again (an offer I most certainly wished I could have taken her up on).

Mom wanted what she wanted for me, which was to talk again. She didn't understand that I needed to have the right to make my own decision, even if it didn't make sense to her. My decision was to stop letting doctors take me around in circles and try learning to live with it, instead of escaping from it. If it was ALS, it was only a matter of time, so I'd just as well make the best of it. If it was something I needed to be, then I would go on and be it, although I didn't perceive it as a need.

Another traumatic change happened when I started taking a prescription drug for my dysarthria (inability to control the muscles to articulate speech). I was taking it with no noticeable effects, until one day as I stood before the mirror at home, an aura passed over me. An electrical surge bolted through my body like lightning. I felt confused and disoriented, as if the room were spinning. I watched my face contort into an asymmetrical grimace with my mouth pulled to one side. The muscles on the right fell limp, while the muscles on the left stood motionless. There were twitches, tics, and little shocks all around my lips. I spun to my bed, rested a few hours, then called a doctor.

I was scheduled for another battery of tests as these symptoms provided new evidence of neurological dysfunction. The office examination revealed a repressed gag, a wandering and tremulous tongue, double vision, and inability to do rapid repetitive movements; and I had difficulty walking a straight line, yet a subsequent MRI was unremarkable. Doctors still had more questions than answers. Another big conference was held and more opinions expressed. Mom's new doctor said it could still be a conversion heightening my sense of guilt and frustration.

While they debated back and forth, I felt like the rat in a scientific experiment wandering through a maze, being observed, tested, violated in every way with no understanding of what was going on. Finally they wrote "progressive neurological dysfunction of unknown etiology," leaving me deathly afraid of what was going to happen next and not knowing what to *expect*. I was trapped in a body that was malfunctioning and out of order. They said my problem was very complex. I guess I just didn't fit whatever it said in their text.

Meanwhile, I was ashamed to even smile for fear others would see how broken I was, knowing how natural it is for humans to judge each other by how we look. To create a smile, there was a terrible war that went on as the right side pulled and tugged desperately, but the left wouldn't give an inch. My head threw back and got caught in their spastic clinch. Tremors and quakes raced across the right side of my face; one eye drooped while the other ogled and stared. My mouth draped sadly to the side, then dipped suddenly in a valley of despair. I looked so ugly, disfigured; there was no happiness there. It wasn't noticeable with my face at rest, but when a smile placed those muscles under stress, others saw the paralysis. I started walking around with my face expressionless so that I could look like every-body else and no one on the street would have to know my secret.

When you're trying to be as normal as possible, you pay a price for it in personal anguish. I remember how I used to scuttle along hurriedly, hoping not to run into anyone I knew. If by chance I stumbled upon a familiar face, I'd cleverly hide my disgrace by sticking tongue in cheek to make a hilly peak. Pointing wildly pretending to have just come from the dentist, I'd scoot on by, thereby avoiding the communication encounter. When I needed something in a store, I searched for one that had merchandise displayed prominently where I could see. But every once in a while, a salesperson would ask to help me. I'd blurt out a little gibberish, and they'd yell back in the back for a Hispanic stock boy to come out and interpret my "Spanish."

Quite amusingly, it brought me to a new revelation that I could face my problems with a bit of humor. Laughter is good medicine for the soul. A good hearty laugh really does help what ails you. I believe God gave humans that special ability other creatures don't have, because He knew in tough times it would get us through. My sister Fay was always a life-of-the-party type, and I began to under-stand why. She used to say, "This ain't no easy life!" When you go through it taking everything so seriously, you begin to totter under the load, but facing it with humor lightens the burden. Being able to cry and let it out helps too!

I thought of joining a support group to try to meet others who had similar experiences, but where would I go, Question Marks Anonymous? For some things there just are no definitive answers. Life is full of mysteries and unanswered puzzles, and I guess I am one. I just leave it in God's hands and believe it will all come clear in heaven one day—why it happened and what God's plan was. The body is still a mystery, and so is the mind. If we knew all the answers, we'd be like Him. Though inundated by adversity, I had a sense of being upheld by His mighty hand. It tended to counteract the yo-yo effect of the experience on my emotions. My countenance, obviously cracked, could no longer be concealed, but my spirit and will actually started to gain strength.

Yet, it was still hard to accept myself. Why? Basically because I found the way I was to be objectionable. Society never says people who have disabilities are okay the way they are and are always devising ways to get us out of it, not putting as much energy into finding ways to help us live more fully with it. In short, having a disability is not what most people would desire because it is projected as meaning you are weak, deficient, vulnerable, and not valuable to have around. I kept holding on to things to remember who I was instead of letting go, accepting the change, and believing it was not because of anything I had done to get this way, to acknowledge God's love for the new me as well as the old me.

There was a commercial that said, "When the tough get sick, they take..." All the while a woman in the picture repeated, "I'm not going to get this!" suggesting sickness is akin to weakness, that it is your will to be sick or lack of will causes you not to stay well, that you are in control. It's your choice to be that way, consequently your fault. You are a weakling because you can't overcome it and refuse its effect on your body.

When we internalize that notion, it's harder to go on. We tend to withdraw, lose focus, get locked into our sense of failure and shame. Failures can be tools God uses to shape us. I came to see my disability as part of His plan. I had to get to a point of realizing if I would just cooperate instead of pull against it, then I could learn from it. I needed to ask Him to teach me, not take it away. Also, I needed to learn to stop questioning and having to know all the answers and what He was doing. And just because I considered myself a Christian did not disentitle me to doubt and become afraid. Adjustment didn't happen overnight. It was a day-by-day process of learning to manage and adapt. Grieving the loss was a natural process that I had to go through, which allowed me to begin creating a new life.

The Bible says, if you have the faith of a mustard seed, you can speak to a mountain and it will move. That doesn't mean it will go away. It means it will move so that it no longer blocks your joy or sense of well-being. I had to ask God what He and I could do with this obstacle in my life, to turn it into an opportunity.

We bring our own personality to the disabled experience. Who we were before developing the disability remains and determines somewhat how we face it. I struggled with wanting to isolate myself and was plagued by social anxiety. Yet with God on my side, I finally felt equal to my challenges.

The thrust of my life before had been to help disabled children. Now my aim was to get help for myself. The mere thought of getting started carried tremendous weight. I guess I always just assumed there was so much out there readily available, having for years watched the telethons sponsored by various help groups. Everyone tends to think there're lots of places for people with disabilities, but when I found myself in the driver's seat, was I surprised to find there wasn't. Programs that existed were geared toward very specific disability groups, i.e., the New York Society for the Deaf or the Lighthouse for the Blind. But when you don't have a slot, where do you go? Not only did these programs operate with a fair amount of isolation, but staff working with one disability group knew precious little about another. If you didn't fit neatly into a given slot, they didn't know where to place or how to work with you. The first thing they asked me was, "What are you? Deaf? Blind? An amputee? A disabled vet? You have CP?" Society should stop the labeling and be more concerned about enabling!

I was mute but could hear, so that placed me in an unusual category, and my abilities didn't match my disability. I had college education and work experience, which should have been a plus, but it was not treated as such because most programs were geared for people who were "lower functioning." In short, I was overqualified to be a handicapped person being more able than expected.

Knowledge empowers. The more we learn about available options and our rights, the better it is for us. That's the information no one wanted to tell me unless it served them, not me. In other words, my participation would bring special funds, benefits, tax credits, or the like. To some the disabled represent profit and job opportunities, to others unwanted expenditure because of the need to accommodate us or increased liability and costly insurance.

Also, programs tend to treat us by symptoms rather than their effect. A person who can't hear and one who can't speak will experience the same kind of isolation and limited opportunity for social interaction, yet the focus of remediation would more likely be for (A) their lack of hearing and (B) their lack of speech as if the outcome isn't the same.

Groupings are set up based on what the person can't do or the problems they have, not what they *can* do. Emphasis is always on the can't. On the contrary, the so-called normal are admitted to programs based on their abilities, not their inabilities with an accent on their strengths. I wanted to find a way to get from can't to *can*.

We had become so specialized and compartmentalized we failed to see that human problems are many dimensional and multifaceted. Each person only knew his particular discipline and failed to see the big picture, how things connected and interplayed. Services were too fragmented—doctors here, therapists there, counselors and teachers over there. The left hand didn't know what the right hand was doing. There wasn't much communication between disciplines in service delivery. Mounds of paper got written up and sent around, which nobody read. A lot of it ended in the round file. There was tremendous waste of time, appointment foul-ups, and delays. It took so long to get anything done. There is a need for centralized dispensing of information about services available to the disabled community and greater communication and coordination. Hopefully, computer technology and the internet will open access and dialogue between groups.

I found myself stranded, didn't know where to go to be accepted, fit in, and find emotional support. I wanted a place to come out of my shell and share feelings with peers. What happens to the disabled is always politicized and made an issue. We end up feeling *powerless* to effect change, just like members of other minority groups. We lack vehicles through which we can be *heard* by politicians and decision makers, giving us little say in how things are done. Somebody else creates "ghettoes" where we are supposed to remain and be happy that we are allowed to be around at all. We're treated like another underclass of "imperfects," burdens to society, that others just tolerate. Most often, decisions that are made regarding us suit someone else's agenda, not ours.

What do you do when you have been living with nothing but remembrances of what once was? I was too frightened to build any new expectations because my look to the future was much too dim. Would there be eminent decline? I thought I saw the death angel standing over my bed at night, smiling at me. What should I do in the meantime? It seemed like nothing could persuade me that part of me was *really* gone in spite of it all. I had to wean myself from the past and start looking at the present, stop dwelling on the pain and turn my energies outward. I have always been an accommodating person, so I just moved over and made room for the disability in my life. Instead of trying to kick it out, I looked for ways to make us compatible. After a while, we became good roommates, sharing the same body. Eventually my speech loss became integrated into who I was and was even embraced by me. As I viewed it, God had simply created a new way of my being in the world. I could still bring good into it as I was not totally incapacitated.

I spent many moments of quiet reflection to find a new path, to take stock of my assets, goals, and dreams, and made a strong resolution to find happiness as who I had become, not who I had been. I tried to rechannel my thinking and my efforts. One good thing about being handicapped is, I didn't have to go around acting "edumacated" anymore because no one really expects a handicapped person to have any brains!

At the Bronx Independent Living Center, I researched to find a company that sold communication aids for people who have trouble expressing themselves and/or being understood.

I ordered things to help me function out in public—a set of picture cards illustrating basic living needs, a wipe-off communication board, and an attention-getting beeper. Then I invited Mom out for lunch to try out my new aids. We went into a diner, and when the waitress appeared, I whipped out a folder and pointed to pictures to place our order, enjoying being like the old Jean who could handle things. She looked on quite baffled as I dealt my cards out on the table, showing what we were going to eat, but said nothing. I suppose her look said it all. She found it really weird, but I was undaunted. Next day, I popped in my favorite junk food joint, stood at the counter holding up a picture of a cheeseburger then a Coke while searching for the card with the fries. I got a lot of rubber necks and rolled eyes from cocky young teens in line behind me. Suddenly, I lost my feeling of victory among their unkind words. The cards were cute, but for the birds!

I didn't bother after a while, just joined the queue and looked for daily specials on giant posters in clear view or some dangling doohickey to point to. I found ways to make things easy and avoided *standing out*! That's what it's really all about. The problem with equipment and aids is they announce to the world our disabled status when most of us love anonymity. It's not because we're ashamed of ourselves; it's because we are trying to fit in and be as "normal" as we can possibly be. Aids force us to reface our disabilities and the public's reaction each time we go out by obviating that which we don't want made obvious for various reasons—vulnerability, unpopularity, appearance, not wanting people to gawk and stare, which can be uncomfortable, especially when you are not used to it. No matter how practical and functional equipment is, it serves no purpose if a person refuses to use it. Willingness really depends on the individual, their needs, quirks, and level of adjustment.

To keep from getting preyed upon, I tried to avoid looking helpless even though I now felt without protection. Lacking a voice in a menacing environment means having no safety weapon. But I put on an attitude like a seasoned New Yorker, which said, "Hey, don't mess with me!" and it worked. A sense of safety built on the inside as I decided not to be consumed by that which I couldn't control on the outside. I had to just roll with the tide, be flexible! I learned to look for ways to get around my disability. I had to come out of the shadows and take the risk of living life.

When we are hurting, we often withdraw and pull back. We live in a vacuum where we feel safe, but this leaves us nonproductive. We do this out of fear of rejection. Everyone has parts of themselves they are afraid of showing people. It is painful and scary to take the chance of unveiling our hidden issues. We question, if you knew who I really am, would you still like me? It's hard to say I am grieving and lonely, especially when you have no words. Being able to connect gives an important sense of belonging.

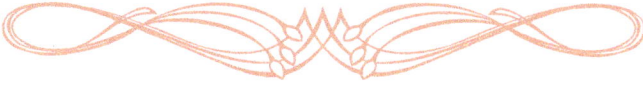

CHAPTER TWENTY-SIX
The Chrysalis

NEVERTHELESS, my twisted visage and lack of speech always let the cat out of the bag. I couldn't hide the fact that I was now a member of America's largest minority group, people with disabilities, 43 million strong.

As a new inductee, I began experiencing the same dynamics, the same struggle for power and dignity African Americans have long been faced with in a society that tends to look down on us, the same struggle to hold on to my identity and be sanctioned as worthwhile in spite of my difference, the struggle to feel okay being who and what I am while in with people who are not like me, the struggle not to lionize my difference and see my common bond with those around me. People similarly try standing in the way of our getting an education, having a career, or living in certain places, even getting goods and services we need. And as some whites view blacks, they think we're all of low IQ and have limited potential.

Americans with disabilities, though a major subgroup, have been controlled and paternalized by a main body who tries to define who we are and what is good for us, a group that has found it hard to convince the world we are just like everyone else in all the normal ways with the same needs and range of abilities, for whom access also is a primary issue; a group walled in or out of society by negative attitudes, images, and lack of opportunities for economic success and social acceptance, trying to claw our way to respectability with the help of new laws and civil rights legislation (ADA). This legislation, like many of the laws enacted to help blacks, lacks an enforcement tool beyond negotiation and education. Therefore, full access and enjoyment of the services and pleasures of modern living are still being denied the disabled. We're seen as irresponsible and unable to handle our own lives, thus infantilized by society at large. In this hierarchical system, our placement is somewhere near bottom. No longer wanting second-class citizenry, we're coming and speaking out!

In the new politically correct terminology, instead of handicapped, we're called physically challenged, exceptional or special, not to mention a host of more humorous ones like "differently abled" or "handicapable." They're changing the names for this minority group just like they changed from using *colored* to *Negro* to *black* to African American so as not to wound us with their words. It all sounds so disingenuous. Someone told me I am vocally challenged and manually communicative in today's new jargon. These titles don't make me feel any better because no matter which they say, we all know what they mean.

People don't even use the word *mute* anymore. Guess that's not PC either. The deaf don't seem to like it since they now stress orality. The speech professionals say nonverbal, so I guess that's what I am. On the street they say, "She cain't talk! She don't have no voice!" That one I don't like, because I feel I speak volumes to those who will "listen."

One long-held view is that the disabled are weak, wimpy, self-pitying, non-goal-oriented folk—a notion that defies logic because given all we have to deal with in our daily lives, it seems obvious that weakness is not one of our overriding characteristics. In fact, I believe strength of will and determination are among our best features as we learn to survive in a hostile milieu. Most people seem to believe what we need is a good swift kick in the pants to get us going and that one should not show sympathy or we will waddle in it and do nothing, that we must be prodded and compelled to do for ourselves at all times. Consequently, many won't lend a helping hand. People are often harsh and strict because they think we need it. Think they must toughen us up as if our lives aren't already tough enough. Let us give the cues for how we want to be treated!

As with ethnic minorities, we are often perceived as incompetent, babyish, needing to be controlled, requiring close supervision and decisions made for us. We are sometimes viewed as having a propensity toward violence, to have little to give and always taking, to be lazy beggars looking for handouts. The origin of the word *handicapped* is related to the image of a beggar with a cap in hand for passersby to drop coins into. Like many other groups, we suffer from the "allness syndrome." All handicapped are…The disabled are thought to be either sexually out of control, completely nonsexual, or driven toward perverted and unnatural acts.

People tend to see us in extremes. Either we are superstars like Ray Charles and Stevie Wonder, possessing some special gift divinely compensated with wonderful abilities to make up for our area of disability, or we are boobs who are absolutely out of it. They overlook individual characteristics, personalities, and varying abilities, not recognizing that we are people first and handicapped second with the same potential to fail or succeed.

We are often associated with behavior that is abnormal, socially inappropriate, and not acceptable to the main group. In short, we don't fit in. We're not thought to be fun to be around or associate with. We make people uptight, and in a looks-conscious society, we just don't look right! Our packaging doesn't give us appeal.

Some feel we need to be isolated, institutionalized for the protection of others, or it just costs too much to integrate us fully into the mainstream. In today's budget-crunched economy, the government is looking to roll back funds, give programs the ax rather than allocate more to meet special needs. The most cost-effective solution is to lock us away and throw away the key or just put us in with everybody else, let us do or die, ignore our needs, treat all as equals. It's costly to try to level the playing field. Some think there's not enough return for all the expense. Attempts are being made to right the wrongs of the past by forcing inclusion in regular classrooms, but as in reverse discrimination cases, there are those who feel disenfranchised. To put it simply, too much is being given to us already for what they feel we are worth, and somebody else has to lose out for us to gain parity.

Negative assumptions about disabled people cause us to be looked down upon, families to be ashamed of having us as members, and businesses to be afraid to take us on as employees because of presumed "diminished capacity." We are sometimes viewed as harmful, dangerous, threatening, and prone to crime and deviance. We are believed to be inherently deficient, products of bad genes, of impure stock with the potential to pass on our ineptitude and create more of our kind, threatening future generations. As a result, people aren't too keen on marrying us and making babies. Advances in cloning animals might mean in the future, efforts will be made to ensure no human is born with a physical or mental impairment. For us it may mean scientific genocide.

Americans with disabilities face discrimination in housing also. You soon discover people are afraid to live around you or fear having you near their children because you might "do something to them." They feel we are destructive and irresponsible and may tear things up because we are "not all there." Something in disability says we are less, subordinate, dependent, incapable, just like being black, unless you happened to be one of the successfully disabled, in which case you become a shining example used to pummel the less successful over the head for their failings to achieve. There's always that crowd on the bottom, a few bright stars above and very few standing on middle ground.

I often felt my blackness was a wall that I was trying to reach beyond to others or that we are somewhat of a spectacle in this society because our ways, communities, and problems are made to stand out so markedly. Now I feel the same way about being handicapped. When you have a disability, there is a similar feeling of being a spectacle, that all eyes are on you, especially if you use equipment like a wheelchair and enter an assembly of onlookers. Often we who have disabilities live with low dreams because of fear of confronting and conquering that intense sense of mockery and rejection. Sometimes I get bogged down in a morass of anger and frustration when nobody seems to really understand how hard it is to persist. No one sees the walls or feels the pricks but me. Morning by morning, I ask the Lord for new mercies to help me carry on. There are so many intangibles to the experience. We need great encouragement to be all we can be in order to live up to our capacities, not for the sake of others, but for our own self-fulfillment.

We need to create doorways so more of us can get in and out of who and what we are and connect with someone on the other side to improve our morale, our sense of cooperation and inclusion, while building better understanding through open communication. We need to cultivate a nourishing environment conducive for all to grow.

Americans with disabilities, like black Americans, have never been properly memorialized throughout history in books and the media. As a result, our contributions have never been fully noted in the record book of time. This has led to poor perception in the public mind. We are likely to be portrayed as villains (Peg Leg Pete), gnomes, monsters, or mischief makers led by the forces of evil (Egor), grotesque pieced-together folk tortured by rejection and driven to acts of violence (Frankenstein), deranged mind aglow with evil intent (Mr. Whitley in the 1965 horror *Die, Monster, Die*), helpless pathetic folk looking for handouts around the holidays (Tiny Tim), angry self-pitying invalids seeking to use the disability to make others serve and wait on us hand and foot (rich girl in *Heidi*), simple-minded people, odd-man-out types, not too bright that everyone affectionately mocks and mimics (Gomer Pile), eternally childish souls, neighborhood dunces who need to be protected and provided for by their families (Nunzio) until the unlikely day comes when being like us works, or a social outcast living in self-imposed isolation, enjoying what meager victuals life allows because he is too horrible to look at (the Elephant Man), befriended only by a creative misfit like himself who finds him gentle but sad (Michael Jackson), even buys the bones when he dies to enshrine him for his difference, marveling this freak was born, thus he lived and…died. And of course there are the unrequited lovers—disfigured maniacs who develop a penchant for murder and mayhem to make the world pay (Phantom of the Opera) for its rejection.

We are used for shock effects in horror films or for amusement; our oddities give people chills or make them laugh. Painful portrayals date back to Greek mythology (Cyclops)and take us into the future in sci-fi adventures like *Star Wars* and *Star Trek*. Hollywood extra-terrestrials and beings from the far beyond always just happen to be hydrocephalic, have speech problems, stand bent over, walk funnily, and have missing or deformed limbs (ET), making them look an awful lot like some of us or at least the way the public views us. This feeds fear, discomfort, and mistrust.

Whoever remembers the fact that the great apostle Paul was nearly blind, or that Moses had a speech impediment when he told old Pharaoh, "Let my people go"? We are more likely to recall the lame, blind, dumb, and maimed who begged Jesus to heal them of their afflictions, as if being handicapped was so terrible. But do we remember the paralytic Mephibosheth, who sat at the royal table, was provided for and loved by King David? Do we know that Beethoven was deaf when he wrote some of the greatest compositions in musical history or that the artist Monet painted some of his best and most famous works when he could barely see? Or that one of the world's greatest scientists, Louis Pasteur, had a brain stroke and was para-lyzed on one side? Or that the English poet Milton wrote the world's greatest epic, "Paradise Lost," and other poems as he imagined with blind eyes? What of the artist van Gogh, who was missing an ear, or deaf/blind Helen Keller, or Charles Steinmetz, the mathematical genius and engineer who was crippled? Their disabilities didn't stop them from enriching the world with their talents.

Indeed we have wonderfully accomplished persons with disabil-ities. In the arts there is the famed concert artist Itzhak Perlman and blind opera tenor Andrea Bocelli. In politics, puny, asthmatic, near-sighted little Teddy Roosevelt grew up to be a leader of the Rough Riders and a bear of a president. A quarter of century later, his cousin Franklin spent fourteen years at the White House in a wheelchair and made a very effective leader of this country—the only president elected four times. There was Charles Ruff, the White House counsel who gave the closing arguments at President Clinton's impeachment trial from a wheelchair; Senator Max Cleland of Georgia and the now deceased Barbara Jordan, who was the first African American woman to address the Democratic Convention, also from her wheelchair. There was also a legally blind runner on the tag team in the 2000 Olympics, and there were two practicing attorneys who were dwarfs. In the business world, how many have heard of John Yeh, a Chinese-born deaf/mute who founded the high-tech company Integrated Micro Computer Systems, which turned into a multimillion-dollar enterprise? And what of the winning Yankee's pitcher Bud Abbott, who had no right hand? Or Dana Bowman, the skydiving double amputee? Or Erik Weihenmayer, who hasn't let his blindness stop him from climbing to the top of Mount Everest? The list is incredibly long of those who have achieved to our credit, yet little recognition has been given to them. Maybe we know of their deeds, but not of their disabilities. Why is that part always so carefully concealed? Can it be that if revealed, society would have to answer for the mistreatment of so many for so long, for doing a deserving group wrong?

It has been said that the achievement of economic status is a prerequisite for any minority to achieve acceptance and respect, that the basis of acceptance of minority group members is economic. However, economic progress has not brought tremendous dilution of blacks into the melting pot of Middle America, and perhaps it won't make a great difference for the disabled either. Old attitudes die hard. They are so ingrained they seem to be etched in stone. We do face the challenge to tap into our self-esteem and empower ourselves, to be determined and open-minded, to turn our disabilities into abilities and show others our competence. This may be a way of breaking down walls and changing attitudes.

A poll by Harris and Associates shows 40 percent of people with physical disabilities live in households with income below $15,000. Other surveys show 66 percent are unemployed, although 82 percent express an interest in working. There is a need to make the workplace user friendly by installing special equipment so that we can perform tasks easily and for support services in some cases to be provided. Because bias and discrimination in the job market often belies our hopes for success, the Americans with Disabilities Act requires employers to make "reasonable accommodations" to help the disabled perform the duties of a specific job by modifying procedures, adjusting the physical environment, and meeting job-related needs. However, sometimes a greater impediment beyond the challenge of getting our feet through the door and equipment needs is the insensitivity and lack of consideration we often face from employers or coworkers who show little understanding, won't be flexible, and are not comfortable working with an employee who has special needs. As with other civil rights issues, we remain far apart because we can't legislate the heart.

For those who receive entitlements, the hindrance to employment is, if they go to work, all benefits and medical coverage within months may be placed in jeopardy. Most are afraid to step out there on nothing, having so little faith in their employability and career longevity. Given the economic blight on our nation, most workers worry how long they will be able to keep their jobs. Moreover, the disabled feel particularly vulnerable because if they can't hold on to their present positions, they don't have lots of career options and will catch heck going back to collect a check.

Moving ahead, of necessity, does involve at times looking back. Sometimes I longed to be normal again and do things I previously enjoyed, such as getting on the phone and yapping with my mother and sister. You know how we women are! But I stopped short and asked myself, "What is *normal* anyway?" Scanning keenly, I decided I'd rather be like me. Besides, it's not what you have but how well you use what you have. Lots of people have all their parts in good working order but don't make full use of them.

In the Bible, God takes credit for creating people with disabilities for His sovereign purposes. In the book of Exodus 4:10–11, when speaking to Moses about his speech impediment, He says, "Who is it that creates the deaf, the blind and the halt? Is it not I, the Lord?" And when questioned whose sin it was that caused a man to be born blind, Jesus replies, in John 9:1–3, it was not his sin nor his parents', but so the power of God could be made manifest. Despite this, society and its ground rules always give the so-called normal the advantage.

Of the millions of Americans who have some type of disability, people with speech, language, or hearing disorders comprise the largest number, more than 22.6 million. Yet and still, public awareness of how to interact with us is low. The average person on the street reacted to me as if I had just beamed down from outer space. Some, assuming I was a deaf/mute, raised their voices like the blast of a foghorn, as if talking loud can make a deaf person hear, or they got right up in my face and enunciated their words with exaggeratory movements so that I could "read their lips," all the while raining sputum into my eyes. I got so sick of wiping spit off my lids. I didn't know what to do, and I couldn't say, "Would you please step back or lower your volume?" At least those people showed a desire to make an adjustment for the sake of my disability. Most didn't even do that! Just went about things same as always and stood there looking at me as if I was crazy. I'm the one who was expected to bridge the gap and do something, not them. They didn't accept equal responsibility to try to relate to me. When I have to do all the reaching out to others, it's unfair. Communicating is a two-way street, and midway is where folks need to meet.

After a day beating about and feeling beaten, I had to come home and find retreat with my old love—moody blues records—and let those down-home boys moan and wail out my frustrations for me. They may have been lamenting about another kind of losing out, but the power of the emotion hit home. I tuned into it, felt released by it. Everything spilled out in the safety of my living room. Music has always been a facilitator and a strong means of expression in my family, so it was natural for me to turn to it to say what I couldn't say. I liked the one that went this way:

> Am I blue? You'd be too!
> Ain't these tears in my eyes telling you?

In passing notes in public, I made a startling discovery. There were lots of folks out there who couldn't read, not even a simple sentence! It's hard to believe in this information age. I don't know how they managed to cover it and keep their jobs, but it made me realize

I wasn't the only one trying to keep my limitations masked. After meeting these individuals, it occurred to me literacy is good ability. I just needed to find what to do with it.

I kept wandering around trying to connect, to reengage myself with others and stay active. I asked my sister for advice for she had already gone through the rehabilitation process, having grown up with a disability. She steered me to OVR, today called DRS. Their main focus is to help disabled people become employable. Every adult deserves to experience the dignity of work, but I think the goals of rehabilitation should go far beyond vocational needs and be more holistic in terms of restoring the whole person—body, mind, and spirit. A career is not the answer, nor is it feasible for everyone. But everybody has something they can do, even those with severe limitations. We all can participate and should have more choices to find out what is right for us. Expanding our horizons through work, socialization, and education while improving mobility and function in the physical environment will meet the needs of the whole person and give us enablement. The purely vocational approach eliminates applicants who either don't choose to or are unable to pursue a career for whatever reason.

I signed up for service and was assigned a counselor. He appeared genial and professional but wasn't the type of person who seemed driven by a sense of mission in wanting to help people. It was more like just a job. There was no apparent passion about my problems. The first thing he did after orientation was to send me down to an agency on Twenty-Third Street, where they typed, sorted, and labeled everyone, placed us in categories, and assessed how well we functioned—saw how good we were at putting square pegs in round holes. The evaluators gave me a variety of tests supposedly to identify my strengths and weaknesses. But testing didn't help pinpoint specific skills for a particular job, so it was of no benefit to me, only them.

We were given so many assessments that seemed inappropriate, unnecessary, inadequate, or meaningless and didn't measure what they purported to measure. Tests were given without regard to individual differences and were not good predictors of how well a person would do on a real job. Often skills in one area can click in and make up for weaknesses in another. In addition, there was so little personal contact and exchange between the evaluators and the clients; things that can be gleaned in a one-on-one interaction or through careful observation were easily missed. The format was basically we were given a test or task to do, and the tester walked away and returned when time was up. That was it! There is a need for better evaluation procedures and communication between service providers.

We consumers worked real hard because it seemed there was more on the line than just our eventual placements. It was our own self-worth. Someone was deciding whether we measured up! I poured sweat each time I went in and had to come home and go to bed because of the stress. That was only the beginning of the pressure to perform, do well, and prove myself useful and capable in spite of my limitations. They told us, "We will *expect* this of you and that of you, and you ought to be able to do the other too! We're not here to wipe your noses!" The system put counselors in positions of great power over us while placing us under the magnifying glass at a time when we were probably at our lowest esteem and very vulnerable.

Today's social theorists harp about having too low expectations for the disabled, but I think it's also possible to have too high! Society often places unreasonable demands on the disabled to use all we have to use, do all we can do, and be all we can be. There are corporate executives and geniuses sitting down on Skid Row in New York City, so why should the disabled always have to function up to full capacity? Don't we deserve the luxury to fail and do what we wish with our lives, even if it is not all that we have the potential to be? Society drives, pushes, and expects too much, when, by human nature, we have the same range of differences as the rest of the population. Some will rise to high levels of achievement, and some won't.

There are many factors that influence what we do with our lives. When the unique combination of ability, circumstances, opportunity, and readiness presents itself, most people will progress, but riding people with the notion that the more we are prodded, poked, and pushed, the further we will go just isn't so. Society needs to make room for individual differences, set reasonable standards, and stop asking people with disabilities not to do what others do themselves, which is manipulate, make excuses, fall back on whatever they can fall back on to get over, flub things up, look for pity from others, take the easy way out, and not do all they are really capable of doing. I am not advocating this but suggesting it is an individual's *choice*. When will they stop asking the disabled to compensate society for being here by proving our worth and our value through achieving what others never do by overcoming every obstacle? We need to have value appropriated to us regardless. Our value is intrinsic and shouldn't have to be constantly proven.

I'm not speaking against expectations, only the habit of holding the stick so high and expecting everyone to jump over it. As in the limbo dance, be willing to adjust the level of the stick, realizing not everyone will perform at a peak. It needs to be high enough to provide challenge but low enough to make it reasonably attainable depending on the individual. Those who work with us can only point the direction and give encouragement but can't create hunger and desire. They can only swing open the doors of opportunity and let all go through, whether they walk through on two feet, ride through in a chair, hop through on crutches, or are wheeled through on a stretcher. Make success possible for us, but don't insist on it from us. In all cases, focusing on abilities rather than limitations will bring greater success.

We can't be expected to live up to stringent demands that are more than we are ready or able to give. What works for one person won't necessarily work for another. It's that human element—the diversity of personality and spirit—that must be recognized along with the effects of environment and conditioning. Our emotional states are very complex. No one holds the barometer to tell when something is just right or when someone is ready for things. And no matter how in-depth one studies disability, you can't learn the full dynamic of the experience from a book, nor can you perceive by empirical observation what it is to wrestle with bodies that don't work correctly, emotions that are out of kilter, and a world that doesn't understand.

I've heard the argument a doctor doesn't have to have an illness to know how to treat it. Before developing my disability, I thought I knew a lot about the subject, but now I see from the opposite end there's much more to it. I don't believe I can adequately put into words all that I go through. There are so many layers, nuances, and things coming at us from all sides and so much stirring within. We need to be the teachers, to tell others what the world is like to us and what works best for us, to give our input into the planning and implementation of programs for others like ourselves. We do make powerful role models, but our knowledge is grossly underutilized and not valued. Like other minorities, we are disrespected.

Ladening ourselves with constant criticism is a problem too. We are more demanding and critical of ourselves than anyone else. Now there's the rub! We strive too hard, overdo, bite off more than we can chew—all to measure up. Our lives are exceedingly stressed, and we carry a lot of excess baggage. We need room to be people and not have extra pressure placed on us. We need freedom to be who and what we are and not have society like parents pressuring us to perform up to their expectations to prove our value in their eyes. Yes, expect us to do what we can do, but relax a little and embrace us as people. Let us come up for air and stop making us jump through hoops! Celebrate small victories with us and help build on them.

With rehab services, there is so much wasted *time*. It sometimes takes years to get our lives booted up and out of stagnation, to see real progress in a case. For one reason, we often have to fight every step of the way to get what we want. Most things asked for will be denied, even if appropriate to give greater functional independence. Strange we have to do battle with them, when they're supposed to be allies and provide a base of support. Even with our own help organizations, we have little clout. They don't put us first, just use us to create jobs for others.

Unfortunately, the training available didn't offer clients extensive learning opportunities. What existed was geared toward the lower-functioning adult with an emphasis on structure and control and not on high-level skill acquisition. The placements after training were generally entry-level positions set up specifically for those with limited proficiency, barely paying minimum wage. They found somewhere to put everybody to satisfy placement requirements and get themselves off the hook. The major consideration in training was first and foremost *money*. The rule of thumb was, spend the least amount, get us placed, and close the case. The client's indigence as well as disability had to be considered, so naturally if you had more than the clothes on your back, you didn't meet their standards of poverty. In my case, having an MA, they were unwilling to pay college tuition for additional education to change careers. Not being abysmally poor and owning a home didn't help either.

Finally they placed me in a computer class set up for "higher-functioning adults" to learn word-processing skills. I wasn't terribly interested in it as the idea of sedentary work for hours before a screen seemed boring. After all, I hadn't sat five minutes in the ten years I'd been a teacher and was adjusted to being in high gear. But because I couldn't vocalize, it appeared I was unsuitable for the board of education in any capacity. There was no attempt made to find another place to make use of my prior teaching experience. As it went, *choice* sailed out the window with my voice. They were now boss, and all my priors were lost.

Rehab workers were not big on imagination and actually weren't that gung-ho to find us jobs. There were so many disincentives to work maybe they figured why push the issue. Counselors were very unwilling to make contacts, pursue leads, or leave their offices to do anything on the client's behalf beyond their perfunctory work. If you didn't call them, they wouldn't call you! Of course if asked why, they would probably have sighted caseloads of up to eighty clients each and emphasize the desire not to "baby us" by doing things for us that we could do ourselves. The problem is, in many cases some do need more assistance than they are willing to give. Most of us have dreams, ambitions for ourselves, and things we'd like to do but have no idea how to begin actualizing them. I saw stacks of printed material and announcements about civil service jobs and special projects to employ the disabled piled high on desks, yet that information somehow never got into the right hands.

To make headway, a consumer had to be very assertive and persist in calling and bugging the counselor to get what he wanted, even to the point of filing appeals for things like equipment that would promote self-sufficiency. I feel sorry for those who don't have the wherewithal or resourcefulness to seek out information and go after help for themselves. So many of us don't see ourselves as *entitled* or *deserving* and routinely discount our feelings, objectives, and desires in favor of others because, in our position as people who live off a government check, we don't feel we have the *right* to demand more. We are made to feel like a pain in the neck when we insist on having our needs met. They expect us to go sit in a corner, be quiet, and take what we can get. Therefore, we often don't end up in places where we can make a significant contribution or see our dreams fulfilled. Rather, we get sent based on our DX to placements where it costs the least money without total regard for our interests, abilities, and needs. They don't look for the optimum situation, only that which would be minimally suitable as required by law. Today they seem to be pushing to close as many cases as possible by rushing to place individuals, often without really exploring the best options for them or investing in adequate education and training, while alleging dedication to serve the needs of the most severe.

I accepted the computer class because, like everyone else, I took what I could get, figuring what the heck! The group consisted of eighteen-to-twenty-year-old high school graduates appearing to be of low socioeconomic level. The instructor spoke to us as if talking to a group of imbeciles—slow, laboriously, word by word—"My name is Mr....! Can anyone tell me my name?" then, "This class is called...! Who can tell us the name of the class?" He continued in this manner, though the answer was posted above the blackboard on a computer-generated banner. One guy yelled out, "Hey, he think we stupid, huh?" causing a gush of laughter. The students were pretty on the ball, but it was obvious the level of instruction was for someone hardly alert at all. The few antiquated terminals in the room, we never got to touch. Veteran students using them seemed to be also collecting dust as they waited for him to busy them, while he tried to busy us.

As he commenced calling the roll, everybody answered to their names, except me. Of course, no one had told him I couldn't speak. Upon making the unlikely discovery, he tapped his assistant on the shoulder and whispered, "Go tell the secretary we've got a deaf/mute in here!" (Like y'all done messed up somewhere!) They, receiving the message, sent in a retarded client wearing a hearing aid, who apparently knew a few signs. Looking on grinningly, he fingered, "My name is Joe!" and gave me that gaze Mighty Joe Young gave Fay Wray in one of the old movies, then suddenly tried to put the moves on me and wanted to give me a big, wet welcoming kiss. Luckily, I ducked and he missed. When I saw the package deal being offered there—he and the class—I headed for the pass, never went back. As my younger son would have said, "It was whack!"

Then it was back to the other agency, this time to go over my medical history. I was seen by a very competent doctor teaching a young internist the ropes, who was a real dope! Fascinated by notes showing I had a repressed gag reflex, he decided to put me to the test. And so he proceeded to see how far he could stick a tongue depressor down my throat. It made me choke. He didn't stop until he had located my esophagus and the things I carried in my belly bag, like my guts, lay strewn around the room like dust. Just because a person has MD behind his name doesn't mean he is altogether sane.

By the mid-1980s, what computers could do was nothing less than astonishing. Most people came to see smart machines as the all-in-all in resolving every problem. OVR decided to get a computer to speak for me, to "resolve" my disability. They sent me to a college speech department for an evaluation where I was greeted first by a therapist with warm salutations. Then out came the old word list I was familiar with. I sat close to her and went down as best as I could. My efforts were no good, nothing but strange groaning. She marveled at my senseless chatter, administered a hearing test, then called in a voice specialist to ask him what was the matter. He slid in and eased down in the seat like he was "the man," all suited up in Pierre Cardin. He had all kinds of alphabet behind his name, "Dr. So and So," head of audiology, who I'm told gave grand lectures on speech pathology. I started from the top, while he looked on discerningly.

She, with a puzzled glance, turned and asked, "Well, what do you think?" He responded with a motion that said he hadn't the slightest notion and sallied out, leaving me. Nothing left, we made a video to use as a resource to demonstrate, I guess, what a mess mutism can be.

Augmentative technology had advanced to become very useful to people with disabilities. She whipped out a computerized voice machine and demonstrated this "wonderful new technology." She explained how words typed in first appeared in the display, then it would say what I wanted to say. So I, using my hunt-and-peck system, punched in, "My name is Jean," and a robotic voice repeated, "My name is Jeen." It was the voice of a *machine*, not a human being, and a male to wit!

She spieled on about how lucky I was that VR would pay the $3,000 for me, as if to say, "You already don't have to work and can live free off government handouts, and now you're being *given* this expensive piece of equipment to which you have no entitlement. It is only the good graces of others providing for you, and you should be grateful!" As the slaves were in past times, the disabled were sometimes treated like less than people as if they had no rights to anything, could make no demands, and were exempt from the protections of the law and the privileges of a civil society. Today's society is just beginning to recognize our rights, because of the Americans with Disabilities Act, to full access to those things that other citizens take for granted. Finally, freedom is ringing in the ears of the deaf, shackles are falling from crippled limbs, and the light of a new day is glimmering from the eyes of the blind. There are many out there who still have a song to be sung, when our rights to full participation are won.

She looked at me inquiring if I would accept the new toy she was giving me. Always hiding my feelings, I tried to look overjoyed but bravely penned, "Can you make me a girl? I don't feel very comfortable being a boy!" to which she plied me with apologies and "I'm sorrys" then promised to see if that can be arranged. They have absolutely no awareness of us as real people at all. To them we're just handicaps in funny wrappers made of flesh without the usual accompanying prettiness—don't realize we may look different, but we feel the same inside. They can only see us as broken, incomplete, dysfunctional, and they're going to use their technologies to "fix us" and make us as close to normal as possible by giving us the human attributes they think we are lacking. Like the Tin Man who needed a heart, if they can just pop something in there, then all our problems will be solved.

I seized the opportunity to get a free computer, but as they say, there are no free lunches. I paid dearly in dignity. Upon its delivery to the office, rehab counselors crowded the room to see my new wonder machine. They encircled me with great curiosity, while I typed in "My name is Jean," and it repeated, "My name is Jeen," this time in a synergized female voice like a nameless, faceless machine with the same tone and inflection throughout—relaxed, efficient, the voice of a voice mail. To me this was the ultimate attempt at destroying my personhood and individuality.

The counselors all clapped, patted me on the back, and said how sensational this was, that the poor little *thing* would now be able to speak again. They reacted as if to the message sent across the wires by Alexander Graham Bell on the first telephone, "What hath God wrought?" But to my mind, this was not what God intended for me. People who don't have a disability rarely understand those who do, don't understand how depersonalizing technology can be. I decided I would not marry myself to a machine, nor would I accept it speaking for me. The Bible says in Psalm 139 that we are wonderfully and skillfully made. That suggested I already possessed all that I needed to get along, just had to tap into it. It is said 90 percent of what we communicate is nonverbal, so to me, a 10 percent loss is really no great loss. I'd just have to deal with what I had left—my body, hands, and face—and communicate in natural ways. In a communication situation, the body speaks first anyway and never lies. So why not try that?

We've all grown up thinking the solutions to our most challenging problems rest with science and technology, so naturally, people believe it is the answer to solving problems of people with disabilities. To some extent, it has in making prosthetics to replace missing limbs, sophisticated iron lungs to help people with polio breathe easier, and telecommunications devices for the deaf. But never should we lose sight of the fact that we are dealing with human beings, not machines with missing parts. Don't treat symptoms and forget there's a person behind them.

I haven't run into too many of those "special kinds of people" we all envision working with the exceptional. In fact, I've met very few. There are more of the opposites—people you have to wonder how they ever got their jobs in the first place. Some came into the field back when all that was needed were warm bodies to fill positions because working with us was viewed as undesirable, emotionally taxing, and unrewarding. The very idea of being in there pitching every day with folks considered hard to learn, slow to progress, difficult to control, and unpleasant to look at doesn't bring the finest and brightest running. Dedication to service has gone out of style.

Poor training, insensitivity, and lack of input from the disabled themselves hinder understanding our experience beyond facts and statistics. Rather than being able to empathize, many workers only add to our frustrations by chiding, deriding, and mocking us while setting themselves up as specially chosen emissaries sent to bring poor heathens into the light, to them be all honor, glory, and praise as if doing the world a big favor. They act as if they have all the answers, know everything, and can *rescue* us from what we're going through, when most often, progress is a slow and painful process. We don't want mommies or daddies, just decent, responsive, and respectful service. Workers should not become patronizers! Rather, encircle us with support and build relationships based on partnership and professionalism. To do this, be flexible and attuned to what's needed and appropriate according to the individual. That would be the ideal situation, but in the real world, even the ones supposedly well trained sometimes say and do the dumbest things, such as making crass jokes that put down and disrespect the people they serve. At a state conference for rehab workers I attended, a longtime veteran in the field did impressions of blind people, making a mess trying to ice Christmas cookies, then taught profane and sexual gestures to be communicated in sign language to amuse staff over lunch.

Often verbal jabs are hurled at us that leave wounds. Once I was told, instead of sitting around being lazy because I don't want to work, trying to collect a check, I should go out and get myself a job. And on another occasion, when discussing my frustrations in getting a diagnosis, a therapist remarked with a hearty laugh, "We won't know what's really wrong with you until you die and we cut you open and do the autopsy!" What tactless things to say to a person wrestling with fears of decline and death, whose livelihood has been taken away. You'd think they'd know better! Such thoughtless comments really hurt!

And there is the issue of confidentiality. Nosy workers having nothing to do with my case would walk up and ask, "What's the matter with you?" like, "What's your problem?" They delve into your business, then add it to the gossip that runs rampant within their circles, thus breaking rules about not betraying our privacy. It's as if they think they can do with us as they will, dissect us, pick us apart, and try putting us back together again. It's about control! Besides those sins of commission, there are the sins of omission, those things everyone knows they should be doing but aren't because "nobody else is doing them," yet they know in their hearts its right.

There are some who make a habit of saying, "Oh, disabled people can do anything everyone else does now. It makes no difference!" Just as African Americans are told there's no longer anything holding us back, yet no one wants to have a disability, and still no one wants to be black. If they sincerely want to do us a favor, let them treat us normally but not ignore or deny our disabilities and the very real problems we face, nor make it more difficult for us by being mean and ignorant.

Probably the biggest challenge for us is not to be deterred when we encounter stumbling blocks in the form of people. Often out there in the public I feel like licking my raw wounds and going home. It's hard not to let the voice of discouragement resonate louder than my own inner voice prompting me to go on. Sometimes I have to shake water off my back and turn up my inner volume.

This raises a question I have often wondered about in relation with the mainstream. Why is it society places the onus upon the minority group member to forge ahead, persist, try to overcome obstacles, and achieve, in spite of people who try to stand in our way, instead of placing the ball in the court of those who actively or passively hold others back, unmask them for their biases, and make it their obligation to change? They're the ones who most often call the plays and control the game, so they're the ones who will have to change the rules by which we play. But I guess that would strike the right people the wrong way.

Actually, a lot of them don't even know when they are doing it. After all, we are all well intentioned, aren't we? Nobody means any harm! Sometimes they even think they're complimenting us, like when they say, "Oh, you deaf people make such w-o-n-d-e-r-f-u-l actors!" and tell blacks, "*You people* are so good at singin', fightin', and runnin'!" implying one has natural expressiveness and the other, natural rhythm. They don't see that as stereotyping. We get tired of everyone else's assessments of who and what we are.

I remember at Columbia University the only time we even heard from someone with a disability was after all the professors had their say at the end of the last class, a lady in a wheelchair was invited in to share a few tidbits like an unnecessary little addendum to the main course of our education. We disabled are viewed as ineffectual even in areas that affect us. The normal have all the jobs and answers.

When I look back on my course work there, even getting an MA in education of the physically handicapped, I realized we learned so precious little about the disabled experience from a subjective point of view, how they saw themselves, what their struggles or needs were, and what it was like to be in their position. It was the so-called normal describing, labeling, and prescribing remedies to suit "our problems" in the same way whites have always done with blacks, giving their spin on who we are, creating for us an identity that often doesn't match how we see ourselves. People in the mainstream are biased against the disabled, not only because we are different, but also because we do things differently, like using all sorts of gadgets and gizmos or just doing things the way *we* do them.

If we get jobs at all, it's usually with others like ourselves, because as with the minority job seeker, we are channeled to our own little ghettoes where we can help our people, as if no one else could benefit from what we know. They discount us for the valuable input we can have in programs and public policymaking in other segments of society. After all, if this society is going to work, it has to work for all of us. It is no wonder self-help groups have sprung up across the country where people with disabilities ban together to advocate and push their own agenda to affect public policy just as we African Americans did to foster the civil rights movement.

Many in the nondisabled community suffer from a mixture of arrogance and ignorance. Attitudes that see us as so full of anger and self-pity still persist and blind others to what our real needs are. True, they can't walk a mile in our shoes, and if they had to, it would be a really tight squeeze. Therefore, there is a need for a teaching/learning process for all Americans to confront issues regarding disability, not only those presently affected. It is a reality many will face at differing points in their lives, so issues regarding it should be a part of everyone's awareness and concern.

We in this society avoid talking about disability just like we avoid discussing issues of race, as if by refusing to acknowledge them, they will cease to exist and give us trouble. The lack of discussion forces us to go on living with old attitudes and fears, preventing our getting to know each other better. Consequently, most of us remain stuck back when we were kids and our parents told us not to point and stare. It is unwise not to talk about it! Frank, open discussion, sharing of feelings, and asking questions, I believe, are helpful to both sides. Although disability is a part of life, we are not out there being seen as people living, functioning, and making it. Rather, we are locked up in the confines of our own private worlds, in the closets of society where others can't interact with us and thereby come to know there is *value* in our experience and it is not inherently bad, that we can feel good about ourselves.

It was ironic that as I worked on this segment, reports screamed from my radio with accompanying shock and regret that the actor Steve Reeves, who played the bigger-than-life Superman in movies, was thrown from a horse and sustained a spinal cord injury, possibly meaning he might never walk again. The reports blared as if ringing his death knell. We all tend to see ourselves as supermen and women, until chronic illness or disability strikes and convinces us of our mortality. None of us knows what awaits us around each corner. Disability can strike anyone at any time.

As baby boomers like myself are starting to gray, many more may find disability a reality, and it will no longer be possible to discount what we know. In fact, the sizeable population moving into middle age can prove to be the greatest boost to opening society to the disabled. As boomers lose their bloom and demand their needs be met, we will sail through the door in the pockets of their vests and reap the benefits. I don't think we should necessarily sit around waiting for that to happen and not champion our own cause, but it is certainly true we have common issues such as nursing home versus in home patient care, payment for attendants, national health care and entitlements, Medicare, Medicaid, SSI and Social Security, our base of surety. While others live with fear of losing their jobs, we live with "the Medicare scare." Because of warnings of drastic cuts in assistance by the government, we worry if quality health care will be even accessible to us in the future.

As America is losing its "kindness and gentleness," concern for the infirmed, the elderly, and the disabled is lessening as evidenced by the hue and cry for full employment for *everyone*, apathy about our plight and condition, cutting back, calls for doctor-assisted suicide, the rise of Jack Kevorkian, lack of giving to organizations to help the handicapped, shortage of volunteers, and harsh insensitivity of people on the street toward anyone who cannot "fend for themselves."

So many today are guilty of blatant lack of compassion. People who work with the disabled are sometimes the worst offenders. It is easy to become numb, especially when you are exposed every day and grow acclimatized. I am not speaking of compassion in the sense of having folks fawning pettily because of our disabilities, but of being sensitive to what the person is going through and setting about to find ways to make it a bit easier. The public needs to stop looking on impassively and waiting for others to take the lead.

Whatever happened to tenderness and gentleness between people? Not only lovers but friends and people who *care* even in the work setting. Why has that gone out of style? Why has everyone gotten so cold-hearted as if afraid to reach out and be nice to one another? Don't they realize their day is coming? In dealing with the disabled, there is a need for persons who will make a personal commitment to do their best, even under stress to deal with us with gentleness, good humor, and understanding. So many disabled people are out there dangling, some with hidden disabilities not easily pinpointed, needing a helpline, an anchor, and a good base of support, who may have to borrow strength occasionally as they struggle to get in the swim of things. Workers should not confuse being a pillar and a driving force with callousness and insensitivity. A gentle prod is not the same as a good swift kick. For the person with a disability, there is a need to hang tough, not be overly sensitive and wear a thick skin. Realize not only we go through this, because people don't care what they say to anybody these days and keep things in perspective.

When we are new to something, it is common to give control over to others. It's difficult to take back control and begin to commandeer your life when so many factors working against you make you feel like, why bother? It really takes some fight and feistiness that we must reach down in the deepest part of ourselves and pull out. It's not just there, and no amount of people spouting truisms like "life goes on" puts it there. It has to come from within.

An ominous problem with disability is having to bear our burdens all alone, having few friends, no support group, and often no one to share the load while trying so hard to achieve our independence and maintain it. It can become self-defeating, and we can easily be overwhelmed. I felt like I had been exposed to some deadly Kryptonite and my strength was being drained, though I was trying with all my might. What I needed were people who could be positive, upbeat, and present to talk me through my fears and lend support while remaining calm. I needed to know those I depended upon would *be there* for me through the long haul. I didn't need others to increase my anxiety. It's hard when you haven't been through it to understand the experience.

The use of our abilities, however small, is enhanced by *love*. We all need kindness and respect, but often a disabled person endures bumps, bruises, scorn, and rudeness. We go without a kind word many days. People rarely care to encourage us with a word of love. In fact, the rehab community takes that as babying, encouraging wallowing and dependency, when in fact, kindness and encouragement are the very ingredients most need in mega doses. We should all try to be a pick-me-up to others rather than a put-downer!

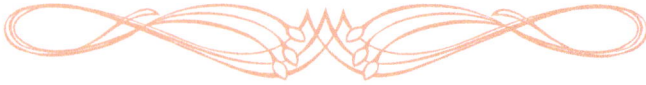

CHAPTER TWENTY-SEVEN
Friends and Family

MONTHS had gone by. I'd kinda gotten used to my body's malfunction, but not to dealing with the external world. My struggle became increasingly nonacceptance by family and friends whom I cared about and depended on in so many ways. They, most of all, were baffled by the malady and couldn't accept this strange new *me*. It brought out all sorts of feelings and unanticipated behaviors. Not only did it short-circuit my career, but it impinged upon my ability to sustain close personal relationships with intimates, thereby cutting me off from the household and undermining my base of support. Everybody did the best they could, what they knew. I don't blame them. It's simply they didn't understand and weren't prepared to deal with it. I can't say they didn't care or that they weren't there. They were there, but not *there*, at least not where I was.

In the ides of the eighties, everyone was on the fast track. Ol' Jim Crow no longer held us back. Down-home blacks had gotten outta those hovels and sad little shacks, done got sumpin' now. My folks up north no longer lived like packrats in steamy tenements. They had moved to high-rise buildings and were paying top rents. Wasn't walkin' up no mo' 'cause they had come up in the world. Nobody had time for the ill 'cause they had to work and pay dem bills. Black families keep on keepin' on come what may. Ain't never had an easy time of it, no way! Often we show bravery when going through pain, 'cause it happens again and again.

Actually what my family members did was laugh, joke, and pretend things were the same as always. They went into denial and remained for a very long time, pretended it was not there, and I mean at all. They continued calling and saying, "Tell Jean to pick up the phone!" attempting to engage me in conversation, not realizing my aggravation. Some acted afraid to draw near, like I had something catching, forgetting the importance of human touch. An arm around the shoulder, a hug, a gentle squeezing of the hand would have meant so much for bonding, affirming, and encouragement.

When trouble comes, it is best to be near the ones we love, to talk about it and share feelings. Being unable to speak, my feelings became so intense and scary. Nothing made sense. I wondered about death, what it is like, and wanted to cling to them for dear life. But they talked at me, not with me, used meaningless words and didn't listen. Mostly they avoided the subject altogether, because they were too uncomfortable with grief. Everyone started whispering—the doctors, folks at home, friends. They got in little huddles and chatted among themselves, as if afraid to speak openly, not realizing I was aware that they were aware of the changes and needed the opportunity to vent. I sat back watching and wondering what was going through their minds as I'm sure they did mine. There was so much secrecy and hush-hush. No one dealt directly.

This led to miscommunication. What I intended to transmit was often not what was heard. Transmissions get interrupted when you have no words. I wanted people to look at me, give me their undivided attention, read my little notes. Some people just couldn't cope with that, and a lot of disrespect got passed around. I needed a quiet room with the TV off, focus on me, my issues, but everyone was going through their problems too!

At the onset of my disability, like with any calamity, news spread fast. Relatives called and came by to see how I was, but soon the newness wore off. I became old hat, nothing to be concerned about. After all, life goes on, doesn't it? It moved in and settled down, friends took off, and family followed close behind. I felt a certain derision and a terrible sense of scorn. I'd catch them staring quizzically, trying to decipher me. Their looks said I was unacceptable or something was *wrong* with me, not that there wasn't, but I mean like I was *bad*. There was unspoken fear I could be accursed, like I had done some God-awful thing for which I was being punished, so they began dredging through my record, what they knew of it, tallied the sins in my dossier to see if they thought I was getting what I deserved. Black folks say, "You must not have been living right!" but most felt I was a nice person, so why me?

Before long I started receiving message cards, prayer cloths, holy water, and sand from "the Middle East" (more likely from Orchard Beach). Our people combine elements of religion, numerology, dream books, signs, and talismans to chart their crafts through life. Having faith in what we can hold is easier than an invisible God who saves souls.

Overnight old friends disappeared, got raptured right out of my life, leaving me alone and lonely. I just wasn't fun anymore because of their discomfort. Imagine, just a few short years ago, we were doing what young people do. Now look at me! They said they couldn't bear seeing me this way. I think they were afraid of being called on to help or felt leery of their day coming. People don't like to be reminded of their mortality. Only yesterday we sat, talked, and laughed. Now I was locked away in what appeared to be a living tomb. There's a lot of pain to that. They wondered how long I'd be forced to linger in cruel estrangement before fate set me free, or if I'd linger forever in soliloquy. They sure couldn't see anything good about it. I wavered between longing for the company of others and enjoying my solitude; I began excluding myself from everything.

Communication instead of a pleasure was now a chore; the tedium of reading and writing, a bore. We couldn't just get together and let our hair down like before. Plus everybody had their own responsibilities and couldn't take on any more. Some hinted if I really wanted to overcome this, I could; thus, it was my fault. They played the blame game. Yet they'd prefer jumping off a bridge than ending up the same. My loved ones wanted the best for me but got tired of being bothered as relating became arduous and cumbersome.

Families get no training in how to relate to the newly disabled member. They see the changes and are left with their own twisted emotions—pity, guilt, shame, whatever comes. Some have low reservoirs of patience and just stay away. Others buzz around but don't quite know what to say. Some vacillate between the desire to protect and the tendency to reject in front of others for fear you'll cast a bad reflection on them. They too need reeducation and enlightenment. It is a slow process.

My folks were ignorant to the medical system and felt powerless to fight for my rights. No one accompanied me to doctors to make inquiries and get answers, except Mama went a few times and did the best she could. But my problems weren't easily understood. She even made a pact with God Almighty what she would do if He would only heal me. Everybody was too busy, and nobody stayed at home. That left me to face my problems alone.

My house got so quiet I thought of calling the phone company to check if it still worked. If they did call, it was to tell me how my condition was hurting *them* and how they wished I was back to my old self again, as if I had cooked up this charade to put them through hell. They said how they prayed daily for me to talk again. It seemed not so much for my sake, but to free them from the torrid emotions ripping them apart in relation to me. It was a self-directed kind of concern; I was not the object. Oh yes, they passed the hat and took up a small collection. Those who had the least seemed to give the most, which I well appreciated. But more than cash, I would have preferred their time, presence, and support, which I never seem to get enough of. I needed to hear them say they still believed in me.

I penned this little poem, feeling cut off from those I loved:

> While I'm here let there be laughter and singing,
> Let the doorbell be ringing,
> And let me know what you are feeling.
> While I'm here.
>
> While I'm here bring tidings and good cheer,
> Everyone please draw near,

To help me face my fears.
Try and understand my tears.
While I'm here.

While I'm here won't you just stop by?
Even if you see me cry,
I promise I won't die, not while you're here!"

When you develop a disability, if the family and friends don't pull together to help, feelings of rage, anger, and helplessness burn out of control. I thought there would be more support and understanding, but there wasn't. Instead I was expected to continue in my role as family rescuer and savior, always putting out rather than receiving. At best, I got a cursory "How are you feeling?" But no one *really* wanted to know. It was hoped I'd nod in acquiescence so they could get on with their hurried lives. They couldn't tune into my needs, and I daren't ask. Turning to them would have made me feel I was bowing or dropping my guard. I certainly didn't want to run to others when I'd made a point of independence for so long. Neither did I wish to walk back through old conflicts or awaken hurts. Doing my best on my own and dealing with professionals paid to assist kept me from having to be beholden for every little thing someone did. We tend to hold on to loved ones to give us strength but sometimes realize latent feelings we have shunned or blocked out before. Hurts, pains, and disappointments regarding family may not be all their fault but get magnified by the situation. Yet I know I can't begin to imagine what it must have been like for my loved ones, what they were going through.

Malik was moving from puberty into the teen years. Changes in his body and interest in the opposite sex were wreaking havoc. He was in a new placement with acting-out kids and didn't feel safe but couldn't come home and talk about it. After school, being there with my silence, confused, wondering what was going on, often looking at me with a glance that said, "Who are you? I don't even know you anymore, and I'm not sure if I like you. I want my mother back!" Poor kid became my protector on mean city streets, accompanied me places, played bodyguard. Just he, I, and it were home now. Hector, laying up in traction after a car accident, couldn't call home and hear Mom's soothing words. He became disturbed at our being left alone, so he shuttled between the pressures of competing in a prestigious all-white school and being "man of the house" on the phone. Must have devastated him the thought of losing a second mother. Could he go through it again? Would he have to?

Both sons were in the throes of manhood; how could they have understood? In fact, I think they did pretty good! Why should anyone expect them to accept a disability that snatched me away so abruptly?

Poor Mom, had already raised one child with a handicap…now this! Two daughters? It was like lightning striking twice in the same place. She must have pondered what she had done that such trouble was visited upon her children.

And my other "mother," that chummy neighbor, it must have cut at her like a knife to be pushed out of my life. No more fence-side chats. No quick popping in and out to shoot the breeze, kids tugging at her knees.

Sis and bro were out there fightin' to survive, had their own lives, couldn't live mine for me. They cared but were not able to be there. More distant relatives were all off somewhere.

My father? Why, before I was his favorite girl, but now I was different, and he couldn't relate to the difference. Daddy was not the mushy, gushy type. He kept feelings locked up inside, but a tender heart lie beneath that tough cowhide. I confirmed it the only time he ever cried, when I left just before he died. He loved me regardless to the distance it created.

It took time for all of us to realize this wasn't going away but would be a part of our lives each day—time before they could give me that full family embrace, welcome me warmly, and be with me comfortably. Death in the family seemed to help them realize I was not gone, that they could still reach out to me and express the things they really wanted to say, that the good times didn't have to be over, but I just needed to relate in a slightly different way.

I've learned life has to do with adjusting to changes, to having things for a while then letting go, like my dolly at six, pickup sticks and my goldfish, Santa and the elves, that cute boy at twelve, the slop, diddy bop, and sweet sixteen, tattered jeans, my first beau, and on it goes. We live happier when we learn to say "The Lord gives and He takes away. Blessed be the name of the Lord!" I learned I needed to be careful about the people I allowed to influence and possibly discourage me. Then I began encouraging myself that something good was going to happen.

We all think our problem is the worst and nobody understands. It's like the joke about the elephant who says to the hippo, "The worse thing in the world is a cold in the nose," and the hippo responds, "Well, you've never had chapped lips, have you?"

Since the advent of email and fax machines, modern people are less inclined to communicate face-to-face. I, perhaps more than most, have come to realize the importance of interpersonal communication and the pitfalls of relating without speech. When you put down words, you don't know how they'll be taken. You have to learn to express yourself in ways that won't be mistaken. It's hard without tone of voice and body language to accentuate them. I had to begin bringing my body into it. Relating interpersonally is a rapidly dying art now that computers have gotten so smart. Yet it is crucial in a business as well as in the family. Maybe that's why God gave me this disability, to make me a set of ears. There ought to be at least one person in every family who will not talk, just hear! The book of James says, "Everyone should be slow to speak and quick to listen."

If family and friends abandon us in our time of need, it leaves us feeling deserted. That's human nature! Even Christ felt abandoned at His most crucial hour on the cross. Somehow onlookers viewed me as a strong person who could handle it. Yet I had lots of weaknesses; I just didn't let them show or sit around moaning and groaning. No one would have guessed the battle that was going on inside to suppress emotions I tried to hide, the effort it took to put on a happy face while my spirit ached. My twisted smile was always there, but it was forced and tired. I looked wired. I'm sure all thought to help but didn't know how.

There are those who don't want to be identified with someone going through emotional trauma, won't get involved, can't deal with problems not easily solved. In this age of incredible medical technology and scientific breakthroughs, folks have little tolerance for conditions that you can't pop a pill or do a procedure for them to go away. Not like in the old days when it was common for family members to take turns caring for a sick, indigent, elderly, or disabled member. Now that everyone is on a treadmill and no one has time, the primary caregivers have become state and local agencies. I had an uncle who asked me, "Do you mean as smart as dem boys is now they cain't make you talk?" We had gone from seeking the Lord for answers to seeking physicians.

Fear of my condition made others want to put distance between us. Of that I had no doubt. But friends saying they'd pray for me while walking through the door seemed like a cop out. To my chagrin, members of my church family were noticeably absent too. Not the elders, but parishioners I sat with in the pews, my brothers and sisters in Christ. Missing them was painful because we had grown close. But all alike stood ready with a pat excuse. Unable to hold on to them, I held on to God's promise He would never leave nor forsake me. Sometimes I wanted to hold someone I could touch and see, but that's the way it had to be.

Like Job's friends, mine made innuendos I must have done something to bring this on myself and sprinkled in a little poison that if God is so good, why would He let this happen? They snuggled up, picked, and said things that got under my mettle. I was very much nettled. Said they were just trying to help, that they were on my side and a lot of other jive. Words can leave deep, deep scars. At times it's best not to say anything; just *be there*.

It's not so much I wanted something from them, just to know they were by my side come what may for support, that I could depend on them, that they assumed the best of me and believed in me, that they'd not be scarce when I really needed them, that they would love me regardless, in good times or in bad, that they would be caring and sympathetic. I didn't need any buttinskies to tell me what to do or try to run my business. Disability hadn't impaired my capacity to make my own decisions or taken away my rights to do so.

I came to see disability creates many dilemmas. Others know the depths of our neediness, especially in social arenas, and use us to serve their own, knowing we don't have a lot of alternatives for attention and companionship. The ones I wished would come seldom did. The ones I didn't want showed up too often, arrived unannounced, abused my time, and stayed too long. Everything was, "Oh, she don't mind!" In my loneliness, I went along with their rudeness. It strikes me funny that they never asked questions requiring a head shake yes or no and couldn't care less if my fingers cramped up and hands dropped off at the wrists. They didn't feel it! I was the one expected to accommodate. They'd do nothing differently for my sake! In fact, they got bugged if I wrote too many notes because they got tired of reading, not of me writing. I didn't show anger or drive them away because if I did, I'd have to deal with the emptiness of no one's presence. People know when they have us at their mercy. On jobs we get used because they know we can't easily go and find another one. In families we get tossed aside, uninvited and not told important things. We become the servants rather than the served.

Sometimes I just wanted to go visit somebody that was not a family member to change the dynamic, be with peers and have a pleasant time. But there was no one, so it was back to family or out to shop or eat. I had no circle of friends. So I tried to be content with food or things to replace people. Needless to say, I put on a few pounds and was no longer a Jeanie Weenie! When I did visit, I didn't know how to project myself. Thought I came across weird or retarded and began to long for the safety of home.

Sometimes I wanted to talk about my disability, share my fears and struggles, but it seemed like that was taboo. People either clammed up and fidgeted or looked like I was getting ready to drop a bomb on them. Some came up with quack cures and said, "I've been praying for God to heal you!" which dumped a load of guilt. Black people especially tend to be very charismatic in their faith, looking for signs and wonders and miraculous recovery. Of course, if you don't get healed, it is your sinfulness that is at fault.

In a constant struggle for acceptance, I found myself insecure and overly tense with each new encounter, feeling unable to handle the experience. My nerves got caught up in knots, giving me no peace. I chomped and chewed on my nails endlessly and drank cup after cup of coffee. I don't know which was worse, being out with others or being alone with myself. We harbor a lot of turmoil inside as we try to make the adjustment to our condition. Those feelings seem never to go in remission.

Anyone who wants to befriend a disabled person should not look at superficial appearances, odd quirks, or deformities. Try to get in touch with what is going on *inside*. Most have gone through a great deal of change and may be only a shell of who they were before. They may simultaneously want to send you away and embrace you. Expectations and feelings get in the way. Handicapped individuals have a threefold battle with their bodies, emotions, and people around them, the attitudes of the so-called normal. Anger may arise and misunderstandings readily pop up. Others can mean well and easily say the wrong thing. Mixed feelings constantly jump back and forth. It takes sensitivity, patience, and an ability to hear even what the person may not be capable of saying in words. Listen for the voice of their spirit.

A call or a visit to one who is isolated can bring cheer to a depressing atmosphere if you bring along a dish of encouraging words. The important thing is to go to serve, not to be served and played up to because of the need. There is an intrinsic reward in showing kindness, but you have to extend their way before you'll receive.

Today humans operate by the law of the jungle. It's every man for himself if he wants to survive. We've made self-concern and self-actualization so paramount responding to the needs of others rarely crosses our minds. A disabled person who requires an assist in some way has a hard way to go. He'll more likely be shoved aside and trampled by the throng in the mad dash for personal fulfillment.

The premier result of my speech loss was the alienation it brought. Lack of being able to connect with others left no sense of belonging. I felt as if I were the only one going through this problem because of my isolation. I came to really, really know something about loneliness, even though I was in the midst of others. I was there but not there, present but unaccounted for. Those I'd been closest too had problems too. Malik didn't read well because of LD, Fay even less due to blindness. My notes to them were almost meaningless. The gap between us became so uncrossable. Mama was getting older, slowing down. How much could I expect from her? And I didn't want to. She'd been through enough already. I wanted to get out from that menagerie of emotions to be with others like me, but there were none I could see. I felt like a refugee in a strange land. It was that same feeling I often got passing through white neighborhoods, like I was an intruder. People grew ruder. It was so hard to befriend and make friends.

It takes time to heal, to find ourselves and pull it all together. There are no shortcuts. We go through a process that is grievous, painful, and hard to deal with. Our loved ones should love us through it, not write us off. People who cry, feel, and understand the pain of healing can throw out a rope and help pull us along. Hope is the rope we hold on to if we want to come back ashore.

It got to the point I was so lonely for a friend I clung to my VR counselor and therapists, tried to engage them in idle chatter before we got down to business during my office visits. I even tried to strike up conversations with the CAs on the other end of my TDD (telecommunications device for the deaf), delaying extra time online after my call had ended. It was good to know there was someone out there I could connect with who was concerned about talking with and for me.

Before long all my relationships were business. I remember how I used to call the social worker for the deaf when I had the blues or didn't know what else to do. She was someone I thought understood and knew what I was going through. Special bonds began to develop with those who came into my life professionally. But then it hurt when I found out they were only doing it for the money and there was nothing personal to our relationship. It hurt so much I preferred not to be attached to anyone at all so I wouldn't have to feel the pain when they left and I was again by myself.

When I had an operation, a home attendant came to visit daily. We became so close, sharing tidbits and little secrets. Then one day she was gone. Time carried her on to another job, and I felt robbed. My days were so empty without her. Workers easily become everything to us. We suffer longingly in their absence.

I still yearn for real friendships but find myself suspicious of everyone's ulterior motives. Wonder why when someone is attentive and nice. We disabled often experience charity once a year at Christmas when people try to score brownie points with God out of guilt. I ask myself if their acts are sincere, heartfelt. What if I begin to care and suddenly they are not there? Impermanence frightens me! Better to walk alone, I say, but it's not possible.

To improve communication with a disabled person, speak the truth but say it lovingly. Stay calm and don't be too overwhelming! Measure your words and your time. Don't run things in the ground or try to insist. Respect the other person's rights to do things their way. Be able to take no for an answer. Don't pour out a lot of anger on people. Express your feelings and your fears honestly but gently. Be careful not to destroy the person's fragile self-image by saying things that are mean or not funny in jest. Take matters seriously! Talk in words that build up and encourage rather than tear down and discourage, especially when speaking of sensitive matters. Try to see from their point of view. Imagine being in their shoes how you would want to be treated. Realize their experience is quite different from yours. It's hard to think like a bird if you are a fish and have never been out of water. Let them tell you what the sky is like. No matter how different your experiences are, in some ways you still have lots in common, so focus on those areas. Remember you're relating to a person, not a disability. Be kind, tenderhearted, and forgiving. Be a listener more often than a speaker. Give that person who is struggling an opportunity to vent. Most of all, acceptance will bring restoration.

When we feel alienated, we need that listening ear. We want someone who can be empathetic and get in our skin for the sake of identifying with us. We want someone we can communicate with and ask questions. We need people who will respect us as people, that we can reveal ourselves to beyond the surface—someone who can relate sensitively and not raise our level of anxiety. We need people who will not tell us what we need (we already know). Others have no idea how deep our shame and wounds are. Don't try and tell what *you* think is right for us. Instead listen empathetically and imagine being in our place. It is pretty hard to do because you may think you know but don't really *know* all we go through. So let us tell you! People have a tendency to tell us what we could have and should have done. As a substitute to preaching, try to make connections in this disconnected world.

Relating empathetically means getting past the small talk and getting down to the heart of things, getting to know where people *are*. The handicapped long for warm friendships, to be comfortable, to be understood, and to feel at home. They enjoy so much the simple activities others take for granted because they can do them so easily, like going out to lunch, sitting and chitchatting over coffee, going to the movies, shopping, and visiting. A handicapped individual desires to relate to those around him but may not have the skills, and those engaging with him may not either. Often neither feels comfortable with what to say or how to act. A lot of emotions become awakened. The normal feel frustrated and powerless. People with disabilities fear bonding because they may be afraid you will go away and not come back. Relationships that are transient bring a lot of *pain*, and they don't want that to happen again.

Sometimes I desperately desired to talk about my fears, the changes in my body, and the struggle to deal with circumstances, but my family and friends didn't want to. They well meaningly said, "Don't worry, don't talk about it! Concentrate on the good things and be thankful!" It seemed better to them not to talk about it, not realizing it had to be dealt with. After all, not only had it changed me, but inevitably it would change the lives of those around me. We all need openness, honesty, and support to help us cope.

When we are grieving a loss in our lives, we don't need lots of words. Rather, we need compassion, someone's presence, and time to work through anger or denial. Also we need others who make us feel safe. Sometimes I wanted to revert back to the little girl who use to crawl up on my daddy's lap and hear him say, "Everything is gonna be all right!" I talk to him in heaven even now and say, "I'm going to look this joker in the eye just like you taught me!" Don't judge us for being weak and frail in the face of a frightening situation. Support and encouragement without the phony stuff people always say will go a much longer way.

Sincere dialogue can help us come to grips with our feelings. We are usually talking to ourselves really but must get it outside so we can hear it and thrash it around, then make the necessary adjustments. Don't come and tell us nice, neat little pat answers and clichés like, "When life gives you lemons, make lemonade." We may be too far down to be lifted by words like that. What helps is to ask the person what they are feeling. Let them vent. Try to get in touch with their pain. Don't say you know what they're going through. Just show you care and are willing to listen. Let them cry on your shoulder, if need be, and not have to walk away feeling ashamed. Make vulnerability acceptable. Christ was meek and vulnerable!

Sympathy is to have a heart to want to gather with another person to share their hurts. Sometimes there is a need for sympathetic *silence*, and sometimes there is a silence that comes from discomfort with grief and not knowing how to deal with it, which makes you feel like you are dangling there alone with no one there to try to rescue you. Books always seem to discourage sympathy, as if it is bad or destructive, and can lead to doing things for people they could do for themselves, or that you might get ripped off because of your tender heartedness. But I think, for certain people, if it wasn't for sympathy, there would be nothing to prompt them to get in touch with what the other person is going through, because of being so locked in their own cushiony world, so self-concerned and not wanting to listen to another person's problems. A person who is suffering is often bothersome, unpleasant, aggravating, and can make you feel uncomfortable and guilty for what you have and what you're not doing.

Empathy is saying to a person that you can't possibly know what they're going through, but you're willing to listen and want them to make you understand. Not you know how they feel and here is what they should do, which is the typical reaction of people to a problem or disability. This immediately blocks off the other person's voice and feelings from being expressed. I think sympathy should precede empathy, because you need to have a basic sense of compassion that will allow you to respond to an obvious condition you know is bad or difficult, e.g., death, sickness, loss of job, and home and family issues. Out of that sense of compassion, which maybe surface or temporary, one can be moved to want to listen and understand more fully what the experience is and become involved in helping. There are crushings and bruisings in life that defy instant cure. Many of those deep hurts are hard to explain. Scarred, bleeding people are the ones others run to for help with real-life circumstances.

As time moved on, things began to wind down, knots untangled, and I wangled my way along but found no escape hatch. The only way out was through it. In fact, disability is something we never really overcome. We struggle to reconquer it daily. An old gospel song says, "Lawd, don't move my mountains, just help me to climb 'em!" Mountain climbers use a good, strong rope. Hope is the rope we hold on to for dear life. When we are at our worse, God is at His best. His strength keeps us going long after ours runs out. He was teaching me to hang in there. From my earliest days, I had creativity. God was now giving me form and solidity.

The world encourages us to hide the cracks and put on a happy face. I found out I could let Him see the cracks and how much I was hurting. He understood. I never felt far away from Him and knew He wasn't ignoring me. We developed greater intimacy as it became my opportunity to get to know Him better. When going through changes, we often need spiritual as well as physical help in order to make it through the pressures. Words from the Bible ministered to me as never before, and I could see their spiritual significance for the first time. I learned there are bonds that come with going through a hard time together, both as a family and when we share a difficult experience or circumstance. My eyes were suddenly open to the pain around me, and I could feel for others who were hurting.

Everyone deals with things differently. Everyone has different levels of patience and strength. One challenge is to lend your particular gift to the disabled person. Not everyone is good at everything, but each family member or friend usually has some special gift or ability that, if put forward, would be greatly appreciated, i.e., some are resourceful in getting information, others are very consoling, others like to talk and listen, while still others have ministering spirits and don't mind helping with dressing, shopping, or chores. The trick is for each person to do a little so the weight doesn't fall all to one person like the spouse or members of the immediate family. For a structure to be solid, it needs to rest on a firm foundation. Family and friends can supply the base of support we need to jettison us back out into the functional world after suffering some sort of setback. The more we feel loved, the easier it is to make it through the process.

When you are grieving a loss in today's society, you are expected to go on with life and not let your grief get in the way. Neither are you expected to let it show. But earlier societies recognized the need for rituals and ways of marking the letting go of sadness surrounding death or trauma to help us move on. There is a need for a time to mourn and then a breaking of the mourning period, although the memories and pain may linger long after. It is best to cherish the good memories, let go of the bad, and they will always be ours. We should hold on to those rituals and keepsakes that bring comfort to us, but tuck them safely away in the attic of our hearts so they don't stop us from going forward. And then every once in a while, take them out, dust them off, take a trip back only briefly to remember and enjoy time well spent. It can be a source of strength and grounding to know where you *were*, but realize you can't *stay* there.

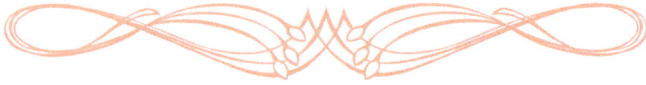

CHAPTER TWENTY-EIGHT
Elim

SPEAKING well is requisite for smooth communication in general society. We are often judged by our speech and language. Society looks down on people who speak poorly or use substandard English, likewise on those who don't speak at all. A good talker has monetary value in the workforce. A nontalker…well, everyone knows in the game of life it's odd man out. But I had made a firm decision not to depend on mechanical wizardry I needed to carry around to speak for me. I wanted to communicate naturally.

Though my vocal ability vanished, in essence I remained the same. I felt God's providential changes were leading somewhere, perhaps to a new career, a new lifestyle, maybe even a new location. Where? I didn't know. My thoughts swirled around rapidly, yet I was moving slowly. Slow is different from standing still. The fact that I was wanting to take back the reins of my own life and jump back up on the horse shows I was headed forward. But I suppose those unanswered questions held me captive. They were like ghosts that kept me tied to the past and didn't allow full closure in my experience with loss.

Everyone goes through a valley experience in life. Mine was with disability. Yours may not be. However, climbing back up has certain constants that remain the same. The first step in moving from *can't* to *can* is moving away from folks who stop you from letting go of the past. You have to get away from the same old people, locked into doing the same thing in the same way, and look for support from others who have made it through trials. Sometimes adversity pushes us to higher levels of performance. Sickness can too! To get up after a fall, we must not let others divert us from finding our direction. We need to hold on to our encouragers and block out our discouragers. Be determined to go on with God's help. Recovery does require the fellowship of persons who pledge their support and walk down dark and frightening alleys with us. Sometimes it does take physical or emotional trauma to refocus us on what's important. The only way I could get on with my life was to spend time on my knees and be willing to go through the difficult process of learning something new. You can't keep doing things the same old way if you want to get a breakthrough!

Folks kept wanting to put me in a box, but I didn't fit neatly into any of them. So no one could attach an appropriate label, except perhaps communicatively disordered. If only they had grasped, it's not about how we transmit, but the message that's being sent, the idea being transferred, which allows people to participate in our world, understand our thoughts, and see things as we see them. It's not about broken ears or a broken tongue or being retarded or any of the other boxes we create for sorting. It's about finding a comfortable vehicle by which ideas and feelings can be mutually shared and exchanged.

People talk to me because I can hear, caring nothing that I can't converse with them in oral language. They look for their comfort zone, not mine. Their need cries out for someone to listen. That's all! They feel I should get a talking computer box, because it's the technology being developed for people who can't speak. But what gives anyone the right to define what I am and say what's right for me?

Nonverbal communication is the first language of all humans and the most natural way to communicate for all people. We do it from the time we are born and continue throughout our lives. So why should I choose something as unnatural as a voice box over my own body? That would only be the choice of a person who feels superior and wants to impose his way on me, viewing himself as normal and right and me as broken and needing to be fixed. But why fix what's not broken? If I am able to communicate just not in an oral language, who is to say I am the worse off? What if I feel okay the way I am? And what if I'm not fixable?

The wonderful mimes Marcel Marceau and the Marx Brothers demonstrated how beautifully the body can speak without ever a spoken word and what can be conveyed and understood through gesture, movement, and facial expression. They used pantomime (talking with their bodies) to entertain. We don't realize how much we use unconscious gestures in everyday living to get across our ideas. Often our body language even divulges that which we try to disguise, like discomfort. "Silence is golden" was proven by Red Skelton and the comics of vaudeville. I doubt anyone who has ever seen them had much difficulty comprehending their comedic parlance.

Driven by yearning emotions, I began to look for a sense of belonging and a new place of identity, for an oasis where being like me would be the norm. I actually searched for another person like me. It's weird thinking you are the only one. At the agency there had been deaf people in my class, but they all sat on one end of the room with the interpreter and I on the other with my piece of paper. We glared curiously at one another. Somehow we sensed we belonged together, but we were waiting for the professionals to pair us off.

I was surprised to find the deaf consumers both signing and speaking, although their voices were high pitched and very uncomfortable to hear. I didn't meet anyone who didn't talk at all. There was one man who'd had his larynx removed and used one of those machines he pressed against his throat. Everyone tended to lump the two of us together. But I felt no fellowship with that guy and his microphone voice. He could speak, just had no voice box to broadcast it. I could make sound but couldn't control the musculature to speak. What a mélange of peoples are in this fix we call disabled. In fact, the normal really should be called "the temporarily abled," for who knows what they will face down the road.

Out of curiosity, one Sunday I found my way to a deaf ministry at a Catholic church in the West Bronx. All the hearing congregants sat on one side and the deaf on the other. Entering the assembly,

I couldn't figure out where I belonged. The hearing beckoned me to come and sit with them; the deaf looked on baffled, thinking I belonged on their side. I was in a straight between the two and didn't know what to do. I saw then what kids who are interracial must go through. As I stood there wagging my head, a proud, dignified elderly little man, totally mute and projecting no shame, took the podium and lead the worship service in sign language. Suddenly something clicked!

The beauty of his signing and the peace and comfort he conveyed being complete in himself and at one with God touched me. I found in him encouragement and hope! I wanted to run up and grab him off the stage, hug him, and say, "Hi, brother!" At that moment I made a decision not only about my seating preference but my cultural preference too. I decided to stop walking around, bobbing my head like a coil-neck doll in a back-seat window to say yes or no. I reasoned if a dolphin who performed in a water show could learn signs, so could Jean the Beano!

I assertively marched over, plopped down at the table for the deaf, and decided I would identify with them even if I had to force myself. Whether or not we want to make a choice, society always chooses for us as in the case of race. I *had* to learn to function deaf because there is no way to be "hearing" without speaking. In fact, the sign for hearing people is made at the mouth to indicate their speaking behaviors. In deafness, the primary disability is inability to communicate with the hearing world, and that certainly describes me. The factor of not being able to hear relates to etiology or root cause.

The real impairment of deafness is communication, not broken ears or tongue. To illustrate, imagine speaking to a person who is profoundly deaf and then to me. In both cases, the results would be the same: neither of us would answer, although in the first case the cause is he doesn't hear you, and the latter, I am unable to speak. Our inability to communicate is the issue, not the underlying cause. As I go about publicly, I am usually identified as deaf because most people connect lack of speech with deafness. Yet few understand how inadequate communication can affect your thinking, behavior, and perception.

I developed an immediate yearning to learn sign language. I became a deaf wannabe, going places where they congregate to try to get practice and hopefully meet people. Thus began the long and arduous baptismal process of dying to the old hearing me and taking on a new identification with the deaf. Acceptance of manual language and willingness to use it in public would become my statement of allegiance to the deaf community and my decision to sign on with its culture and struggle. It was a privilege I relished, to be able to say where I belonged and not have it dictated to me. Sure I got tired of being an anomaly, but it gave me an identity that set me apart, made me feel special. I saw it as an opportunity to concentrate and accomplish a goal that had become important to me.

My first attempts at learning sign language began at my local library where I saw a poster advertising a free workshop for kids. I stumbled in and sat in the back of a circle of first graders buzzing about, eager to learn to talk with their fingers. The group leader began by introducing the finger-spelling alphabet and got us to sign our initials. She moved on to simple object pictures, gave a sign for each, then asked that we make a short sentence, i.e., "I like apples," as she went around. But when she got to me, I couldn't even create a three-word sentence or remember any of the signs taught. Suddenly I was the worst student in a group of youngsters like those I once taught. How humiliating and confusing!

God sent another resource, an interpreter who agreed to take me on as a student for private lessons. Every week we met in a back booth at her office and went through the trying emotional process of rebuilding self-esteem and beginning to dream. She helped me visualize myself as a signer, set some goals, and get back into the rigors of travel to study and learn. She gave me her company, became a sounding board for my frustrations, and made me feel no embarrassment as I fumbled along. Her acceptance of me, as I was, helped reinforce self-acceptance.

It is good to have something you need to prove sometimes to give you drive and energy to apply yourself. It doesn't have to be related to the disability, just a dream you've had and want to pursue. When it is achieved, you can look back with a great sense of pride.

Success will bring faith that other things can be conquered. It will help you look past the dark clouds of today and glimpse a brighter tomorrow.

The next step was to register for a beginner's class at the Society for the Deaf. There my classmates were basically young hearing adults attracted to sign language for the novelty of it, perhaps aspiring one day to work with deaf people. But I went in, heart in hand, wanting someone to teach me how to "talk" again, how to be deaf, like myself, and to identify with others in the deafened community. I found only social isolation and mockery. They kept standing me up in front of the group to do what signs I knew. When I faltered, it was like, "Wow! You're a poor excuse for a mute! This is supposed to come natural for you!" Classmates didn't realize I, like they, needed to unlearn dependence on my ears and increase visual acuity, nor did they understand the psychological impact of being cut off from being able to have a comfortable conversation.

There was no attempt by the staff to bridge the gap between us because of the notion we should all be treated the same. The reasoning was that since no one in the sign class was allowed to speak, we were all on a level playing field, but that ignored the full scope of my experience, which goes beyond dysfunctional body parts. I am a whole person, and a malfunction in one part of me affected my total makeup and outlook. I could barely focus on learning because I felt under constant scrutiny and my insides were in mutiny. Hearing students temporarily pretending not to speak did not make us alike. For me it would be a lifestyle, not just a game to stop playing when class was over. I was painfully aware I was in no way like them even though I could hear. The philosophy of being blind to difference can really undercut the minority group member because we have real issues that need to be addressed to undergird our success. It can't be handled by simply pretending problems aren't there and everyone is equal.

In that group, I felt like the village idiot. I was so out of it—so lacking. It was as if I couldn't retain anything or keep a complete sentence in my head. I'd start to sign the beginning but soon lost the sense of it and couldn't complete the end. Everything was fragmented. My ability to concentrate was badly shaken. I don't know if I had gone stale mentally or if there was really something wrong with my neurology, but I was suffering cognitive as well as speech loss.

My sign name became *J*, drawn in the dimple because others commented regularly on my "beautiful smile" in spite of the fact it was slanted. Little did they know how I wrestled to keep up the confidence to let it show. After sweating it out in class, I'd stop off in Wendy's and unwind over coffee. Fighting back tears, I'd sit and wonder if the world is still beautiful to those whose blind eyes can't see it. And if there is music in the hearts of those whose deaf ears can't hear it. And if my spirit still had a voice, even though my tongue could not express it. Had I lost that part of me that made me, *me*?

I'd gone there thinking I'd get treated right, that they'd know what to do with me. Come to find out a lot of deaf people were very conflicted too, went around emphasizing orality, suggesting deaf people are better who talk and appearing to look down on those who didn't. I didn't know they were being torn by hot debate over whether to speak or not to speak and were in a dilemma.

Instead of being consumed with my physical appearance, I decided to let what was on the inside come out, let my inner voice speak and a smile from within show through. It took the inward power of God working in me daily as I applied faith to my pain. This made me not want to lose heart, drop out, and quit. I tried to fix my eyes heavenward and began to imagine what could be, not only what was. Our physical bodies are fragile and transparent. But it is in our brokenness that the life of Christ can be revealed.

At first, it seemed so grotesque to talk with my body. Americans tend to find a lot of expressiveness with the hands and touching, during conversation, ill-mannered and for the less erudite classes. I found an awful similarity between myself and a big hairy ape on the public broadcasting channel who had been taught a few basic signs to make his beastly grunts and groans understandable to a female scientist. In my son's generation, hand jive had become an important part of the urban repertoire of street language associated with black identity. But with it I certainly felt no affinity.

To learn sign language was only part of the challenge. Joining the deaf community was the larger feat. Deaf people have a strong cultural identity, ways of behaving, and attitudes that are hard to adopt. You really need to have attended a deaf school, have deaf parents, or at least have moved within their circles to gain acceptance. In this country, there are such clear divides racially, economically, and culturally. Most people stay where they "belong." So what do you do if you don't exactly belong? It's difficult to go and just *join* a group. The deaf, like everyone else, have strong ties and are leery of "others." How would I let them know I was not an other? First, I'd have to be fully convinced myself.

As the express bus whisked to and from the Bronx downtown for classes past Central Park West and its fabulous addresses, I was swept back in time to when I was a small girl from Harlem being brought down to the other side to get my teeth filled. I was filled with the same emotions—powerlessness, inadequacy, distress—that *they* had all this and I, like the wheels of the bus, was still going round and around in my quest to turn ambition into success, still revolving, unfolding, asking myself, "Who am I?" while hurriedly finger-spelling licenses on cars that zoomed by. Thought I'd have been better off with broken ears and wished my hands could flow as fluidly as my tears. For some reason, I always sat in the very last row. The law didn't require it though. Guess it had just become a part of my consciousness, like a habit of mental secondariness. After all, the back of the bus has long been the place for us—all who are not full fares in this society.

I pressed on, attended a catholic church in Manhattan where I met another interpreter who taught a beginner's sign class, and joined. She, seeing my needs were different, introduced me to a nun who offered to practice with me for a small donation. Soon I was off to the Catholic archdiocese on Mondays, VR on Tuesdays, Deaf Bingo on Wednesdays, my class at the society on Thursdays, and an evening class at NY School for the Deaf, in the time I had left. On weekends, I came back down to catch signed performances in the park and tried to race home before dark. That grueling year was full of angst and anxiety as I tried to take responsibility for what I said

I was going to do. Yet with all my efforts to gain admittance, I was still a lone wolf skulking about the purlieus of the deaf community, unable to find my way into the camp.

New York City has a terrible legacy of controlling power groups and divisions. When you try to get involved in the deaf world, you meet small groups of folk who seem to have the field sew up in terms of jobs, programs, and money. So if you want to study or be a part in a closer way with its workings, you have to go through them because they control the happenings like a clique. You need a nod from one of them to be "in." And every program you go to, you are guaranteed to find the same people associated with it. It's like a country club heading major corporations and deciding who the players will be.

It was impossible for me to break through the barriers to enter deaf education there. Certain ones felt African Americans are not intelligent enough to develop fluency in sign and are disinterested in the cultural diaspora across America. At interviews they'd say, "It will be really, really hard for *you*!" I questioned whether their comments were based on a reasonable assessment of my ability or if it was an assumption that we are all linguistically deficient, culturally dead, and unconcerned about other groups outside our own. The history of divisions and control goes back to the deaf schools where white and black deaf were segregated, separate signs evolved, and deaf clubs and ministries catered to one race or the other.

Communication is a very important issue, whether between two hearing or two deaf or one hearing and one deaf or whoever. If there is no other benefit to being as I am, it has been to understand this. Today there are so many issues surrounding everything we do—so many things coming at us from all directions. Relating interpersonally has become pretty complicated now, especially in the development of intimacy. Yet it is critically important that we learn to communicate more effectively and tear down walls between men and women, parents and children, ethnic groups, deaf and hearing—wherever barriers exist to our understanding. But instead of getting better at it, we are getting worse. Communication styles have become very confrontational and in your face as hardening has taken place.

Hardness is often directed against those most in need, not those consumed by greed.

Today we function at a maddening pace. In our race toward upward mobility, we've lost civility, charity, and the ability to take it easy. We've become more like machines than human beings. Beepers at our waists keep calling us back to work, while relationships in our homes, communities, and cross-culturally are badly in need of repair. We keep trying to deal with our problems through technology, i.e., video cameras allowed us to witness the beating of Rodney King and be jurors in the OJ furor. Yet we remain as divided as ever in experience and outlook. A growing number of Americans can't get their heads in the trough to eat and lay sleeping on downtown streets, while the better off build hideaways in neat little communities far away. In these dream palaces, family members exist in separate rooms, have separate everything. There's so little sharing…seems we've completely lost our souls. Technology has brought advancement and power, but it has also brought estrangement from the natural world and each other.

Communicating for most of society is largely verbal, but relating is nonverbal. It involves taking time to observe, be with and get to know one another by participating in activities that build strong relationships, which make us feel whole, safe, and valued. We all need people to care about us and show interest; all need affirmation and appreciation. However, we are losing our skills in how to talk and what to talk about. Folks are either yelling at each other or sitting watching TV and saying nothing. This has affected our ability to get up close and personal with those around us.

Instead of looking to talk TV and its insanity for answers, we need to regain the art of silence and take time to know our children and God well. We need quietness and solitude more often to get back in tune. In place of going after more and more, there is a need to slow down, downsize, and learn to unwind. Low-income families especially need time for leisure and enjoyment as so much energy is consumed in just trying to make ends meet while our kids roam the street. A lot of it has to do with what we have come to value: a luxury car, an expansive house, a position, and what has now become disposable—our marriages, morals, and kids when they no longer serve our agenda or fit into the schema.

Psychologists say "Talk to your kids!" when most parents I know have plum talked out. Relating is what we should be concerned about. You don't need a working tongue or ears to see when they are hurting and wipe away their tears, to understand their fears and *be there* during those rough growing up years, not only present, but there emotionally, showing you care. We don't always need to be going, saying, doing as most of us think. Looking back, I now realize how times spent with Mama and Daddy doing family things and laughing anchored me. It gave me stability knowing I had them to lean on. So many kids don't *have* their parents today. Some never even knew them, and others know them but don't really *know* them.

I've discovered being quiet and having solitude can be very constructive to the spirit, to allow one to find oneself and see things otherwise missed, like the kiss of frost outside the window on a chilly winter's morn or a wily chipmunk cleverly hiding acorns. Everyone needs to get back to enjoying simple pleasures, spending time together, taking in the beauty of the natural world, and communing with our maker. Today even the youngest schoolkids know how to curse and espouse angry, hurtful words yet would be hard put to make a sentence to describe the beauty of a flower, many having rarely seen one. They are growing up with so much material wealth yet lack activities that are wholesome and healthy to make them spiritually rich and stable. Instead we serve pabulum mixed with sex, vulgarity, and violence at our tables.

Until I lost my ability to say and do a lot of simple things, I hadn't *fully* known how meaningful they really are. More than the "big things" I used to wish for like nicer clothes to put on, a house in the Hamptons, and a Magic Kingdom vacation. Now I stop and think of all the things I should have said to my sons when I could have. I write long letters and insist they be read aloud in my hearing so that I know that they know what I am feeling. Most of the time I write "I care!" and also "I'm here!" Try focusing more on what they hear than my own words, as what we intend to say is often not what's heard. Becoming speechless helped me realize the importance of using words nicely, of saying "I love you!" and "I am sorry!"

If I could, I'd probably run out in the backyard, fire up the grill, make some good ol barbeque, laugh and joke like we used to do, and renew bonds between my sons and me. Let them feel rooted, grounded, and loved unconditionally as they are now out facing life on their own and living in a different vicinity. Wouldn't matter what we had or what anyone was wearing as long as we had each other for a time. That's the real quality of life. We don't need to go back to the good old days, but we do need to not lose connection with from whence we've come, and in our lust for good and plenty, to be careful not to lose our identity. As families and whole communities, we need to do some cultural reconnaissance to preserve and restore our strengths, traditions, and values.

Working on reestablishing connections, linking back up with each other, our kids and God maybe the answer to curbing some of the violence and restoring our urban habitats into a giant network, a functional organism to provide a web of support for America's human ecosystem in which black men have become an endangered species. In fact, there has been a call to place them on the endangered species list, like animals, so that land can be set aside to restart their lives. It was heart rending in 1995 to see an estimated 837,000 black men converge in Washington, DC, for the Million Man March, a day of atonement to recommit themselves to family and community, bearing their young sons upon high shoulders, a sight reminiscent of the march in the '60s yet markedly different. Similar in illustrating their plight now is not much better, with the then president a distant thousand miles away, talking about the depths of white fear. But different because this time they were not asking something of America, rather making a public statement of determination to take back headship of their homes and restore the spirit of communal living to our neighborhoods. As a black woman, it indeed sparked great pride and hope.

Successful membership in the human family is predicated upon our ability to build relationships and solve conflicts. The sad news is, not only is racial tension on the rise here, as evinced by the senseless crimes done by young black and Hispanic gang members and destructive acts of white supremacy groups, but serious ethnic conflicts rage across the globe. So for all our technological advancement, how far have we really come? Instead of more technology, we need to learn to build better bridges to human understanding and open channels of dialogue by improving communication techniques, looking at what and how we relate interpersonally and cross-culturally. Only then can we, as they did in Nehemiah's time, rebuild our homes and cities using bricks of faith, family, hard work, and valuing every human being as having something to offer. We need to restore trust and responsibility.

To connect me back up with the world, VR gave me a telecommunications device for the deaf, which allowed me to have a conversation over phone wires that are typed rather than spoken. It operates by converting electric impulses into acoustic signals and transmits them through the telephone receiver to be printed out on a small screen on the receiving end. Thus, communication can begin. I could call anyone who had a similar device. The problem was, no one I knew had one or could afford the $250 price. So who was there for me to call? How was I to get *on line* with society? Didn't do me any good at all, not at first, only reinforced feelings of isolation and exclusion.

A phone is no longer a luxury but a necessity for convenience and to get a response quickly in an emergency. It makes it possible to link up with someone across the street or across the world. Today Sprint IP Relay makes it possible for me to make a call without a TDD. Relay service operators give us access to the hearing/speaking world by acting as go-betweens in our conversations, but this brings with it other complications.

Always in dealing with the outer world, I must now talk through an interpreter. To even go for medical help or get counseling, somebody has to be in there with me. There can be problems here too. The person interpreting may tend to evaluate and sift out what they think is important out of what I have to say and not always express it my way. If they are not faithful to the spirit or meaning of my message, it may not come across like I meant it. It's difficult to convey someone else's emotions. This at times diminishes my sense of self and of being in control of my own affairs. Others are always in my business, whether I want them there or not. They gain access to every intimate detail of my life, because I can't *directly connect*. In the small sphere of the deaf community, gossip spreads like wildfire, as one might expect. My privacy is constantly being placed in jeopardy. People who communicate by email and computer suffer the same malady. It's like virtual reality. It gives the illusion of inclusion, but not really, and can create confusion in the wrong hands.

I think everyone today feels somewhat "excluded." We live in greater isolation due to crime and lifestyle changes, each functioning as if we are on remote little islands separated by uncrossable shark-ridden reefs amid our own families, as we lose the ability to establish and maintain intimacy. We are all stranded, scared, and finding it harder and harder to let others know what we are feeling, all suffering a lack of "community." In that sense, everybody is just like me! Technology has produced very sophisticated machines, but none are as complex and mixed up as human beings. Trouble is that most of us have problems understanding the manual that came along with us to tell what can go wrong and how we can be fixed. Our spiritual repair centers need to put their technicians to work to fill the vacuum in this area.

I struggled along daily with my limited sign language skills, trying to communicate and make what used to be words into pictures. I always think so much faster than my hands can move and, being rather wordy by nature, find it hard to reduce what I have to say to a few simple signs. That's the problem with verbosity; it all just wants to come pouring out, and I ramble on and on like teachers are known to do. I have to consciously slow myself down, try to think visually, and make my fingers coordinate with my thought processes. In sign language, one picture is worth a thousand words. In English, we search for more and more words to paint a picture.

I don't feel right in either world; I continuously face discomfort and rejection. I want to be in with the group, but I'm not wholly suitable either way, especially in this day when blending isn't cool because everyone is so "culture conscious." This trend is helped along by the notion that I am a *this* and you are a *that*. People who are *this* are like this, and people who are *that* are like this, that, or the other. Everyone is forced into their separate corners. I want others to just accept *me*, not the label that goes along with me…which would be…speech impaired? Vocally challenged? Word incapable? Really, it's political stupidity! Instead of creating so many catchment areas to dunk people into, our most important label should be *human*! If we could just understand that notion, the barriers and walls to communicating would begin to implode.

Hearing people who know how to sign sometimes flutter their hands as if sending some sort of Morse code, forgetting there is a human being on the opposite end, that they're not talking to broken ears or tongue. They miss what is at the core of the exchange—the desire to communicate and share ideas or experiences in a common language that affords ease of expression and description, a language that embodies beliefs and ideas about the world around us. It is not just a matter of filling in for some "deficiency" the person has, something they can't do. Rather, it is a meeting of two minds trying to link up for a common purpose or goal. When interpreters act as go-betweens, they should never forget that it is a human bridge they are building, not a link with some unfeeling depersonalized object, part of a rehabilitation project.

I get rather perturbed by people who know sign language yet still insist on speaking to me because I can hear. I prefer they communicate with me in the same way I communicate with them. It seems an acknowledgment of who and what I am when the person puts himself on my level, thereby entering my world. In regular discourse, one person wouldn't ask a question in English and the other reply in Spanish. That's not the way it would be. Doing so speaks to my disability but denies my humanity.

I liked communicationg by TDD because it placed the caller and me on an even playing field. We both know the language and can discourse easily. We mutually accept the vehicle through which we are making our exchange as sufficient for our needs. There is no bias or prejudice in it. Now they have VCO or HCO, which focuses more on one's disability, i.e., if you can hear, then you only need someone to speak for you. It allows the caller to hear a relative's familiar voice. I guess it's an individual's choice, but again I find it ridiculous to switch back and forth from auditory to the visual mode. Things get lost in the confusion…Boy! Inclusion, inclusion, what is the solution?

I decided to just accept being a hyphen, a connector between two seemingly very different worlds, and be flexible enough to deal with both to the extent I had to. Like a skilled acrobat, I walked the thin line between the hearing and deaf, carefully balancing on the rope for fear if I swayed either way, there were pitfalls. It's lonely in the crevices and gray spaces.

I began staying away from my home church, couldn't take that feeling all eyes were on me, as if I were some kind of oddity. I didn't want to cope with what they must be thinking, like maybe I would all of a sudden do something dramatic—jump up, run around shouting like a fanatic having been miraculously cured. I didn't want to be a hindrance to anyone's faith and probably felt mine was no good. I used to get so choked up sitting there, especially at that point in the service when the minister invites those with a special need to come to the altar and leave it, knowing I'd laid mine down so many times before but grabbed it up and scampered back out the door. I never sincerely prayed to be healed, but to be able to deal with it. I just couldn't take the high emotional level of the black Baptist church; I was trying too hard to hold it all together. Guess I was so overwhelmed by feeling I had to go through it alone and that no one really knew what I was going through. There was nobody else around exactly like me that I could see. I was a real curiosity!

Performance in this society determines to a great extent whether we have or have not, win or lose, graduate, get the better job, acquire trophies, rewards, money, and status. In families love is sometimes given or withheld based on performance. We live in a performance-driven world! If I perform better than you, then I feel I am better than you. If I can't perform, I feel guilty and inadequate. For persons with disabilities, performance becomes an exaggerated and painful issue that affects how we evaluate and view ourselves. When you go to school and become a teacher, you build up self-esteem, have a title, earn income, have a job where you serve others, have kids look up to you, and you gain satisfaction, reward, and feel that you have value. But when you get to the point you can't do it anymore, you constantly look back and cling to trophies from the past as proof of your worth. I battled strenuously not to slip into an abyss as a result of no longer having anything to "show" to make me feel worthwhile. Most of my mental work went into just survival. Daily I rehearsed in my head, "I have my education, a house, family, and sons who need me. Life is not over!" then I dusted off my collection of teaching memorabilia. But when I finished my nostalgia, I had to face the nagging question, "Where do I go from here?" Each time I saw someone with the job I used to have, I still felt that ought to be me. Finally, I came to the reality someone else could save the children. I wasn't God's only hope!

Then I decided, instead of attending classes with the hearing to learn about deafness, I wanted to be in a class with the deaf. Sometimes we bumble along until we stumble upon the right thing. God makes it happen, if we just hang in there! I'd heard of a program for newly deafened adults at LaGuardia Community College in Long Island City. It's a pity I hadn't thought of it before. I didn't know what lie in store when He brought me bleeding to that door.

LaGuardia had an assistive and supportive staff dedicated to helping students become all they could despite our disabilities. They gave us guidance and pointers; supplied lots of encouragement, rewards of praise, verbal pats on the back; and even held award night ceremonies in recognition of each participant as we progressed toward our goal. My first certificate meant almost as much to me as my college degree for it was just as hard-won with all I'd gone through to get there. In the program I found "listening ears" readied to hear. Most important, I found a classroom of peers going through the same pain as I was.

Immediately we became a little rat pack spending most of our time together, enjoying each other, cementing ourselves in oneness against the world. Like early settlers, we circled wagons and sat around campfires, telling stories of our escapades and laughing at the ignorance of the "enemy." It felt so good to be able to laugh and get all that anger and frustration out. It was as if a heavy and intolerable weight got lifted from my shoulders. Open, honest dialogue as we practiced signing convinced me I could get back in the game. A tremendous improvement in morale came. Apparently, though I was locked out of society, I was not locked out of God's mercy and His love, for He provided a place of rest, comfort, and resources. I no longer felt like a *Star Wars* Wookie! Yet and still, there was an incredible disparity between who we said we were and what society and the media projected us as. We'd been culturally processed to feel abnormal and had been drowning in pressure to live up to false standards to prove our worth. Our minds needed to be literally transformed through reading and studying about deaf history and culture and sharing with one another. We affirmed ourselves where the world did not affirm us. A word from someone who means something to us can mean a lot more than a thousand from people out there pulling us down. Having that circle of friends, a group who stood with us, a support team as we moved out into uncharted waters, put us on more solid ground.

The role of praise and affirmation was so important in our nurturing. So was good advice instead of worn-out platitudes. Some even needed a loving nudge in the right direction for their own protection. One participant wrestled with deafness and substance abuse problems and had ended up in jail before coming to the program. We took him under our wing like a family and coaxed him to do the right thing. The message was he was still loveable and that there was hope. We achieved intimacy in laying our problems on the table and collectively brainstorming ways to handle them. This process legitimized our right to feel aggrieved yet took away the tendency to sit, sulk, and sour; it made us feel we could fight back and do what we needed to do to get on with our lives. Relationships took priority again, where before I had been locked into going through it alone. Strong building blocks in those relationships helped develop a healthier mental attitude in realizing I was not the only one with this problem and that it could be *worse*. Others were struggling with circumstances much more compounded by financial difficulties and personal problems than I was. I found with them renewed sense of community and a degree of sanity.

One of the hardest things to learn was to slow down and take it easy in my zeal to get moving, to realize set goals would not be accomplished overnight. Disability very often is a lifelong experience, and coping with it is a process that develops overtime. There was a need to continually build up my spirit, as my physical self began going through alterations, so that I could face my challenges and not get stuck in the mire. When you get tired of whining and crying, you usually end toughening up and growing. And when you reach the point you don't care if God leaves you this way or not—accept it—and are ready to move forward, it's usually at that point He starts coming through for you.

It's good to be out in the flow of things. Work is highly therapeutic for whatever ails you or obsesses your mind. Sitting at home only reinforces the feeling of uselessness and that your life is on hold. Even if it is not paid work, being involved in constructive use of your time studying, learning, and being among people keeps up the self-discipline to not just lie in bed and do nothing but brood or vegetate in front of the tube.

I looked back and wondered why I was so reluctant to get involved with the deaf in the first place, why I clung so tenaciously to my own. In spite of living in a multicultural society, most of us have a low cultural IQ when it comes to knowing about and feeling comfortable in groups outside our own. It reminds me of the problem I had as a child. I was quiet, gentle, and imaginative and did well in school, whereas the stereotype said black inner-city girls were loud, streetwise, ready to claw someone's eyes out, and not very bookish. I therefore reasoned I was supposed to be another color because of my "white ways." Thank God some of those stereotypes are breaking down these days. We all carry with us notions of what we think members of another group are like. I don't know what I thought of deaf people, didn't really have a mental picture because I didn't know any growing up. But I felt defective speech in any form was ugly and an awful stigma to bear even though I had none at all.

Today image is so important—how we look, present ourselves, and "come across" as opposed to what we are. Bad speech and talking with your hands looked deficient in my mind. I'd been afraid to come too close to deaf people because I didn't know how to *be* with them and how they would be. Language is such a reflection of how we think and who we are culturally that when you alter it, it really is like becoming someone new, like being a fish out of water. It was a whole new environ to get to know with different dynamics to get used to. We naturally fear moving beyond the boundaries of what we feel comfortable with in expanding our circle of experience with folks we think are not like ourselves. Being sensitive toward those who are "different" is very important when it comes to disability.

We tend to think we are all so different, when in fact through exposure we find out we are more the same than different. If we remember that instead of emphasizing our differences, perhaps we could find common ground. When we move into unfamiliar surroundings, we are bound to be consumed with fear initially. Branching out culturally moves us out of our comfort zone. When we go someplace looking for that cultural embrace, we are often easily offended, feel rejected as we read cultural cues that tell us we "don't belong." Everyone wants to be part of the group. No one wants to stick out like a sore thumb. Branching out takes effort, and we run the risk of being put down by our own and take a lot of flack from those who tell us we are not like *them*. In a sense, we feel like traitors.

The main thing is to get out there, to go and to seek. It can bring more than culture, which you'll see later. Most of us cling to the safety of old routines and haunts. Strange people bring out fears and attitudes that we are often unaware we have. But once we get around people and see them with their masks off, we usually come away with greater appreciation for who and what they are and how they live their lives. Most often we fear what is new and we don't understand. It causes us to build up a lot of discomfort. But we don't have to be afraid of the unknown if we view it as a learning experience and keep ourselves open. We need to be willing to take risks in searching out the unfamiliar. It takes courage to step out of your own box and try on someone else's. It's intimidating, but it helps you to expand and learn about others and about yourself as things in you become awakened in response.

The best place to learn about anyone is on their own turf. Neighborhoods are living museums that charge no admission. Seeing what goes on behind the scenes can help our understanding. Rather than just looking at the surface, look at the human playhouse of characters who make up a cultural milieu. Getting close to someone different can help us see their beauty and look past labels, then we will not feel so threatened. Celebrating difference is not wrong, but making it our excuse for not coming together is. It makes it harder to break down walls and bridge the gap. As long as people believe to be black or white or whatever group it is by very nature means I must be…and do…and dislike…our individuality will get lost in our group identity.

To be honest, I haven't made a lot of inroads into the deaf community. I still remain very much a loner, avoiding assemblies of deaf just as I avoided being in the crowd before this. Guess that shows who we were before developing a disability is essentially who we remain afterward in quirks and idiosyncrasies. Who we are individually is more compelling than who we are collectively. Seems I'm talking in circles, but not really.

Nevertheless, where worry, fatigue, and stress had been constant companions, LaGuardia provided me with a *safe* environment to let go and gave me a cadre of friends to hold my hand. They were a tremendous source of support. My anxiety decreased and loneliness ceased. All the happenings kept me from sitting around dwelling on things.

At home my coping mechanisms were prayer, listening to gospel songs, and seeking quietude to sort things out. It is amazing what comes to you when you finally sit and begin to focus. I sensed God was getting ready to do something, that He had a plan and wanted me to cooperate with it. Feelings of rejection had set in and killed my confidence, and I couldn't see my capacity or potential. But self-confidence isn't that necessary if we have confidence in God, for He is the source of our enablement. We are nothing in and of ourselves. Trusting Him can lead to a whole new self-image. Only He can use bad experiences to accomplish our good. In hindsight, I see that I needed to be humbled before He could unveil His plan, for I probably would have been too haughty to accept the wonderful deaf man He placed right in the next seat. I was being prepared for a new phase of my disability and to deal with what lie ahead. He was in the process of strengthening and refreshing me for battle by giving me someone tangible to hold on to.

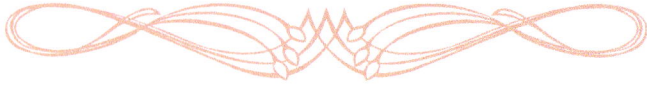

CHAPTER TWENTY-NINE
Marah

THINGS had been going quite well, fun and laughs, goofs and gaffs between us friends, lightheartedness, and the feeling of a brand-new start. The weather even seemed warm and friendly for January, didn't blast with its usual bombast for that time of year. Maybe because a handsome Jamaican guy had caught my eye. And his body language was coming across loud and clear; he liked me. How weird! At the age of forty, I likewise liked him. It was a real-boy-meets girl thing, a sudden fling. It had me going around acting silly like a young philly. (You know the story!) Cupid arranged for us to be seated not far apart, and he completely sabotaged my heart.

We began gravitating toward each other, eyelids a flutter. He watched me intently, and I followed him coyly, pretending to just happen to be around playing the clown. Others made the link up too, saying, "You two look good together!" and called us man and wife. That really spiced up my life! Even the teacher whispered to me that we made a perfect match and he'd be a good catch. I agreed, and thus began planting seeds for him to harvest me. You know how us ladies like to let the man take the lead.

Our first project "together" was to help a deaf immigrant get along and adjust to the customs here. We both volunteered, having in common the desire to help someone, though outwardly there were many dissimilarities. I was a tall-backed woman on the lighter side;

he, a short-legged man on the darker side. His body bore shocks of hair like a bear; I was smooth as a pear. His voice resonated loud and clear, but only I could hear. I was a citified American woman with a low-key manner, while he was agrarian, salt of the Earth, and tough as the coconuts that fall from the trees in his native West Indies. While I saw visions of a better world in my head, he was "by the sweat of your brow eat your bread." And where I was quiet, reserved, he was spirited and impatient, full of tropical fire, had a Rastaman's ire. In style, he was a rabble-rouser, wanted to tramp down Babylon for injustice against the less fortunate. Therein lie our underlying bond.

In a lot of ways, we seemed a study in contradictions, yet each had what the other needed, which made us both complimentary and supplementary, not only in our disabilities, but also personalities. The Lord is good at casting us for roles, knowing well how to create balance. Through signed conversation and writing, I discovered he'd had a curiously similar experience with loss of his hearing, no answers as to why, frustration with doctors and myriad of tests, and had gone through extreme isolation and loneliness. Now we were both feeling a wacky kind of happiness whenever the other was around. I knew a good mate I had found. He used to ask me out to the cafeteria for cookies and coffee. Neither of us had much in terms of money, but it sure was lots of fun. From simple beginnings our relationship sprung. I felt like his "lady" when he escorted me down the street but got sick before our relationship had a chance to peak.

In class, we started talking about what we wanted to do with our lives, our dreams and aspirations. I pondered anew upon becoming a writer, a thought I'd entertained long before but kept tucked away since teaching days. Writing for me was a chore, not a pleasure. I didn't see it as a treasure chest to open and explore because that same old haggard spirit was knocking at my mind's door, calling me back to where I'd been before. Suddenly creative writing harangued in my head like an alarm after blowing in on a petulant storm. Yet I didn't pursue it zestfully. It was more a whim and fancy from childhood that barreled back in on the warm winds of love; it became all

I could think of. Was it borne out of necessity, since the pen was the primary tool keeping me in touch with people? I don't think so!

No, I believe it was actually the hand of God guiding me to use my disability rather than be consumed by it in some way to help others. In the book of Exodus, God asked Moses, "What's that you have in your hand?" It was his staff. He then instructed him to throw it down and pick it up again. God had touched it so it could be used, and Moses went forth with power. Likewise, I believe He touched my infirmity to make it a strength.

But as usual, I wanted to make my program His program, to tell Him what to do with me instead of waiting to see what He had for me. I thought I knew what was best, so as I began to make progress in my signing, I decided to go back to teaching, this time in a school for the deaf. I would just recycle myself in that direction. A school in Westchester had even promised me a job if I got some course work under my belt. I'd heard about an MA program in deafness at NYU, thought signing up would be a cinch, since I already had two degrees and experience. But I was about to get caught in a clinch. Like Humpty Dumpty, who had climbed the wall, I was about to take another great fall.

I recall my trip that day down to Greenwich Village on Fourth Street and the shopping spree weeks before searching for just the right look for a fortyish woman carrying books. Back in the '60s, we wore dashikis and opal beads, but now colleges were overrun by yuppies trying to get their tickets to the land of opportunity. Trick was to spend a lot of money and still look sorta bummy. They called it "dressed down" and casual so you didn't let show how materialistic you were. It was almost like our '60s stuff, just wasn't mix matched or colorful enough, but perfect for an age obsessed with appearances. Most of it was baggy and ill-fitted, yet women tried to make it work, just like they tried on the high-powered career-oriented lifestyles that were so popular and equally ill-suited, as voices of those who enjoyed home life, marriage, and motherhood became muted. So many were now answering the call to have it all.

At that interview, for the first time in my life, I faced questioning about my academic ability. They asked me if I was the same as I was before, implying my inability to speak had somehow diminished my mental capacity. I had to admit I was not the same but felt I could still get back in the game. They didn't agree, rejected me. Said I needed to be able to speak to work with the deaf so they could learn how to speak themselves and function in society. I wanted to ask them, "What about me? Aren't I functioning?" There I was, Ms. Former A Student,—it meant nothing to them though, because I stood silent and none believed in me. Both NYU and Hunter said, "No!" Even the Center for Students with Disabilities told me to go.

Education and achievement had always been vehicles I used to help define my worth. My degrees were like trophies I racked up. When those things slipped away due to my disability, I struggled to hold my head high and keep a positive view of myself. This prompted a pretty hopeless attitude about my future. I found it hard to sleep, stay motivated, and not give in to hostile or negative emotions.

The process of life isn't always an ally in what we want to do and often undermines us. I took two steps forward and was about to take three steps back. In fact, I would soon find it hard to take any steps at all. Just when things seemed to be going good, my disability took another turn, and again I would be locked out of society.

When storms occur in our lives, they test our convictions, what we really believe about God. They try and prove us. God says in His word that He will supply all our needs according to His riches in glory. We hear that and we say we believe it, but it is only when we go through a storm that we see our belief system tested. He wants our convictions to be based on experience. It is people who have weathered storms themselves and have scars to show that others will listen to.

It is only in the storms that we get to know the sustaining power of Christ and sufficiency of God. They become training periods to equip us to help others. The world looks to people who say they know God to see what we do when strong winds blow in. Will we be overcome or dig in and hold on? Often He chooses not to change our circumstances for that reason, but He changes our attitude and response to them. Remarkably, He helped me spend time at home wisely, focused me on developing my writing gift, and enjoined me to use it as a channel to vent all the new emotions that came along with my situation.

When bad things happen, we all tend to try to excise great meaning from them, to ask why. Sometimes there is no rhyme or reason we can discern, except the hand of fate that randomly crushes God's creations, only to restore them again at a later date. God's heart is probably as grieved as ours is with what we go through. Repeatedly, He responds to our circumstances with mercy and compassion.

The wind blows where it wills, and the Lord works in mysterious ways ever His wonders to unfold. Through coming difficulties, He gave me the humility to understand I wasn't going to make it on self-reliance. At the same time, He had already plotted out a new way for me to matter, to do something of value to others. He would show me that I didn't have to, just because of an inferiority complex, limited funds, and feelings of helplessness, give up on my unspoken dreams of writing. In fact, He would make disability an important part of my treatise based on personal experience. Through it, I found richness rather than weakness of spirit, as I learned to live along with it, not fight against it. What was so important before I began writing was to get clear on what I really had to say, to move from what I had learned in books to sharing my own empirical observations. Disability became an asset to me; it made me believable. From God's standpoint, it positioned me where He could be demonstrative of His great love.

It came upon a day so fair, Hector and I went way out there to Long Island, shopping for his first new car. You know how young college guys are! Anyway, we had to walk way far after getting off at the station. Perspiration dripping down, we made the long trek across town looking for a bargain. That's newspaper jargon for a chicken in the bag, one of Nissan's latest gags. When we arrived, it was a rip-off according to me, but Hector couldn't see that; he swore he swung a major deal and bought an automobile. Sure was pretty—all shiny and raced. Shone as brightly as the glow on his face as we left that place.

Tracing our steps back across a wide boulevard, my legs began to give way. I felt faint and confused too, thought it was the hot sun I wasn't used to. I stumbled on, holding his arm as he bore me along. By the time we reached our destination, I was dazed, out of it; I needed to sit. Through the entire ride, I felt really bad but tried to persist. I had to take a cab from my stop to the door, went in, and threw everything on the floor. I took two aspirins and hopped in bed, expecting a long night's rest would clear my head. The next day I had the feeling of having lugs in the bottoms of my shoes. I could hardly move. My legs were shaking unsteadily; something was very fishy. For the life of me, I couldn't walk across the room, whereas before I used to zoom. I'd always been a brisk and energetic walker. Mom used to joke that I covered the whole Bronx on foot, didn't mind taking it on the hoof. Most of the time I lacked money to pay my fare, so there was no other way to get anywhere. I didn't care, for I loved to dawdle, dream, and look.

But now, wow, something had gone wrong with my legs. They were just like powder kegs; I could hardly lift them. My balance was way, way off, and my coordination was poor. I didn't know what lie in store. I looked like someone who'd been drinking, teetering badly from side to side. It was a problem I could no longer hide. I took out Dad's old cane he used when his bunion swelled up big and his foot pained. Gout was wearing him out because he'd taken too many swigs from the jug he carried in his pocket and wouldn't stop it. But I had no doubt mine would go away in two or three days. I couldn't figure what it could be, thought maybe it was all the stress finally catching up with me. Seemed of late I'd had problems persisting in walking, feeling fatigued, sweating, having a strange wobble in my stride, but I wouldn't let it hobble my pride.

Days stretched into weeks, then months, and still I could barely walk along with being unable to talk. So what was I to do? First, I had to get rid of all my cheap plastic-soled shoes. Anything that wasn't skid-proof and flat, I chucked in the trash. Instead of fashiony, they had to be wide and stationary. Suddenly the whole world became one big obstacle course. Ambulating on different planes was a pain, and stairs, forget it! Even with a cane, I could only take one or two baby steps.

What was there to do but go back to Bellevue? This time they thought they knew what was wrong as the new signs were a definite indication of a neurological dysfunction. (You can probably guess the rest.) I had to undergo test after test and more conferences. When you go to a city hospital like Bellevue, if you're not crazy when you go in, you'll be crazy when you come out. The process makes you crazy—all the sitting and waiting, seeing different doctors, being told so many conflicting things, bringing home brown bags full of pills and fat medical bills.

Finally, I got a diagnosis. What was it? Multiple Sclerosis. It was incurable, they said, meaning it wouldn't go away. It felt like doom fell on me that day. How would I tell my family the score, especially Malik, who was so close to me?

I got on the phone and ordered a pair of crutches, finding myself in the clutches of something I knew nothing about, except the person I grew up wanting to be like, Annette Funicello, had it too. We were alike finally! I called MS Society, and they sent a social worker to sign me up for PT. A suffocating feeling came over me, like I was holding my breath. I was scared to death, because *death* was the only way out of this one. Of course, they told me it goes into remission, which means remitting and relapsing are part of the condition.

Naturally, I immediately denied it to myself, said "Ah! I'll be running about soon." I left no room for doubt I was going to snap out of it. How we love to kid ourselves when the truth is hard to face. I felt I was a disgrace—twisted, cracked, no speech, a wobbly body, and lugs in my feet. My muscles had taken a sudden shift, and life, another unexpected turn. I'd come to a new junction of malfunction. Now I couldn't get my feet to do what I wanted them to do, and my body was moving in ways I didn't want it to move. My head control began to falter; I was extremely out of kilter. A smile triggered my head to lock back into spasm, and standing I couldn't break my dystonic pattern. It was go-go like a yo-yo, while my feet were as if cast in blocks of cement. If I closed my eyes, I'd hit the ground. *Boom!* And I would crash into things in my room. Add to that double vision and a great deal of derision. Didn't come on all at once full force but was a slowly progressive thing, and there was no remittance.

They told me some white spots must have taken up residence in my brain, the little buggers causing all this trouble. Said they needed another MRI to get a picture of them 'cause they're sometimes hard to pinpoint. Meanwhile, my whole life had slipped back out of joint. Each time my feet hit the ground with a thud, it was like driving into a pothole. My body reverberated to try to recover from the shock. A few steps and my brain, my whole constitution was pretty well rattled. Needless to say, my ability to walk was going, going, going.

It became hard to remain within my energy level for the day. I was always knocked out tired, constantly overextended, heavily breathing and winded. I needed to learn to budget my time and effort. It was hard to stay energized because a lot of fatigue comes with muscle immobility. Suddenly, I no longer had land legs under me, went around walking along the walls and holding on to furniture. To stabilize, I needed three points of contact, to be grasping something and my feet far astride, to form a base good and wide. Couldn't bring them into midline, and I bounced up and down all the time. Fluctuating body tone was giving me a strange new rhythm. I had gone from woman to rubber band in a very brief period. My problems were myriad.

Loss of head control caused me to tilt sideways, and I was unable to sit up perfectly straight as I did back in grammar school days. All I could do was cruise, like I did before I was two, and pretty soon even that I couldn't do. So I crawled and crawled until finally nothing at all. It's hard when everything you have worked so hard for is slowly taken away and there's so many little things you can no longer do. Yet no one even knew what I was going through. I looked back and could almost remember taking my first toddling steps with Mama standing behind me, holding my hands high. Letting go, away I went, legs straddled like a tent. Everyone clapped, then, when I hit the floor. Now I hugged the wall, afraid to fall, knowing no one would be there to help me up. It became like a slow death, losing a little more of myself each day as muscle strength slowly began seeping away. I tried to exercise my will but got tired of living with "at least I can still…!"

Around that time I became more keenly aware not only of my increased discomfort with others but of their discomfort with me. It is different when you have an obvious physical disability as opposed to a hidden one. People found it hard to veil their reactions. For me it was hard to seek help or admit that I needed it, because there was so much riding on it in terms of esteem and because I had reams of stuff wound up tightly inside that made me sensitive. Besides, everyone acted so unaffected.

One family member affectionately nicknamed me Crip. It didn't bother me. It brought levity to the situation. Making jokes helped me to cope as long as they weren't malicious. It's good to nurture a sense of humor.

As I was unable to gad about, I became cloistered in the house. I began to look for expeditious ways of getting around and doing things on my own. Gradually I had to make an adjustment to all the paraphernalia of disability and that type of dependency. Crutches proved tiring, so I switched to quad canes to improve my balance. Then I bought a walker to pull me along. Next came a scooter with an electric motor. And finally the biggie, a real set of wheels, a wheelchair! Never, ever thought I'd end up there!

I went from vocally challenged to speech incapable in a very short time. Likewise went from physically challenged to walking impossible in an equally short time. I began slipping into depression. I was grappling with so many strong emotions I didn't have the faintest idea what to do with. I had the feeling I was dangling from a cliff and there was no one there to help me down. It was hard to cope with the bluster of emotions that regularly blew through my psyche. I found out when you have a disabling condition, it is easy to lose a sense of purpose, meaning, and usefulness.

Death is something we don't think about when we are well, but when faced with the reality this could be the beginning of the end for me, it brings changes. Life takes on greater urgency. It makes all the things you always wanted to do an emergency, and you think about them with greater frequency. Some of us die while we are living for fear of dying. I didn't want to be like that. I knew I wasn't going anywhere until it was time and God would hold me steady.

Daily I endured the humiliation of crawling on hands and knees like an animal around everybody's house as that was the only way to get about without aids. You get a real sense of lowliness when you exist down there with the dirt and dog hair. It became very hard to maintain a positive attitude as it appeared I now had even fewer options. I began to feel poor, poor me. Luckily, I didn't stay there.

A natural part of me had been stealthily stolen away *again*. And I didn't know when something else would happen. I was afraid to look forward or back, didn't know what to *expect*. Once more I felt cheated out of full participation in life. My problem seemed all so consuming. With inability to walk came confinement and loss of freedom. I became housed in the house because it was so hard to go anywhere, especially in an old city like New York, where hardly anything is made for a wheelchair. Again I was out of my support network and had no peer counseling, no one to communicate with. I struggled to take charge of it on my own; I didn't know how to receive help gracefully. I guess I did begin to expect more of others because of my disabilities, but it didn't happen. I learned quickly not to need assistance when I saw it was not forthcoming.

It was as if the family were saying to me, "Come on, be brave, be strong! Show us you can get along. Make it easy on us!" while my insides were about to burst. So I bit my lip and held it rather than commit the cardinal sin of having to depend and let people know I am human. Let it be known that there are some things that, even for me, are hard to handle. I remember one day throwing myself on the bed in absolute despair, not being able to get anywhere on my feet. Malik stood at the door, looking on helplessly. I didn't realize how much he was going through, seeing the person he had depended upon falling to pieces, wanting him to be strong for me, perhaps wanting sympathy. I must admit my anguish was more for myself than for him.

The MS Society distributed a book designed for use with families when someone close has multiple sclerosis. It described quite nicely in simple terminology what was wrong. Malik read it orally then said absolutely nothing like a boring story he'd just read had bounced off his head. Really, what could he say? I mean, being barraged with words and nothing in his experience to connect them to. How else could he be expected to respond when lunged upon and robbed of someone as precious as a mother by an unseen foe he didn't know? Did I expect he would glad-hand this stranger?

First, I couldn't talk; now I can't walk? He was losing his mother a little more each day. And I say it's not going to go away, but maybe I will a little sooner than he thought. The whole subject was fraught with pain and trepidation. I understood his hesitation, although I did want him to give me the embrace I needed. But there was only distance and silence. I am sure some of his feelings were scary and conflicting, sure guilt and over-responsibility impinged on his free advance into maturity, which always involves letting go. In those situations, it's not the words that count. It is the presence and the support that make all the difference. The Scottish say, "Some things are better felt than telt!"

The specter of no longer being strong and healthy brought me face-to-face with who I really was again and again, forced me to concentrate on substantive things. Confronted with continual loss of bodily function, I asked myself regularly, "What good am I? What is my *real* worth? I am so imperfect now. Am I still loveable?" I felt so deeply ashamed when others had seen me struggling to put one foot in front of the other. I was so broken, so defective. Again came those excessive feelings of insecurity and hopelessness. There was so much I couldn't do and needed to adjust to. My spirit cried out, "Enough already! Enough! My cup is full!"

Before long I became fully incarcerated with three cell mates I really didn't enjoy being with. One was named Guilt, another Shame, and the other Blame. I thought I'd gotten away from people like that, but guess what? They were back! I sat pummeling myself daily, saying, "You lazy bum! Now look at what you've done!" Used that to overdrive myself to do things around the house to cancel them out. I still can't sit back and relax. It's like I got ants crawling up and down my back. I end up overtaxing my muscles and depleting all my resources of energy. At night I can't fall into that deep, restful, and restorative kind of sleep. I wake up at the slightest peep with all sorts of bugaboos in my mind. Happens all the time, so I pop pills for strain and pain.

When you strip away everything that you lean on that makes you feel worthwhile, you get down to that helpless, vulnerable, frightened child in you. We all hide behind the busy things we do and tell ourselves they give us *value*, make us what we are. Take them away and we are left with the feeling of terrible inadequacy. We drift. We try to shift into new gear, do a lot of self-evaluation and inner searching. It really throws you out of circulation, knocks you off the path. Makes it hard to laugh and play normally. Life feels weighted.

I began leaning on the one foundation I had, which was my family. Maybe they weren't all I wanted them to be, because they had to learn too, but they started coming, showing they cared and wanted to support me. I learned instead of being so critical when they didn't help or show concern, to be thankful when they did. I also discovered I had developed inner resources that kicked in that I didn't even know I had. I was stronger than I thought. I found I needed to be more preoccupied with Christ and lean on His strength rather than depending on my own, which was waning. My physical circumstances began to take me to another spiritual level. I came to understand what this verse means: "I can do all things through Christ who strengthens me."

Illness can alter our relationship with God by pushing us away or drawing us closer. It was important for me to be able to say God loved me unconditionally, that I didn't have to prove anything or measure up, didn't have to be *perfect*. We often turn to Him when we are in over our heads, seeking answers to life's incongruities, like how is it the God who loves me stood back, let this happen, and meant it for my good? It's not easily understood. I just accept it. His sovereignty must be resolved in our minds. We don't have to be able to explain everything and know why. He doesn't ask our permission.

When faced with chronic illness, you have to have inner strength, which comes from developing your spirit man. I tried not to focus on my incapacities but on the Lord's ability to keep His promises. It was important for me to *know* He was with me. It helped me through the fatigue and depression. When you lose so much of yourself, it's hard not to also lose your heart and soul.

A bump in the road of life can become a pothole if we allow it to be. We can't go from the cradle to the grave and never have any pain. Even if we smile and think positive, we still have times of suffering, lack of money, and hardships. It may be due to sickness or another kind of distress. There are any number of things that can bring hurt and suffering. But God has a purpose in allowing it. He moves into our weaknesses and areas of need with His *power*. He abides with us and carries us along the way. When we reach a bend in our lives, we need to realize that God can glorify Himself through us, in ways no one else can. When others see the manifestations of His power in our insufficiency, they can't deny it must be the hand of God upon us. My limitations kept me on my knees and in constant touch with Him—forced me to lean on Him. Disability has been good training ground and helped develop prayer discipline. I look back and say, if I could go back to the way I was before, I wouldn't because of what God has done in me, through it. But it took a long time to get here.

Despite effort, my vim and vigor petered downward. When muscles aren't used, they atrophy and become weakened. Yet I came to realize loss of vitality and physical mobility did not necessitate loss of creative freedom to think, to write, to express what was within, to try to understand who I really was spiritually as well as physically. It gave me time to be alone with my thoughts and not be afraid of them. If we get alone and quiet long enough, we can ask ourselves, Why did God give me this, and where do I go from here? This time I was not so resistant to the process my body was going through, but I accepted it as the will of God, who gave it to me for a reason. Quietness made it possible for me to hear the Lord's still small voice whispering He was there, that He did care and would not abandon me. The more torque or pressure life applies, the tighter we need to grip our faith by opening ourselves to the power of God and letting Him take us where we are supposed to be. I was compelled to write as a way of laying things out, organizing and finding direction—a way of answering many hard questions.

But I was stuck at home, and my budding romance with Howard was placed on hold, hurt me to my soul. I didn't know if he'd even been told what was wrong. I went on thinking about him day after day. Didn't want what we had to slip away. God gave me thoughts of him as an incentive to keep trying, since I'd never see him again if I couldn't get back to school. Life seemed cruel, placing me over here and him there, with that big ol' East River keeping us apart. It would be a new year before I returned to LaGuardia.

My immediate family and enduring friends, the Johnsons, began pulling together and became a small nucleus of love and support. Though they didn't understand, they at least tried to lend a hand. We don't need a crowd; just a few will do, as long as we can count on you! Family members need education and counseling, too, to better assist in what we go through. If only they knew how important they really are to us and that we're sorry to have to cause them so much fuss.

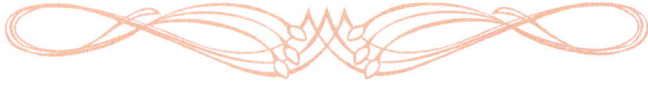

CHAPTER THIRTY
The Winds of Change

CHANGE will come as sure as we live. How we respond to it makes all the difference, whether we make peace or go on resisting endlessly. I decided to be at peace with my wheelchair, but the happenings in the community destroyed my sense of safety and security. There were harbingers of change everywhere—dope dealers, unruly juveniles, barred-up windows, car alarms whirring in the night. Neighbors gave up yard beautification, and long-time residents were taking permanent vacations. A Jamaican posse patrolled the block. Every other car quick-stopped to buy crack or ganja. There was an uneasiness in the air; folks lived in fear. Friendliness was replaced by coldness and suspicion. The grim pall of violence and destructiveness had spread over our area, while denizens suffered inertia. Good businesses, hit in their pocketbooks, booked, leaving pawnshops, discounts, cash-and-carries—a bunch of crooks. Meanwhile, scared residents did nothing but *look*.

Back in Africa activities of daily living and rearing of children were communal experiences, and each person shared in the responsibility for the welfare of the group. Americanization, urbanization, increased isolation, and unfortunately criminalization by some of our youth robbed us of that very basic concept. We came to lose *respect*. Where my generation believed there were things "to die for" like freedom, justice, and equality, the new generation saw things to kill for, like gold chains, sports jackets, and leather sneakers. It was no longer a neighborhood, just "the hood" with hooded black criminals, as opposed to white ones, as our victimizers. But whites were still the drug suppliers. Instead of talking about the brother man and the motherland, it was "Yo, man, don't dis me!" by young punks with pants drooping to their knees. Seemed they were the ones undermining their own success in the way they acted and dressed. Whites no longer lived in the area but were now cocaine commuters traveling in from the suburbs to buy drugs and leave us with the filthy bugs.

Drug hawkers are as resilient as roaches. Around the clock they're on the job, but when cops come, they quickly disperse and run. Calls to law enforcement were as ineffective as household sprays. It was said some officers secretly got paid to allow them to ply their trade. Wakefield, like other black communities, became infested as society no longer invested and cut funds for programs that brought positive social change. The cultural pendulum swung backward. The tide crested. I often wonder what would happen if all the initiative and hard work those men exhibit to sell drugs, at risk of life and limb, could be harnessed and real jobs that build up the community rather than tear it down were found—if there were real opportunity. America cannot stand without impunity for this waste of human life and increased strife within her borders. This system is its chief supporter. When you don't provide people with viable ways to earn their keep, you open a door through which vermin easily creep.

The madness came home to me so horrifically one day when I was home alone and a strange knocking came at my door. Somehow I sensed danger when I looked through the peephole and saw a menacing stranger. I listened closely as he disguised his voice like a predatory wolf. I, the timid piglet, was overcome with fear knowing I couldn't defend myself if he got in there. Just then, I thought to bang things around in the room so he would know there was someone home. In utter panic, I sat on the floor with my back pried against the door, straining to cry for help but couldn't even manage a yelp. I heard him fiddling with the knob and began to sob. My heart pummeled, knowing I was about to get robbed. I don't know what it was that made him suddenly change his mind. Perhaps a passing stranger gave him a curious glance, and he decided not to take the chance. I can only say that God, who indwells every circumstance, watched over me!

I sat alone, but not in a field of flowers, whiling away my hours, like the crippled girl in "Christina's World" by Andrew Wyatt. My world had lost its beauty and color. Everywhere there was a grayish pallor, the shadow of hopelessness and lack of power. Everybody threw up their hands, saying, "What can you do? Who even cares what we're going through?" Night shift, boom boxes shattered the calm and stillness, so no one got any rest. Rapid-fire lyrics shot through the darkness rat-a-tat-tat, cowboy-style like back at the O.K. Corral. Our home got to sounding like Old Tombstone. Days, the streets were swathed in ghostly silence, while drug dealers crawled in crevices to catch a wink, leaving chicken bones from takeout dinners on the sidewalk to rot and stink.

There were still those who remembered how life used to be in the uptown community and carried on valiantly, like my neighbors next to me in their sixties. They are the threads that hold our communities together. Like trees planted by the water, they're not moved by the winds of change. I wanted to take a stand, but it just seemed nothing could withstand the force of the raging gale. Guess I was still young and bendable, a bit too frail.

I started having those inner promptings that said perhaps it's time to move on, believing there was yet a May Berry, Walnut Grove, or some sleepy cove where I could grow old. I kept having the feeling an explosion was getting ready to go off, and I was flinching and cowering, waiting for the blast. I lived with the nervous expectation of eminent destruction, being so bombarded. It's hard to know what I was reacting to. There were so many things stirring my emotions, all minced in together. I just know something was always bothering me, making me edgy. Maybe it was living life in the trenches. Maybe it was feeling helpless. Maybe it was just the times.

Shut in the house, I spent a lot of time watching TV. Everything I knew about it had changed too, so much sex and violence, sitcoms with families dysfunctioning, and talk shows that used people's pain to entertain. The values of the normal were not being sent down to us by Hollywood. Instead, we were being inundated with thousands of images of promiscuity, incivility, and rough force. Reality TV, they called it. The abnormal were being heralded by the media, while women who cooked three meals a day, 365 days a year, and considered it an honorable profession were visibly absent from prime time. Social practices such as behaving like a lady or gentleman, dating and waiting until you marry, kissing goodbye at the door, and nervously blushing on certain topics had become old hat, as if people no longer believed in that. Decency was now part of a time past and gone.

We were being told what to think about and what we needed to go out and buy to feel good, look good, or be in with the popular culture. The image makers themselves were a lot less than wholesome. To me, this was shocking and scary, especially since kids were coming up without the strong teachings of morality and chastity my generation knew. They weren't coming home to the church because they hadn't grown up in church. Not knowing where "*home*" was left them robbed of their spiritual roots and lacking the religious resources to become what they wanted to be. They didn't know the language or the literature of the church, and many were led astray.

Home entertainment centers were becoming family altars everyone bowed before, mesmerized by video and audio equipment that brought quick, filthy stimulation. It was a challenge not to just tune in and turn on, rather than exercise my body and mind.

Focus often strayed to my sons during those long wasteful days. They were just at the age where they were making life-changing choices and there were many pressures to conform to the popular culture. It became increasingly difficult to retain respect for the old values and the church. Although I felt I'd done a pretty good job of rearing them, I feared the effects of negative peer influences. But I was grateful they were not on drugs or in lock up and were nice human beings. They had beaten the odds so many young black males had succumbed to on the streets. What else could I do except hold them tightly, try to model good character, and pray to be a strong factor in their continued growth?

We live in a world of *change*. We must manage it or be changed by it. We go through change from birth to growing up to the unpredictable events in life and finally to death. We need to recognize God is the force behind the changes. He always has a good reason for allowing them to happen. When change occurs, we can face it with optimism or despair. What I had to do was make an appraisal of what I had left and who would help. I tapped into those important connections of resource people placed in my life, made sure I remained connected to God Almighty and continued to hold tenuously to the values that had brought me through. His spirit gave me the power to just keep going.

We were headed for the '90s, a time when change would be even more rapid. The outside was getting very scary. I needed resources on the inside to help me adjust. The one thing I could rely on is that God is constant. He never changes. And I tried to keep a strong home base. When what we perceive to be negative changes surround us, the great challenge is not to be changed by them, to stand firm in who we are and what we believe. I extremely resented my inner-city community being referred to as "the hood," a term associated with criminals. Many earnest, hardworking, goal-oriented families lived there. It caused people to overlook us in our struggles to rear our kids well.

Today I hear a lot of discussions about protecting kids from things that are harmful or objectionable. But what about us old kids who do not like the so-called adult trends? We have to be so diligent in choosing this and staying away from that; it's so easy to get off track! It's so hard now to maintain the heart, mind, and religion of our heritage, which taught us we could still stand tall and strive to be all that we could be by standing on the promises of God. I feel myself being deluged by a nasty cold rain and would like to come inside and be warmed again.

The most difficult part of the day for me was in the morn when everyone was gone and suddenly I was home alone. It was like being stuck in a *Home Alone* movie, except I was not a kid but still had that sense of dependency and exaggerated fears. I worried if I'd be safe in that place, if anyone, even God, were on my case, until I got into the pace of the day. In the AM, I watched poor jerks heading off for work and tried to make myself feel "lucky" to have nothing to do.

But then I started to get cabin fever. You know, how the walls begin closing in on you?

Spending a lot of time alone, I was always afraid someone would break in and do me harm. Wondered how I'd get help if I really needed it and sat devising a way to emergency exit. It's scary to have no one to depend on, when you can't do much to defend yourself. Every creak in the house and every time the wind hammered on the window, my spirit quaked. No one was there to hold my hand but the Lord. In my weakness and vulnerability, I held tightly to His. I learned it was okay to feel afraid, but I didn't have to be helpless, that I could still go on and do what I needed to with His help.

The worse disease of the disabled is isolation because of limited opportunity for social interaction. People in wheelchairs don't associate much. We lack that sense of community the deaf have. Therefore, we have no way to validate the commonality of our experiences and few ways to get together to share. Just being in the midst of people who know what it is like is empowering. Being together gives a charge that lets us go back out and face the world.

We often prefer isolation to the general public that leaves us feeling not like people but like things to be crushed, pushed aside, and stepped on or totally ignored. The rudeness and inconsideration gall me. I sometimes say they need to be brought down a few notches so they can see how it feels to be me. But maybe I'm the one who needed to learn humility by having limits placed on me.

When "exceptional" became what I *was*, not whom I worked with, there was a big difference. It was no longer something I just took a few classes in, attended some training workshops and got to say I was "knowledgeable on the subject." It's a lifestyle I can't put down or take off when it gets uncomfortable and no longer cute, when I get tired of bearing up under the meanness and insensitivity of those around me. Some people think they know all about disability just because they've read a few books written by other unimpaired people. To really *know*, you have to walk a mile in these shoes and get a deeper understanding, which comes from personal experience. Not that I am saying my experience makes me an expert, but that I now see there are many dimensions to this that I hadn't realized before.

The disabled need a voice, a spokesman, and an audience who will listen, people who can be instructed and corrected by folks who communicate clearly to give insight.

Loneliness and isolation can easily lead to paranoia. Wheelchair users tend to be reclusive, not only because we can't get out and join society, but also as a protective device as we are often targets of crime and intentional mischief by juveniles. Today wheelchair status doesn't exempt one from the violence and cruelty of the times. In kinder days, it wasn't this way. In the past, being in a chair or having a disability would be thought to have provided some sense of safety or security, because after all, culturally a person would have to be a real heel to do something bad to a "defenseless disabled person." It just wouldn't be thought right. But now, so many people have a predatory mentality. Not only criminals but just in general, people are looking for whom they can get over on or sock it to. It's every man for himself and God for us all.

When you are a person with a disability, you really have to have your wits about you. Sometimes you need to have others intercede to protect your interests, especially in business dealings because of often getting ripped off or taken advantage of. Folk tend to view us as perfect patsies, always trying to hoodwink us, bogart us, or beat us up. I often felt violated and pinpointed because of my disability. I feared people would single me out and pounce on me, knowing I couldn't give it right back to them or tell them where to go. That's an area of struggle I still have—how to stand up for myself—although I'm finding new ways to express my displeasure. Moreover, we practice careful avoidance for safety's sake.

We live in a time when people see but don't see circumstances and won't get involved. Let it be somebody else's problem to solve. To have a heart of compassion is considered a sign of weakness, so people look on and see others in distress but don't bother helping. I've had to use the police as a constant resource to keep others from taunting me. Communication problems often lead to conflicts as things can't be talked out easily. The emergency number 911 is a number I've called much too often. Yet I've found officers and medical service providers, although willing to help, are poorly trained in how to relate and respond to us in a crisis. Certainly very few knew sign language.

Initially there was no direct TTY access to 911 in New York. I had to call the NY Society for the Deaf and have them call for emergency assistance, creating a delay in response time. When they instituted a direct access number, it was often broken or busy or employees didn't know how to answer it and wouldn't pick up. I ended having to or dial 911, leave the receiver off, and just pray they'd find me. Of course I didn't get to tell anyone the nature of the emergency.

Most of the day, I left the radio on to outshout my orating emotions. That was the only way I could get a little peace. My nerves were in a state of commotion just trying to deal with what everyday life sent me. God knows my problem wasn't the worst, yet sometimes I felt I couldn't take it anymore. I still have moments of lost hope, when my spirit needs to be rejuvenated. Living in the shadows of life rather than the sunshine, I spend a lot of time telling myself I can handle whatever comes up, but then some little thing happens and I lose it.

A sense of morbidity and downtroddenness can hang over a person facing a health crisis. You wonder if life is over and how you are going to make it through, wonder how you will pay the bills and the mortgage. Decisions seem so monumental. Your whole world and lifestyle change. The pace slows; changes are traumatic. It's easy to become embittered when changes are forced on you. Instead of getting into physical fitness, I had to build spiritual fitness to be strong enough to make it.

Confined at home, the telephone became the link between myself and the world I saw outside my window. It was the only way of getting needs met like shopping, but it meant paying whopping amounts for things plus shipping and handling. My pocketbook began to rail about not being able to catch the sales. A ten-dollar delivery fee to have my groceries dropped off caused it more to scoff. And opening the door to strangers brought tension, and thoughts of criminals dressed as service providers, greater apprehension. Supermarkets are such giant stores they're hard to maneuver a wheelchair over. Additionally, there's the problem of pushing a cart and getting through the checkout line. I faced those barriers all the time. A few stores had electric shopping chairs, but finding one in a black neighborhood was rare. The phone was actually the only way I had to let folks know I still existed. So I sat waiting for it to ring and quickly checked who it was, hoping to find a friend on the other end. Wouldn't you know, most of the time it was a salesman.

Quiet can be very disquieting. It sometimes seems to rage in your ears, causing uneasiness. I always feel like someone is coming and keep craning my neck and running to the window to check. Whom do I expect to see peering back at me? I hold my breath because I think it is death. I wonder if I'll be ready to welcome him and if I'll go peaceably.

Facing the fear of being alone with myself, I was isolated, cut-off, felt detached and abandoned. I had to deal with the silence and thoughts that regularly invaded my mind—guilt, rage, bad feelings I'd never put to rest from the past, replay of events, old memories and hurts, good experiences that I wanted to reach back and recapture. But I knew they'd been snatched from my grasp forever like events in the classroom that were rich and warming, that made me feel successful and able, not sitting, fiddling, and twittering. I began to doubt if anything I said or did really mattered, because I had so little effect on the world around me.

I also had a real battle with letting go of my sons. I suppose when you begin losing body control, you try to maintain some measure of control of things around you to create balance. But as time progressed, I realized I couldn't protect, shelter, or baby them and I had to release them to that big, ugly world out there. It was frightening, and I didn't feel ready. I had to let go and let God! But I still needed to be needed.

It got awfully depressing sometimes, especially when I flicked on the TV and saw news reports about "wrongful life lawsuits" by parents suing their doctors for not telling them their child would be born handicapped, thus denying them the opportunity to kill the baby before it was born. Said they loved little so and so but wish they'd been spared the anguish of having him or her in their lives because it cost the government so much to provide for its care. It made me afraid my loved ones would decide one day I was too much of a bother and want to have me "terminated" if I became severely incapacitated. When are we too expensive in dollars and cents or time and effort spent? Families speak of what it costs them, what they go through, and all they have to do. But who speaks for the disabled person that can't speak for himself, even for those who haven't come into the world yet? Who protects their rights? Laws don't seem to be doing an adequate job!

Is it right to say a disabled individual is not contributing to this life if they're not walking, talking, working, and paying taxes like everybody else? Is our value to be measured strictly in those terms? I can think of a number of people who do all those things, but it seems the world would be a lot better off without them, because of the pain and suffering they inflict, like those responsible for bombing the Alfred P. Murrah Federal Building in Oklahoma. Yet they have a right to remain here and eat and sleep at the government's expense.

By this time Mama had gotten old enough to have graininess in her voice, the kind of texture you find in well baked bread after it has set for a while. And I myself, though still young, carried a care-worn look from staying awake and worrying about things, the changes life brings. I had good and bad days and a lot of sleepless nights. I'd been so active and had a zest for life, but now my life was placed *on hold*. I was being kept in custody by my disability, warehoused in the house. At times I felt useless and forgotten. It hurt being disregarded, uninvited, not included and made to feel diminished in importance, like I no longer mattered and had to prove myself worthy of being here. It's easy to build up a lot of petty resentments toward others because of our limitations, to sit, moan, and gripe in our spirits and allow it to steal away our joy. But God sent His spirit to encourage my heart in special moments of relief and refreshment, when my troubles were lifted and He shined light into the dark recess in which I found myself.

Confinement can be suffocating when there is emptiness and idleness. Life takes on a frightening futility. Hope can turn to disillusionment and dreams to dust. But there is a difference between being alone and being lonely. Everyone needs time for contemplation and meditation. Sometimes being alone is very necessary. I began experiencing its power. I had time to spend in intercessory prayer for my loved ones. Radio ministries became a tremendous source of companionship and instruction. I didn't see the value of the time spent, not at first, but it has been a period of growth and testing, an intense time of questioning my own worth and finding substance beneath my girth. Now, when I look back and think things over, I can't complain. I'm learning to be more thankful.

They say we who sit in wheelchairs make eagle-eyed nosy neighbors, and perhaps I am one. But really, I felt a sadness at seeing the community change, the steady decline of our culture and family life. I still had social consciousness and wanted to do something to stop the mudslide. I didn't want to simply hide or play dead.

It was time to start anew, bring closure to that chapter of my life when I was a well, strong person and usher forth a new beginning of life as a person with dual disabilities. Time to publicly join that group of often career notables who are Americans with disabilities. Curtis Mayfield, Richard Pryor, and Lola Falana all had MS. Mohammed Ali, Michael J. Fox, and Atty. Gen. Janet Reno had Parkinson's disease. Singers Ray Charles, Stevie Wonder, and Jose Feliciano were blind. Actress Marlee Matlin and Miss America 1995 were both deaf. Hershel Walker had a speech impediment, and Whoopi Goldberg was dyslexic as a child. And as mentioned before, Franklin D. Roosevelt rolled through the halls of the White House in a wheelchair due to polio. Historical figures also: Sir Walter Scott was crippled, Picasso was said to be a distractible dreamer, and Albert Einstein was labeled a slow learner. The first man to fly an airplane around the world (Wiley Post) was missing an eye. I certainly don't belong in stellar company, but it's good to know a disability doesn't mean I have to give up on my dreams. Trouble in the form of a disability often impels us to become our personal best.

Instead of moving away from change by reacting with anger and rejection, we need to finally move toward it and look with anticipation for positives that it can bring into our lives. That's the only way to really resist the drift of tide. When change comes, we need to *embrace* it and not try to hold on too closely to the past, whether good or bad. Trust God to work things out for your good, knowing He has your best interests in mind. Give up control and let Him be in control. Be flexible so God can lead you, mold you, and make you into what He wants you to be. Changes can help us see and understand things we never could before and grow in maturity and inner strength. We need to try to see old things in a new way. It can actually enrich our lives and bring rewards of personal satisfaction. It can bring new experiences and new relationships to cherish. And a crisis can deepen our faith as God shows us He can bring us through.

When change comes, hold on to some roots and some anchors. Make real commitments to strive for excellence to be your personal best. That's all anyone can ask of you, to do the best that *you* can do with what you have left. And be humble. Change humbles us and helps us get in touch with those less fortunate than ourselves. It makes us thankful! It helps us believe in recovery, restoration, and renewal, also to understand suffering more and gain patience to meet problems. Life isn't always fair, and people can be mean and hurtful. But be kind, even to those who aren't kind to you, like Jesus taught us to do. God's sovereignty is over all adversity and impediments. Though we can't understand why He lets bad things happen, He knows. Whatever comes to us in this life comes through the filter of His grace, and He will hold all things in place if we trust Him.

I've learned change can be positive as long as I make plans and good decisions to determine how they'll affect me so that I'm not just carried along or swept under by them. Once we learn to accept change and manage with it, we will no longer sit singing, "Down in the valley, the valley so low. Hang your head over and hear the wind blow!"

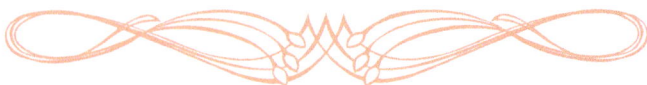

CHAPTER THIRTY-ONE
Chaired but Not Floored

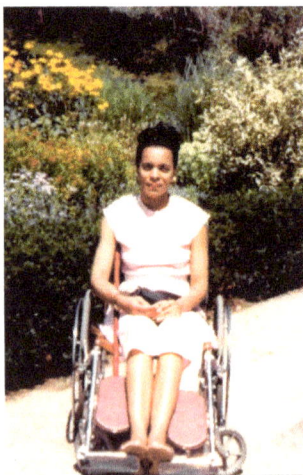

When I first started using a wheelchair.

FROM the standpoint of using a wheelchair, my life changed markedly. I was no longer able to walk or stand. I lost its medical benefits and the self-image that comes along with it. I could never look anyone in the eye anymore, except kids. The change of mobility made me more dependent on others. My life went from standing still to revolving on wheels. Yet I was to discover, a wheelchair, rather than an instrument of confinement, is a tool of freedom and independence. At least I could get around, and I am a lot more independent than most people would think. But I found myself once more on the brink of something new.

I'd always been so active and still had a good mind, so what was I to do? I wanted to move on, but what was there to move on to? The only person in a wheelchair I saw frequently in my community was a young black man missing lower limbs, who sat like a cigar store Indian in front of a little bodega on the edge of the projects. Customers greeted him warmly as they breezed in to buy beer and drop a spot on Lotto while in there. Derelicts, seated on crates nearby, passed out wine to him and stories spiked with juicy lies. You know, the kind of stuff they tell when things haven't been going so well! He was half a man but nonetheless gained their acceptance as life had cheated him also out of "success." It was a strange comradery, he and them. There looked to be more to him.

As a physically challenged person, I began looking around for a leader, but there were no champions for our cause who came quickly to mind, no Malcolms or Martins who regularly pricked the conscience of America about what was fair to us, except perhaps Jerry Lewis, no one at the battlefront to raise moral and ethical issues concerning our rights. And so we got kicked around like political footballs depending on how we made a candidate's heart look big and when being kind wasn't popular.

The pace of the world was quite different for me in the chair. In many ways I was thankful for it because it forced me to slow down. I still struggle with knowing how to pace myself, preserve energy, and not go beyond limits. In fact, it's hard to know what my limits are. I haven't yet learned to hear the voice of my own body, which likes things broken down in shorter steps and timed segments.

Because I was not ambulatory, the city had become a difficult place to live. Every chink in the sidewalk was now a major obstacle. Bronx streets are labyrinths of bumps, hills, and concrete impediments. It is easy to become overwhelmed by cars, people, flashing lights, the teaming throng. I asked myself how on earth I would get along. Uncomfortably I stood out, something I didn't like to do. I couldn't get lost in the crowds. Eyes are always watching you! I needed to learn how to win the game of survival against gargantuan rivals. People rarely think of us as heroes, despite the private battles we face.

When you go through life in a seated position, your perspective changes. Your eye view is everyone's behind, and that's what the experience of being in a wheelchair often feels like, that everyone is giving you the rear end, both figuratively and physically. I asked myself, "How will I face the crowd? How will I make it back?" Suddenly disability forced me to have to rewin everyone's respect. I'd seen wheelchair athletes in competitive meets and hadn't realized, when your muscles are weak, just crossing the street can be a major feat. I would have to pay the price to learn, because I was being required to do so. Abruptly I got up off that "There, but for the grace of God, go I!" Now it was "Here, by God's grace, I go!" Getting down to the mechanics of functioning in my wheelchair, I found out God's desire was to make me tough.

It was hard rejoining the giant public arena with all the comings and goings, the bumps, the kicks and bruisings, the tripping over me, the sense of helplessness in a sea of humans who turn their derrieres my way and look away, having to face down my fears, stare 'em in the eye, and not let them stop me from attempting to do what I had to. What pain I felt inside being on display and in everyone's way. I hated taking centerstage before being incapacitated. It hadn't suddenly changed because of the chair. If anything, the feeling intensified, making me nervous and shy. The first time out was so unnerving, all eyes on me scanning to find my deformity, looking for what's wrong to see why I belong in a seat while they are on their feet. Easily intimidated by a group, I made a lot of silly bloops like a real nincompoop! People actually walked up to me and said, "Lucky you! You ain't got nothing to do!" If they only knew what I was going through! I became an object of envy in a crazy sort of way. There's weird psychology operant today. One goof acted as if he was Jesus and commanded me to stand up and walk. He was lucky I couldn't talk, or I'd have told him to get the heck out of there! Seemed he thought he had the power to heal and that it was my lack of faith that keeps me in this state. Some stared really hard to see if I looked like a "retard" or had gross peculiarities, and not seeing any, they told me I was too attractive to be a handicap. Imagine that! I now know it's not what others think of me or of my externals, but what I have down on the inside and how I play the hand I've been dealt with God's help.

For some odd reason, dogs love barking at rolling things. They chase my wheels and growl at me 'cause I seem strange. I can't help fearing fanged teeth and claws, and I am stifled by all the attention it draws. Understanding how I might frighten others was hard at first, since I also got locked up in my own world, until I looked back and remembered how afraid I was of a handicapped person as a schoolgirl, especially those I thought were "not all there." Folks tend to view us as not being in possession of our faculties and stand back, or they go to the opposite extreme, which is to make no allowance for difference whatsoever, thereby providing no assistance. Most of us need help, but not overly much, just in those things not easy for us. It's hard to find that balance in public attitude between "Yes, I do need help with some things, but I can still do lots of things." So often we feel the pain of rejection for being as we are for no apparent reason. Tolerance is definitely not in season!

As a nation, difference in color, shape, size, and ability still divides us and pushes us into our comfort zones where we know how to deal and what to expect. We speak politically correct and posture when put to the test but still tend to operate within our comfortable boundaries.

Predictably, everyone pretended to ignore the chair, just as they pretended not to notice my lack of speech. It made me feel something was terribly wrong with me, that I had to be approached privily, or even worse, that I was accursed. In the Bible, when people were demon possessed, they often became unable to hear or speak. That doesn't mean everyone who suffers those symptoms has a demon. But being viewed as taboo can certainly hinder you. When folks saw me coming, they behaved as if I had leprosy—walked in a wide arc around and averted their eyes, carefully avoiding me. I don't know if it was fear we would collide or just of my condition, since there's never any admission. There was just a hard glance, a curious stare, or that menacing look teens practice today intended to hold weaklings at bay. Some refused to move, as if to say I was a nobody and should give them way because I was of "lower estate." In other words, I didn't rate. Right away the area I needed around me to feel comfortable changed, and people were always violating my space.

As such, I needed more room to move around in and more space between myself and others. This made large assemblies nerve-racking. I experienced paranoia and claustrophobia, the feeling I couldn't maneuver if something happened. And I was always "in the way" no matter how out of the way I tried to get, which made me anticipate gatherings negatively. It was not only an issue of access, but how I felt when I got in there, all choked up, sweaty, needing air, unable to relax and enjoy myself.

I still suffer social anxiety, get very tense and self-conscious around others, can't stop wringing my hands, and look wired up. I hold on to myself for comfort and survey to see who's watching me, but I keep that smile on my face cheesily. It's a mask, a phony facade. God forbid anyone should know this is hard. I want to measure up, fit in and belong, but that sinking feeling comes so quickly. No one wants to be left out of the act. Being disabled to the so-called normal seems to be my whole person. They can't see past it in the same way they can't see past the fact that I am black. Think it's all I am, and I struggle to let others know there is more.

When I am alone and isolated, I long to be among people. Spending so many hours in isolation, it's hard not to go nut. But when I am out with others a short time, I begin to long for the safety and security of home. It's such an emotional roller coaster I live on. I frequently run out of steam and need refueling. It's especially difficult when people turn their backs and converse among themselves, viewing communication with me a chore, as if I am a bore. I have become effectively left out by my inability to join in easily. We all have a tendency to cocoon ourselves to escape the craziness of these times, yet sometimes we need company besides our own.

It's amazing how resistant people can be to learning sign right down to this family of mine. Basic knowledge would make communicating a whole lot simpler, and we all wouldn't feel so lost without a pencil and piece of paper. Historically, hand signs were used by American Indians for communicating between tribes, and it is an amusing part of our national pastime—baseball. But with exception of rappers and perhaps those of Italian descent, manual communication isn't very popular at all. Hence, it remains for me a nagging pitfall.

To complicate matters, I find it hard sometimes to express the things I want to say—even in sign—the organizing of it in my mind. Something just seems to get in the way, a blockage, especially under pressure. At times, I perseverate or meander, and in my writing, so many misspellings, goofs, and word substitutes. Have to go back, rub out, and scrub out, use an awful lot of Wite-Out. Writing can be frustrating, yet it provides a new way of revealing myself to the world, albeit a scary one, because I still feel like a fright-filled little girl.

As I finally surmised I was no longer free, that this would be my world, I fought it in my own way by tending to reject the equipment I felt announced I was a cripple and made my status visible. I went out seldomly, satisfying myself to sit there, go nowhere, and avoid the stares, but at intervals I just had to get air. In time, it got easier as I began to realize I didn't have to look into all the inquiring faces. A broken body can break your spirit if you let it. Love and acceptance help us to be strong in our broken places.

I've learned everyone has a problem with brokenness these days. Everyone is going here and there, trying to find what will make them feel whole and complete, trying to fill a need. Everyone is in pain over one thing or another. We all see ourselves as cripples because we focus on our inadequacies and imperfections. We need to get our eyes off what's wrong with us and focus on what's right with God. It is only when we seek the Lord and restore our relationship with Him that we experience His love, which puts our brokenness back together. Only He can heal our wounds. As dark and as difficult as life may be, our only hope is when we bring the light of God's love into it.

Contrary to those oft-heard words, that I had it easy, my life became characterized by hypertension. Pitted at odds with the environment, I struggled heartily to do the mundane, while multiple factors warring against me brought added stress and strain. It's easy to become oppressed by intangibles, the pressures of time, space, hostile attitudes, mixed messages, and our own unreal expectations coupled with inner turmoil. My battery needed recharging and my spirits fresh oil, this ol' body, some brand-new coils. I was about to stall, but there was no one to call. It was difficult not to lose heart and get stuck in a rut. We conquer the disability before overcoming all the *stuff* inhibiting us.

My first wheelchair was a big old chunky thing with a plastic seat and lots of chrome fittings donated to me by the MS Society. That ugly chair by Invacare made me more reluctant to get out there. Problem being, it took so much effort and planning to go anywhere—all the dressing and preparations beforehand, the transportation nightmares, the concerns with exactly where I would go, what I would do, how I'd communicate, knowing the logistics, coping with insensitivity and rudeness. Oh my goodness! I've heard other chair users report folks falling over them offering help. That hasn't been my experience. Can city living alone be blamed for their unwillingness? No! I see a general disinclination by the public toward acts of kindness.

For the average New Yorker, winter storms and natural calamities can create travel nightmares, but for a person in a wheelchair, everyday maneuvering in public can be a tremendous if not insurmountable challenge. Every break in the pavement, every gully, every gulch in the road impedes movement, not to mention steps, curbs, rocks, grass, and gravel. Fortunately, I now have one of the new lightweight, high-performance models in a rosy pink that makes me feel well and sporty, not fat and portly. Dubbed the "Quickie," it's the industry symbol of movement and action and gives better traction. So much of society is uphill or down, while chairs move best on a level grade. Certainly a strong foundation of new technology has been laid.

By the eighties, America had become a foulmouthed nation lacking consideration. Pedestrians would not move out of my way. They went first; I was last, not like the past when folks would let us ahead. Common courtesy was dead! People could be as threatening as a darkening sky. Some acted as if I was a *what*, not a who.

For example, they stopped and said, "Look what we have here!" The fact that I was human and had feelings didn't seem at all clear. My neurologist even referred to me as "it," as in "What is *it* here for today?" and deferred to my escort rather than wait for my retort, as if I was not a real person. It's no wonder folks walked up, babbled, and cooed like the wheelchair was a stroller and I an overgrown tot. Boy, did that make me hot! People feel if you don't talk, you can't be too intelligent.

With use of a wheelchair, a bevy of new problems came to replace the old ones. When Malik was young, my problem was protecting him from hazards around the house, to try and hem him in as he toddled about. But now it was me in a seat being pushed up and down the street and a mass of mixed emotion I did meet. People in public often feel all at once protective and rejective of someone who has a disability. The disabled must get over the attitudes of the abled community, first by achieving higher visibility and moving on to viability. And we must get over those low-down attitudes that cause us to discount ourselves.

There are so few places we have access to. Access to me means more than doors I can get my wheelchair through. It's what happens after I come in. We need full participation! Curb cuts and accessible bathrooms are a start, but that doesn't get to the heart, which has to do with attitudes as well as physical barriers. There are so many obstacles to overcome; it seems this society is not meant for and even hostile to us, as if we shouldn't exist. If you're paralyzed, that's your problem! They've got problems of their own. No wonder so many of us just stay home! Thank God Jesus isn't like that or like friends and family who often hit the door running when trouble draws near. He is always near, speaking to the needs of the crippled both physically and spiritually.

Former president Bush (senior) spoke of a "kinder, gentler America." It's not happening. The bottom line is, today people ain't nice. They're getting crueler and more thoughtless each day as moral restraints are taken away. Gone are the time-honored values like "Do unto others as you would have them do unto you." Gone is compassion for the blind, the halt, and the lame. It's a new ball game. Hardball says it all!

It's hard to live by the brutal rules by which we play in this day and difficult to see those vistas that are potentially ours if we stick with it. Power-driven, self-concerned individuals step on anyone to get ahead. The person who has a disability or is unable to compete really gets little mercy from them. It takes great strength to persist and become people of grit. That "just pick yourself up and start all over" stuff is phony! You'll be weak as baloney if the reason to go on isn't found within you, if you don't have a dream strong enough to motivate you, and if there isn't something you really want to do. Also, there must be something down on the inside that sustains as well as people who say "Don't quit! You can do it!" The role of significant others should be to support and encourage rather than prod and push.

At times I get fed up and want to lash out on paper, but loved ones, not wanting to make a fuss, say, why cause a ruckus? They're not trying to be mean. Everyone is confused as to whether we are entitled to special privileges and what those privileges should be. We have ADA on the books, but there is a great need for clarity. So I go on feeling like an obstacle and a burden, like a problem to others, while they're the ones violating me, until social mores catch up with what the law says. It irks me when I move and the other person spouts "You're fine!" as if the offense is mine, not that they are annoying me, impeding my liberty or functionality. I'm stuck at the end of the line still awaiting my proper turn.

Most everyone is unclear what a "reasonable accommodation" is for a person coming into a business as a customer or employee. Staff is not well prepared for what to do if someone with a disability enters the door. Accessibility generally means you have a right to come in, so now we're in. What happens next is where we need to begin. Many businesses are afraid of insurance liability and see our presence as a monetary threat if something should occur. I was abruptly asked to leave a store once, just leave, without an explanation, but I believe fear belied the situation.

Since ADA rulings primarily affected buildings constructed after a certain date, New York City, being very old, was largely inaccessible to a chair, and it was tough getting around there. The subway was completely off-limits to me, most buses too. Toss on that pile the miles of tenements and high-rise buildings so germane to city living. Few older dwellings had handicap entrances, access ramps, automatic door openers, handrails, or special elevators. And when there were curb cuts leading to a little cement path just for us, it was often barricaded by vehicles, people or other encumbrances that blocked our way. Always something or someone impeded progress. There were so many barriers, i.e., steps, narrow doorways, carpet, revolving doors, and overfilled space lined with things impassible.

Stores displaying blue wheelchair stickers had handicapped parking areas in compliance with the law. But of course, folks figured, why should we get the space right in front of the place? So they parked there and didn't care. They've got to do what they've got to do, so later for you! Those spots became catchalls for junk, shopping carts, and other gunk people wanted out of the way, just as they tended to stash us out of the way. Those who survive the battle over parking, for that alone, deserve a Purple Heart.

If I wanted to get down to midtown, I had to make an appointment with the New York Bus Service to be picked up on a specific corner, at a set time, by one of their buses equipped with a special lift and needed to have someone to go with during off hours, after nine and before three, so the public wouldn't be inconvenienced by me. At first they didn't have lift van pickup service through the NYC Transportation Authority, and when they did finally institute it, it was based on the lottery. Only if your name was pulled out of a hat, you got a ride, and Lady Luck has never been on my side.

On the streets I couldn't do something as vital as stop and ask directions. My lack of speech and the wheelchair put a whole new complexion on things. In the din of car horns, I rolled along silently, feeling very vulnerable. Trouble is, I couldn't stockpile confidence to help me face the world. My emotions were always in a swirl. Plus I lacked physical strength and stamina.

The city had become a battleground, a killing field if you will, and I was very frightened still. The one powerful thing I had going for me was my faith. I believed God would give me the ultimate victory over my disability. Weakness of upper body caused me to slump and sag as my arms flapped wildly to push the chair everywhere. Instead of physical fitness, I would have to build spiritual and emotional fitness to steady me. Self-help is good, but God helps those who know they can't do it by themselves!

Urban living spaces are like tiny rat mazes with bulky furnishings and things in the way. Everything is either too tall or small, and there are lots of places I can't go in at all. When I did enter, I stayed in one place as if entombed and prayed not to have to go to the bathroom. That room can be one of the most frustrating and dangerous zones in a home for a person in a wheelchair. To start, I can rarely get in because of the narrow doors, then there are slippery surfaces and floors. Porcelain is slippery too when wet, and don't bet on finding grab bars to ketch on to. Next, there are the switches and towels I can't reach, faucets hard to turn on, and the mirror that holds its face so high I can't peek. Toilets are always waaaaaay down there, and I've got to slide and, when finished, try to get back up in my chair. Once seated, I can't make a full turnabout to get back out!

Even public toilets supposedly designed for wheelchairs are sometimes so small I may be able to get in but can't close the door of the stall. Prying eyes get to see my all! We lose dignity and privacy just to eliminate, because they don't investigate properly. To add insult to injury, ladies go in the one accessible toilet, sit, defecate, and make me wait. Never mind the rows of empties they have that I could never use. But we get accustomed to their being rude, take it casually with a smile. Not complaining seems to be our style. We're lucky if we don't find a receptacle or large equipment stuffed inside, making it impossible for us to fit, or they make it so high you'd have to be an acrobat to jump up on it. There should be a disabled manifesto that reads, "We have an inalienable right to go to the bathroom and will fight to do so!"

Public sensitivity and awareness of our needs is so poor. I guess we will have to wait until more of my generation grays and begins using walkers, canes, and chairs before attention is paid. Americans appear to buy into the concept of diversity in theory, but in practice, live, hire, worship with, and marry those who look like them, whom they feel most comfortable with. It's difficult to be an American and make no distinctions, to just take people as people, to be accepting and genuine with all we encounter. Harder even to get past deformities, mangled limbs, drooling, sometimes offensive odors, and the equipment used, to just see people—human beings who need respect and affection from those around them. Ironically, those who work with the severely disabled sense needs of their own being met, perhaps a need to be needed and accepted unconditionally. "Our kind" seem to be very good at greeting all with a simple welcome, appreciating that you've come, you care, and most of all that you are there. Another person's total neediness links up with something in each of us that wants to serve and give.

Much of society remains insensitive to the needs of minority populations. That is why without the law to enforce and the commitment of schools, organizations, and individuals, I feel we will likely go backward. Equality for African Americans and Americans with disabilities is more a wish than a reality. Neighborhoods are still basically black or white, schools are becoming resegregated, and black unemployment is still twice the rate of whites. The majority of the disabled population have no jobs at all. The road to employment for both often ends in low-paying, dead-end jobs with little future. More than half of the nation's maids and garbage collectors were black. Only 4 percent of the nation's managers and 3 percent of the nation's doctors and lawyers are black. The number of people with disabilities who hold professional positions are a mere pittance. The government is presently cutting funding for programs that give disenfranchised groups greater access to jobs and higher education, despite the fact diversity has brought positive change. It's indeed a tragic situation! In the future, I fear my grandkids won't have the opportunity to attend a university like I did, which makes me feel pained. I hope schools and employers will see the benefits of inclusion and continue the practice even if quotas are removed and the law maimed.

I find many of the same dynamics I've experienced over the years as an ethnic minority at work in my encounters as a person with a disability. People tend to take our feelings or the things we say and trivialize them or not give them as much weight as the "normals" in the group, be it in a family or in other social situations, causing us to feel diminished in importance and to self-doubt. It has an ongoing damaging effect. What's right for us always gets minimized so that we don't even give ourselves permission to stand and take action and make changes about the things that bother us. We need support in finding ways to break negative behavior patterns on the part of those around us.

Although some now show greater desire to know and willingness to learn, others continue to demean, diminish, and dismiss those of us they come in contact with. Addressing these problems requires that we practice self-advocacy with diplomacy in talking with the business community and public about what modifications are appropriate. The crux of the problem is, accommodating not only means different things to different people but can require varied arrangements in individual cases. Like other civil rights legislation, ADA emphasizes reeducation and depends very much upon the cooperation of all parties involved using incentives as a rule because it lacks a strong enforcement tool. My hope for the future is to see folks come together to meet our needs for dignity and compassion. Hopefully, ADA will "handicap" society and equalize the competition.

Bringing things back to home base, it was especially painful to discover that home I'd been so proud to own was now structurally inadequate for me being so tiny. But I couldn't just get up and go as I hadn't any place to go. I couldn't afford expensive modifications either. Bills kept rolling in, and there was never an end to them. It was a struggle to go on keeping the few possessions that I had. Getting my house modified meant having grab bars installed on the shower wall, that's all. Costs for equipment and treatment are astronomical, abuse of the system, phenomenal. Disability is an expensive lifestyle, which only the wealthy can live comfortably. Things like in-home nursing care aren't covered by Medicare and Social Security.

That's why so many of us live with the Medicare scare, afraid it won't be there if we need it and nothing else either. We've turned to support groups and politicians for help in getting our basic needs met. Fortunately, the MS Society gave me equipment, provided therapy, and dispensed information, which made me feel I wasn't out there all alone. Independent living is difficult for people with disabilities because we don't have many options, except to live at home or be warehoused in high-tech facilities we don't want or need. So each time I sneeze, I get scared to death and hold my breath, afraid somebody is going to say "No!" or that I'll need a doctor and can't go because there is no coverage. When we need help, we find again and again the government isn't there, unless you are the poorest of the poor and qualify for public aid through Medicaid. That too is being scaled back these days. Stranded at home without an assistant, I had to make it on self-will and persistence. In the coming days, I learned to do ordinary things in extraordinary ways.

The really hard part was trying to be a mother on paper with my sons, to keep open lines of communication in spite of the situation, to be constant and consistent in dealing with them. With all I had lost, I didn't want to lose the two who meant the most to me. I kept wrestling with that feeling, "Am I all I have to depend on?" especially with so much of my body function gone. Without support, it was hard to convince myself that the essentials for wholeness were still present. Parenting is one of the most important jobs we have, and to be able to remain home and keep a handle on things was indeed a blessing. So instead of lying around brooding about what I was missing, I told myself, here is where God wants me and He will keep me.

Nevertheless, I fought a daily battle with low esteem, feeling I was nothing. As an African American woman, I'd tried so hard to achieve respectability through education and employment, to develop a career where I could make an impact. Now I was just sitting back, which is a no-no for the ego. Being out of the work environment made it hard for me to sustain feelings of self-worth as work had become the basis of personal identity for many women in society. Most women contend with issues of respect who don't bring home a paycheck. For me, it was hard to maintain a sense of mission, keep alive my passion, and not feel my degrees had gone to waste—harder even to believe I was winning at life and was still somebody in their eyes, that they looked up to me otherwise.

Disabled men and women who are largely unemployed suffer wrongs for lack of success. They face prejudice based on ability and productivity. If you don't "do" anything, people really won't respect you. Therefore, it is said education and employment are the paths people with disabilities will have to follow to find status. Similar to other minorities, however, when we get jobs, they are often the least desirable with the lowest pay in positions no one else wants, and we're told to be glad to have a job at all, not to mention the use and abuse we often tolerate because of having few employment options. Yet it's still important to get a foot in the door of a position and be able to function and hang in there over time to achieve longevity so that others see us and work with us regularly to bring about a change of attitudes. It is also important to note that a person's worth is more than in the holding of a public job, and one can contribute to the fabric of life in countless other ways.

In reading about talented disabled workers who have done very well in the job world, I've wondered what happens after five. How many get invited to the social gatherings, the parties, and really join the inner circle or marry the boss's son or daughter and have kids grandma just adores? Despite strides, we still struggle socially to overcome the stigma of being halfwit, burdensome, or incompetent and, like other minorities, find congeniality at the office but after work hit the door and head on back to "our place," to loneliness, isolation, and social ostracization because of the depths of fear. For many, the challenge so often is to just lead normal lives, to pal around with close friends, date, marry, start families, and stay involved in the functioning of local communities.

We all sit and feel that terrible sense of inadequacy and self-pity in our lives at times. But we must find peace on the inside that gives us the courage to face our guilt and fear. Fear stops us from setting goals and realizing the full potential we are capable of. Faith helps us get through those struggles and rise to face our challenges. So often my circumstances seemed to tower over, overwhelm, and render me powerless. At times it did help to get angry, to adopt an attitude of "I'll show them a thing or two!" while stirring up juices down on the inside. But what really helped most was *love* of family and of things I enjoyed doing, which could motivate me to go through whatever I had to for its sake or theirs.

You will never know what it is like to be in a wheelchair, the impediments and difficulties until you live in one, not for just a few moments to sit and glide around. I mean, day in and day out, in season and out of season. After a time, that chair becomes a part of you! You suddenly become broad and can't fit through hallways, aisles, and openings. Your heaviness makes floors rumble when you come gambling through. Say goodbye to the missy, prissy you, 'cause you are a big ol' thang now. Whew!

People tend to overstep our boundaries physically as well as relationally. They grab on to the wheelchair for support or use it as a prop, not realizing it is like holding on to a person's glasses. Or they violate us by inappropriate touching, fondling, hugging, or kissing in ways that are not welcomed. It's hard for us to learn how to be assertive and set limits on the negative behaviors of others toward us, i.e., saying "I don't like that! Please don't do that!" It is an art in itself to do it without coming across as a pain in the neck or being overly demanding. It's often said we take ourselves too seriously at the expense of others. But we've got to stand up and show we have our druthers! Some people view us as miserable whiners and crybabies harping about every little thing. Perhaps some do take advantage of their status, causing folks to hate us. But maybe they'd be like that even without the chair. It's just their personality. There are lots of people who seem to derive pleasure out of complaining. However, that stereotype certainly doesn't apply to all. Like everyone else, those with disabilities come in infinite varieties.

When you have a physical disability involving muscles, all the little things that you once took for granted become hard, like putting on your clothes, cooking, eating, going to the toilet, taking off your jacket, putting on pantyhose, and applying makeup. You don't feel like washing up and gleaming up your teeth, combing your hair, or dressing in nice clothes. Those personal care attempts are not only physically challenging but emotionally challenging as well, because we fall in a rut and figure, why bother? There's so little motivation to do anything, to fix yourself up and try to look attractive. Besides, whoever looks at a paralyzed woman and finds us pretty? Whoever expects to find us all decked out? How many suitors stop to take a second look? It became hard to believe in my sexuality. The media never projects people with disabilities as sexual beings, except in some sick or perverted way, so I didn't see myself as desirable.

And of course, came the difficulty with doing household chores, like sweeping, dusting, and making the beds. With lots of equipment around, things easily fall into a mess, and keeping things tidy becomes major stress. One thing you quickly learn is how to make do with less to preserve space. What you do or can't do has a big effect on those around you because of your dependency on them and on equipment and machines. It's so easy in a household to let the focus become attending to your needs. It can deteriorate family relations, if things get out of balance, especially if overattention is given to the special member at the expense of everyone else. Disability has to be a family-assisted effort, but all responsibility should not fall to one person because they may become overwhelmed. In fact, giving a gift of time off to care providers can be one of the most appreciated gestures of care and concern.

When disability becomes chronic, people always just assume the family is going to step in, pick up the slack, and do whatever has to be done. But, it ain't like that! Urban families are often not close-knit and function as isolated units. It's a tough adjustment facing new responsibilities never held before. Family economics change, and relationships may become strained. Lifting, toileting, dressing, helping with cooking, banking and chores, while coping with a cornucopia of new moods, shifting behaviors, and volatile attitudes, can cause eruptions and the spewing of words not meant, breeding conflict and discontent. Unbaled hurt has been our substance many wintry days. Happily, most make it through this period of foul weather to practice warmer ways.

I found it strange to be "touched" by my sons, to be hoisted into the car and back in my seat, having long acquiesced to their march into manhood by keeping physical distance, save for a peck on the cheek. As big, strong fellas, they found it awkward to be gentle, to render love in handling me, to behave patiently. In fact, the Lord had to begin teaching us through our distress to dress wounds with tenderness.

Not only is there a reconfiguration of living space, but there is a shifting of power in the family. Paralysis doesn't give pause to family wars. It can often start or exacerbate them. Those sibling rivalries, accusations of being Mom's or Dad's pet. It can be as bad as it gets when someone thinks you now have an edge or this is giving you special favor and jealousy savors. Don't dare bring up your problems and expect sibs to jump in and try to solve 'em! They'll say you're playing on it to make others feel sorry for you and to get your way, taking unfair advantage of your condition to make loved ones pay attention or give affection. Even doctors sometimes view it as a tool by which we manipulate others, reaping benefits of sympathy, thereby feeding repressed or unmet needs. While it may be true some of us have a "sick mentality" and go around sucking up attention like a wet sponge or use it as a crutch, I don't feel I do that very much. I am too busy about the business of surviving to be sitting back whining.

It's humiliating to have to depend on family members for every little thing, like getting out of bed, putting on your clothes, and even exposing private parts of your body in order to potty. Sometimes we want those who are close to us to just *understand* the drain and strain everyday activities are both physically and emotionally. When they seem not to, what can we do? It's easy to become acclimated to feelings of anger and hostility within ourselves because of hostility around us. It was hard to just *accept* that I needed help. But I learned not to feel bad about having to accept assistance, because really, we all need each other. No one gets through this life *alone*. The typical image of a woman in a wheelchair is a real pain, like Danny Devito's mom in the movie *Throw Mama from the Train*. It was important to me to go on doing things I always did with family and friends who remained. It's amazing how that sustained, made me feel I was not alone though locked in at home. We so long for others to come alongside, be there to shore us up, keep us going, help fight the battle and not give up. Burdens don't seem so bad when shared. Family and professionals can serve us best by listening, being reassuring and walking with us through it. We will be so much stronger with you holding our hand. There are some things worse than physical disability, such as the lack of love relationships. Many people who can walk and talk don't have anyone to be there for them. Mother Teresa spoke of loneliness and emptiness as the most prevalent disease the world over. It's easy to see and feel its terrible impact though impossible to gauge in effect.

That's why it's crucial to marshal up whatever support you can. Having friends and loved ones around makes all the difference in the world. Support can also come from unlikely places. There are still good, caring folks out there needing to be needed. Making others aware of what we need and how they can be most helpful is the key. We all need a balance of challenge and support. Tip the scales in either direction, and it's not healthy.

When going through physical changes, it's best to have a spiritual attitude. Draw closer to God in dealing with the problems and circumstances that mount up. Inevitably, we ask ourselves if God is still good when life no longer seems to work. Don't try to go through debilitating situations alone. Relationships provide companionship and compatibility. Reach out to those who touch your life and borrow faith. God can move into our lives through family to bring goods and resources. Sometimes family is the only one we can depend on when in need.

People often think of religion as good for the lame, the sick, and the grieving, but assume strong, healthy people who have it all together don't require it, other than to use as a crutch. Contrarily, I've learned exercising active faith is only for the tough and is not a good place of hiding because God will find you right where you are and force you to come to grips with things.

It's been said, "In life's battles, it's not how many times you get knocked down as long as you get back up!" Although that sounds very noble, it gives very little to look forward to, especially today when there is so little tolerance for failure. We can be so afraid to fail we refuse to try, because we just don't know how we will handle it.

Trying to cough up more determination to persist is taxing and robs one of their sleep. Fear of failure can be completely limiting. Most of us tend to hone in on what we can't do and go to therapy and focus all our energy into regaining that which we have lost. Sometimes it helps, and sometimes it brings frustration when we only see slight improvement for tremendous effort. Instead, we need to identify and build upon our God-given strengths, focus on the positive, and reward ourselves for small steps of progress toward our goals. This isn't easy because what we can't do becomes a billboard sign, so over-powering we miss talent, which is like fine print you have to squint to see. Inner strength, coping skills, and positive attitude can help one get through anything. What counts is resolve and tenacity. We must get to a point of understanding and acceptance that we can glorify God by health and by sickness, either one, as His great spirit becomes magnified in us and enables us to live and carry on with complete surrender.

This isn't a cure all, and being seated and halt didn't bring daily responsibilities to a halt. Still life goes on and bills have to be paid, even though fortunes sway. The role as mother at home never ceased either. Neither did the demands my family placed on me to meet their needs. A mother is like a spoke in a wheel. Everything revolves around her. She is the home manager, the meal preparer, the bill payer, and the kids' problem solver. There was so much pressure to perform, so I wouldn't let them down and fail to meet what they wanted me to do. I still had a learning-disabled child and felt obli-gated to see him through. My neediness went unspotted, same as before I entered disablement's door, because of the tendency to put everyone's needs before my own. God forbid it be said I was rolling over, playing dead. I wasn't about to cop out, so I hung in there for the bout.

I tended to push my body to its physical limits to keep up and paid the price for it in being exhausted, worn down, and even sick because of this. I really didn't know how to let myself off the hook, when everything in life had taught me to *perform*. Now more stress was placed on me by society to not sit back and feel sorry for myself, to do something in spite of my disability. They didn't know just getting up, fighting with my body, and making it through the day was a battle in itself that should have been commended. There is so much stress on persons with disabilities to live up to someone's expectations and prove ourselves, when we are the ones who really do face tremendous daily challenges.

I think we ought to succeed and become what we want, not to prove something to others or make ourselves acceptable, but out of our own ability to dream and go after our dreams, for personal satisfaction. Folks tend to look to us for inspiration, to give them courage to press on. But I don't need that aggravation! I can't always be upbeat. Society says run a race with one foot tied behind your back so normal people can be inspired by it. But I say we are not here for your inspiration. We don't live to prove things to you. We live because we live! God has given us life just as He gave the flowers, each having a unique and special appearance and way of thriving, yet a part of His lovely hand-tended garden.

We can do with our lives what we chose just as "normal people" can. If we chose to take our wheelchairs and go up the side of a mountain, hooray! But if we chose to sit near the mountain and admire its height and majesty, that's our prerogative too. Why place unreal expectations on us to be superstars? There is no special compensation. We don't have those amazing gifts a lot of folks think we get the minute a disability happens, beyond ingenuity and hard work. We are human first and disabled second. Give us the right to succeed on our own terms! We can also begin to succeed on God's terms when we stop, ponder, and ask ourselves, Why did God allow this in my life? What is He doing? Look for His hand at work.

Despite our physical limitations, our spirits still respond to the challenge to live our dreams. Most of us are starving for stimulation and challenge. When you present yourself to the world every day in a wheelchair, the message constantly comes back that there is something wrong with you. That's very stressful in itself. I needed to have something to combat that, needed to hear a different tape inside my head to fortify my self-esteem and have dollops of encouragement added on by family and friends without being condescending or insincere. We all have things we are good at in spite of our disabilities, and helping us to identify and focus more on them rather than what we find hard is critical. People with disabilities are unique, albeit imperfect patches in the quilt of the human community deserving equal opportunity.

Regardless of our status, life doesn't stop calling on us to do. And when we do well, people get excited and say how w-o-n-d-e-r-f-u-l it is. Underlying that is a believe or lack of expectation for our success and achievement most normals have about us. Yet we have feelings. We laugh; we cry and still climb mountains in our minds. This is not a participatory democracy that includes all people. Americans with disabilities, as the largest minority, still suffer bias, prejudice, and extremely limited choices in jobs and economics. The public's perception vacillates; either we are specially endowed superhumans possessing unique gifts, or we are incompetents, taking up space that the world and our families would be better off without. In utter hopelessness we can either call Dr. Kervorkian and arrange to check out, or change our self-perception from unable to handicapable and exert power to positively impact the public's view.

There are one and a half million people in wheelchairs in America. Paralysis is seen as permanent, although there is tech innovation that holds out hope of enabling wheelchair-bound persons to walk again. With the passage of time, I no longer concerned myself with walking, just developing my level of independence, seeing really it was not the end of the world. I wasn't going to hang my hat on what I'd lost to try to regain it. And I wasn't sitting around praying for a miracle, for God to do something to zap me out of this "cursed predicament" as most imagine would be my lament. For me, small gains and simple joys became important.

Gradually I adjusted to the reality of what was. Disability is not a condition to be rescued from but a fact of life, and the only way to get along is by the principle of simple dogged endurance. You can't be a weakling in your spirit! Most of us get by on guile and whatever resourcefulness we can summon up. Surviving becomes a battle of the will. You lose some rounds and win some with yourself. Sometimes you wallow in self-pity. Sometimes you're indecisive. Sometimes you feel guilty for wanting the world to cry with or for you. Sometimes you want to nurse your mother and crawl in a cocoon and be a baby again. Sometimes you demand special attention and pampering and then think that means you're a wimp and can't stand on your own because you're not facing this like a "real" man or woman. I never dreamed this would happen to me, but it did. People forget they could end up in the same position.

Going through a transition is stress, stress, major stress! For a while, it makes your life a mess. The only way to make it less is to identify what you can do something about and leave the rest to God to work out. Then marshal up support from others who know answers and can lend assistance. One must carefully separate in mind the facts of life from its problems. For me, it meant separating the fact that I was black, female, and disabled from the problem—how to achieve greater independence and mobility. Often we waste countless hours and emotional energy worrying over the things we can't do anything about. Instead, we need to focus in on what we can change and take positive steps toward that. Having the feeling of being able to move when I wanted to is a freedom that came with the chair, made it possible to get from here to there. It became like an extension of me, and I learned to live in it. Slowly I came to view myself as distinct rather than disabled, which made me feel more capable.

About one out of seven in an estimated 35 million people nationwide have a long-term disability that limits their activity, according to the National Center for Health Statistics, and as America grows older, those numbers are increasing. It will be interesting to see what changes will be brought about by the graying of our nation, when we as a people can no longer climb the stairs to world dominance, fight the cause of democracy on every foreign soil, and sit crippled by our own insensitivity to Americans with special needs, be it the old, the poor, or the disabled who have not yet gotten their feet beneath prosperity's table.

It's not easy, what families go through, coping with the changed or changing you. It is as if an alarm bell is sounding and all attention is on you, but no one knows what to do. They feel scared and helpless. You're the loved one they adore and wasn't like this before. It's hard for them to accept this is all that's left. They feel bereft and grieve, missing you! Conversely, it's not easy for us to understand why they don't *understand* and continue e-x-p-e-c-t-i-n-g us to be and do the same as always.

There's a culture in each family—ways how you do things, who is depended on for what, and how you interact. When that's affected, they feel neglected and out of sync because this isn't like you. And when the process of the illness is so mysterious as mine has been, it's easy to suspect foul play or think you're crazy. There has to be some explanation for the situation. How do they make application when they have no facts? How do they learn to use tact in dealing with you? This is all so new! Where does one go to learn disability etiquette like whether to bring up the person's condition or avoid the topic, or whether to volunteer to push the chair or pretend it isn't there? No one rehabilitates them like they work to rehab you! That's why they go on behaving as if nothing has changed, and though you explain again and again, it does no good. Families need reeducation and new information before they can behave differently. There's a need for open lines of communication to help foster good relations, but when speech or hearing is impaired, those avenues get logged up. I felt cut off and distant even when in the same room—so near yet so far away. Almost as a survival mechanism, I let go a little too, because in order to adjust, I knew I had to be with people who only knew the *new* me and were more accepting. Letting go can be an act of love.

Most people with disabilities, even if not mute, have problems with communication. Families just have to learn to live with that and recognize the person's style and ways of letting you know what's going on that's unique to him or her. Because I can't speak, I sometimes feel like an animal around the house. People talk and yell at me; I can't answer back, so they look at me and watch my ways for clues to my mood. Dogs perk up and wag their tails when happy, go lay in a corner when sad, and snap at you when you cross their lines. I find I also perk up and skin my teeth happily, I retreat when down, and when really upset, I fluff my feathers, cackle, and rail like an old hen. And I'm told I fire off looks that can kill you. Anyway, those around me get the point! But through our squabbles we learn to cooperate and interact. That's why it is very important to build your own bonds and ways of relating. My sons and I related a lot through music, which had always been our love. We ordered tapes and CDs from the music club, and when they arrived excitedly, we cracked open the wraps and enjoyed together our favorite artists. Sometimes we battled my generation of stars against theirs to see who had the latest hit that really did it for us. Sometimes things said in song can help folks get along.

In changing times we need to be sensitive to misunderstandings as our emotions are in an upheaval, or there will be greater conflict. Don't over react until you have all the facts and try cutting others a little slack! Sensitivity needs to go both ways. You're not the only one going through changes. It's all around us. Even though we have disabilities, we need not be wimpy and pathetic. Fight the temptation to treat yourself like an invalid. You have to make a decision where you stand and make some choices instead of sitting around vegetating and mulling over the past. Get out into the flow of the culture and times, but don't become just like it. Become a part of bringing about positive change to help others live more hopeful lives. By making plans, choices, and being serious about our priorities, we can affect change positively.

We can be mobile, get a job done, and organize others if we decide for ourselves not to be "crippled" in our attitudes and become masters of our own destiny. Disability actually makes people strong and resilient, not weak and dependent. New technologies are changing what it means to have a disability. It has helped us become more freely integrated into the community. Being able to live in the community, exercising control, and making decisions are empowering. Society has low expectations for people with disabilities, just as it has for other minority group members. We must go through a similar process of changing our attitudes toward ourselves before others will change their view of us.

One of the best ways to empower people is to convince them of their worth, by ascribing worth to them by your words, actions, and deeds. It's no good to say with your mouth we are equal and have potential if the message we get back from you by your actions is we are second class, barely pass, and won't last. There's a stark contrast!

Neither should the message be that you pity me, rather that you believe in me and my ability. Partner with us in pursing goals that will bring greater independence and dignity.

ADA bars discrimination in jobs, education, and housing, but we all know that as in the case of race, laws are one thing in this country, and actual practices are another. Disability teaches us about ignorance and prejudice, just like race. As a disabled person, I couldn't get into schools I could have easily entered before based on score, like what happened at NYU. I would never have imagined that type of situation until it happened. They told me I suddenly wasn't qualified to be a teacher; I guess 'cause I'd become this strange new creature. Yet I viewed myself as a potentially positive role model for students with special needs. Obviously, the powers that be disagreed.

There are a lot of analogies between a disabled person and a racial minority. We are segregated from society because of stairs and architectural barriers and left out socially and in jobs due to negative attitudes. We have to really strive to prove ourselves and be self-advocates. Unfortunately, the situation calls for a fight from folks who, to a large degree, are not always able to take a stand and hold forth for their rights, and thus we need those who will join us in the fight.

However, we don't want to be given something just because of the disability as in the affirmative action controversy, but because we are capable and deserving of opportunity. It is important for people to see us functioning and doing things. The disabled also feel a keen sense of injustice, which can be harnessed to propel us to act and do for ourselves. I try not to think of myself as a "crip," but as a person of strength and ability, out to write my own life story. Only I can fill in the ending. And I can make it either exciting or dull. It's up to me!

One thing I've learned is that we need to keep a mind toward fairness and work to bring it about but really can't live with the expectation of fairness everywhere we go. It simply won't happen, and we will be left bitter and upset constantly. Fair play just isn't a part of today.

Disability is an obstacle, but we should not let it become our excuse. Just because something is hard to do is not a reason not to try it. We need to develop a policy of determination! Most problems can be overcome with time and stick-to-it-ness. No matter what kind of obstacles life throws in front of us, they can be overcome with hard work and firm resolve, whether they are physical challenges or other kinds of problems. Endurance and a dream are the keys to staying on the winning team. The great Wilma Rudolph overcame childhood polio to become a six-time Olympic gold medal winner. Crippled in her left leg as a child, she wore a leg brace and learned to walk, then run, leaving a marvelous example of striving against the odds to be an overcomer.

We are all cripples spiritually. Only Jesus can lead us to heaven by grace. We became this way because of Adam and Eve and a "fall" in the garden. In the Bible, Mephibosheth also became crippled because of a fall. His name means "a shameful thing." He lived in a place of emptiness, yet he was being sought by King Saul so that he could show grace to him and bring him into the palace where he would enjoy many blessings. Likewise, though spiritually crippled, we are being sought by the Lord to live in a place of blessing.

It's weird having defective parts. You feel all at once sorry for yourself, helpless, and yet gutsier because often it is when one's back is up against a wall that we come out swinging and put up our best fight. You get to a point where, like Mao Tse Tung said, you "turn grief to strength." One thing for sure, the experience is lonely and humbling because so few wheelchair users are out there with you, at least that you are in touch with. You have to go through it alone. The discipline to go out and do comes as you go out and do; it's in the process. The worse thing is to sit at home and say you can't. The thing about staying home watching TV is, it's so very easy and requires nothing of me but leaves me feeling bored and empty. Everything else is hard, and it does take a lot of heart to get out and make a start. The challenge is to not let crime, senseless violence, and insensitive imbecilics impose on us too many limits. A sedentary lifestyle is also not good for your health. We have to keep moving and working our muscles.

The more flexible we can be in accepting the alterations that come with life, the more peaceably we can live in spirit. But how do we cope with changes occurring around us and in us, so much of it for the worse? What else is there to do but hold on to the tried and true, things we've always been taught and for which battles have been fought—the right of every man to live lives of freedom, justice, and equality with as much dignity as possible. If we believe God is the author of life, then we can trust Him to be our sufficiency and accept what life gives us and what it takes away.

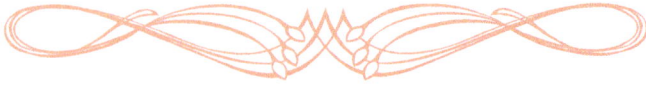

CHAPTER THIRTY-TWO
Take My Hand

THAT time in my life was full of changes and challenges. But in every challenging situation, there are miracles and rays of light. Sometimes we just need a special someone to bring the sun out in our dark and lonely world. Serenity came into my anguish in a most wonderful way. Not that my problems were gone, but God provided someone to help me along.

I knew I had to find a way of making it. I kept saying in the back of my mind, "I'm gonna do whatever I have to do to pull us through!" But the biggest problem may have been *me*. Lack of real motivation stagnated the situation. It was so hard to get past it and really *do* something. The trouble with doing nothing is, it's so very easy; you fall right into it. And if you're not careful, you'll stay stuck, like a stick in the mud.

I tried to escape loneliness and boredom by running off to TV land by way of the morning, midday, and afternoon movies, thinking I could break free of the emptiness and uselessness that bedeviled me. I tried living vicariously through them. But I couldn't flee, for as soon as the credits rolled and the orchestra played the final score, those old bandits broke back in and tormented me even more. Once again there was no phone ringing, no one at the door. The mailman came and went. I was frustrated and guilty, feeling there was a lot I should be doing but I was not. That's a tough spot to be in. It's like you'll sit there until you rot!

I remember Christmas that year. Loneliness draped over me like garlands on a tree. Then came January and my New Year's resolution to seek a solution. I would return to school and find that guy of mine—at least the one I wanted to be mine. What else? I was tired of sitting like a toy on a shelf!

It was a tough choice to follow a different course and set a new direction. But it was the only way of bringing my season of solitude to an end. I made the decision to take a *chance* and move forward by faith.

God knew I needed that time of being isolated, of being alone all by myself so that He could show me, because as I looked inwardly and wrestled, I saw things in my life I wasn't pleased with. I took an honest look and didn't hide my weaknesses. Instead I offered them to Him. When God makes changes, He does it from the inside out. I came to realize scholarship and teaching did not have to be my only sphere of influence. There could be other platforms of "respect" for me. I was still a mother, a daughter, and a sister. But I really desired companionship and intimacy, to have a husband and be a wife, to be affirmed as a woman in a very traditional way. More than being a high-powered career woman, I wanted to cook, clean, sew, and be content with things like crafts and gardening while in pursuit of creative writing.

This seemed good, in a way I never understood, because of taking someone else's values rather than mine, never really taking time and not having much of a selection. Some people find it hard to believe you do not lose your sexuality or your interest in dating when you develop a disability. Others are very surprised to know disabled people marry, hold jobs, buy houses, have families, and travel like everybody else.

Falling in love is one of those weird, warm, and wonderful things many disabled never get to experience, and if they do, it rarely leads to dating and marriage. Many are doomed to go through life alone, with only family members as companions. But if you are fortunate enough to fall in love with someone who loves you back, you are truly blessed. A relationship can become a ladder to success.

I went on a mission to get back in commission and bring fruition to my desire. I just knew the Lord had put that person in my pathway from the time we sat side by side and laid eyes on each other. But so much time had passed. Could what might have been a momentary attraction really last? I needed to know! I was so afraid he was a fair-weather guy and almost let him slip by because I had lost self-confidence. I thought perhaps, if he knew what happened, he would no longer have an interest. I didn't know if he had even been told or if that affection would endure a frosty winter.

It took tremendous effort to get going initially. But I called the director and told her I was on my way in to school. And she said the most surprising thing, that he would be there *waiting*! I was unaware he had been coming and asking where I was. For confidentiality reasons, she wouldn't dare give him my number or a reply.

Funny, isn't it, when someone becomes the object of our strongest affections, how we get so timid and protective of our hearts? Happily, our relationship didn't need a jumpstart, for as soon as I came through the door, we were right back where we were before. Howard showed right away he still cared and was indeed a treasure. He greeted me with open arms, immediately grabbed the handles of my chair, and began pushing me everywhere—to class, for lunch, to the van at the end of the day—never letting a moment of time slip away. He came close to me and listened to what was in my heart. He answered my need for communication as we began sharing our dreams, hopes, and desires.

We were great friends before we became sweethearts. We shared our frustrations, fears, helplessness, and guilt in the face of being late-deafened adults. Before long, we were never far apart. There was no condemnation or putdown for my feeling weak and vulnerable, for my shame and sense of failure, only understanding and support, only his saying, "Let's be *partners* in this! You help me and I'll help you!" Whenever he needed to know what was being said, my fingers quickly danced and fluttered. And he spoke words for me that I couldn't utter.

We began climbing up the ladder rung by rung. For example, to use the phone, I'd dial, then he'd speak, while I listened and signed the reply, and he'd speak again and I'd sign what was spoken on the other end. We put ourselves together to deal with the reality of pain and loss in our lives. We began to *thrive* and discovered what fun real closeness can be. It gave me comfort to be able to express my struggles and problems to him. Sharing who we are takes courage, but he made it easy by not judging me. When he would say, "You've been going through that? I have too!" it was so encouraging. Sometimes we need to hear that others are struggling. It helps us to open up. His presence was like a balm in my wounds—it made me feel I could *heal* and rebuild my life and my self-image.

As we moved closer in the relationship, I became more confident and less fearful of what lay ahead. My sense of doom and dread lifted. Knowing he understood how I felt heartened me to take those steps I was afraid of taking to face the world. I knew I had him to lean on and felt *safe*. Sometimes what we view in life as another problem being tacked on and we wonder how much more we can take, it is actually the Lord sending us a solution or answer to our prayers, for it was in the wheelchair that I developed a relationship of love and care with my special someone. Howard could no longer hear the sounds of everyday life, and I was mute and crippled. Gradually, the reason God made us that way became perfectly clear. It was so we'd know how much we needed each other and draw near. He created interdependency. I have no doubt getting back to doing the ordinary things in life is what our relationship was really all about.

Yes, God put a rainbow in the clouds. When it looked like the sun wouldn't shine anymore, that's when He placed Howard right there to be my life partner. He immediately just took up responsibility for me and I for him. I became his ears; he, my legs and tongue. Together we made one whole body. We shared the laughter and the tears. We began to unveil ourselves and got right down to the marrow. Most importantly, we practiced *teamwork*, each contributing our strengths, each compensating for the other's weaknesses. I dreamed big dreams, but he had daring. I had imagination, and he the strong back and determination to see us through. I possessed wit and he true grit. Where I was cautious, he was courageous. I practiced a heady believism, and he, fundamentalism taught by a strong mother, who struggled to raise six kids in a poor island economy. In some ways I was stronger, but he had been facing really tough times longer.

Over the years the women's liberation movement and careers had not brought satisfaction and security for most black women. They had just moved from white women's kitchens to other forms of labor and were often tired, frustrated, mad, and upset. Most still didn't have the men in their lives sharing the load and meeting needs. Children were still being raised by female heads of households, with the added responsibility of work and career demands vying with commitment to family. Many kids were being raised by the streets out getting into crime and violence.

I felt it was time for me to look beyond things I wanted to *have* and make family and kids my top priority, time to get out of "the war of the sexes" and pull together to form a support base for my kids and community. Marriage and family are spiritual institutions. Ultimately, we must look upward for direction, teaching, and grounding. A rebirth in individual homes can affect neighborhoods, cities, and our nation. This may be the only hope for improving the situation. Thankfully, God provided a companion to share my struggles with me. For Howard it came so naturally, since he has a helping gift. The relationship freshened my spirit. He didn't open an escape route but made a way to work it out by teaching me to dig in and hold on. Then He gave me someone to hold on to, knowing the only way around was through.

The relationship quickly accelerated to its zenith. I found him responsible and protective, felt I could securely place myself in his hands. To me he was a real man's man. Friendship quickly blossomed into romance; our lonely hearts never stood a fighting chance. He enjoyed being needed, liked having me to depend on him. And overnight I switched from R&B to hot reggae, from Mickie Ds to rice 'n' peas. But those are the adjustments you gladly make for love's sake. One might think it was loneliness and desperation that made our feelings shoot through the ceiling. But I don't.

I truly believe God placed him there just for me and opened my eyes so I would see clearly that we were right. He gave me another kinda sight and confirmed it by everyone around us acting as if they saw it too. It was kinda like some crazy glue stuck us together. I wondered if he wanted a paralyzed woman, and he wondered if I'd accept a broken-eared man. We ended hand in hand, with his other hand pushing the chair. I'm sure he hadn't figured it into the equation when we first started. And I was all ready to say, "I understand!" After all, what man wants a woman in a chair? But regardless of everything, he was always *there*. That Valentine's Day I gave him a little lacy heart, just a symbol of the one I had given him right from the start.

Time moved at high speed, and when my wheelchair van started feeling like a horse-drawn carriage, I knew it was time for marriage. I felt like Cinderella going to the palace ball; I still didn't have it all, but in the relationship I'd found, I gleamed like a princess wearing her royal crown. With new underpinnings, my sense of security abounded. Now I wouldn't have to face trials all by myself. He and I had what some would say was a whirlwind romance, got hitched after only four months of dating. However, I viewed it that when God shows you your mate and you know he is the one, what's the use of waiting? So I made a decision. Yes, I was scared that day, but I just couldn't let that big fish get away.

What we need when we are in the eye of a storm is a person who will come into the pit to weep with us, to care, and to walk alongside. Having nice talk isn't enough. We need real flesh and blood, people who'll share our grief and loss and help us as we grapple with problems, uphold us as we creep along, until we see some type of relief. That's what Howard was to me. Finding someone who has "been there" is really important, someone who doesn't know all the answers and is willing to let you go ahead and cry rather than treat you like a wimp or a whiner. Sometimes the best way to climb a mountain is along the rough side, because if you ever make it to the top, you look back with great appreciation for from whence you've come.

Persons with disabilities shouldn't wait for others to do for them what they can do for themselves. But some things we just can't do for ourselves, and that's where we need people who will come to our assist, to help us have our dreams realized through interaction to bring information, respect, sensitivity, and a positive outlook. If these relationships are not romantic, that doesn't preclude our need for them. What's done should be done for our sense of hope and the building up of character. It's enough if you can provide a little buffer from the storm and make our hearts warm for the time you're there. We really do carry your kindness with us everywhere once we've been touched by your compassion.

Sometimes when God tells us to do things, we don't feel ready and we hold back. Insecurity, low self-esteem, and the history of an affair and alcoholism in my parents' marriage caused me to fear taking the chance, thinking maybe he'd only want me then but not later. I'd seen my mother's suffering and felt it so much. I didn't know if in marriage I could learn to *trust* and operate in a balanced way. But I was dying to *live*, to be free of old demons and insecurities as a woman. Most of my cousins' marriages had already ended in divorce, and this would be the second time around for me, of course. It would indeed take a leap of faith. The fact that I was older and he younger troubled me yet the more. Should I listen to fear and caution, or obey the voice of my resounding heart crying love, love, love?

Instead of the usual, sometimes we have to do the unusual to make progress and to propel ourselves out of a rut. Even disabled people have to learn to take risks and hope we don't go belly up. Howard's family was in the process of relocating from Coney Island to Atlanta, the "black mecca" of the South, seeking to take advantage of the affordable housing market opening there. But Howard wasn't moving with them. He'd remain behind and we'd go on as planned, but he needed to go down to give his folks a hand. And guess what? He wanted me to come with him!

I had gained confidence, but I wasn't *that* confident because I'd never been on a plane before. I was still as phobic and timid as ever, especially about going up in the air. He reassured me he would be there, and Mama said, "It'll be good for you!" It's very embarrassing being hauled on a plane like a lump of flesh. This would be the first of many tests. I went and had the time of my life. It was at that point I decided to be his wife. Spring blossoms and I were all in bloom. Within a week I was on the phone telling Mom I'd be married by the time I got back home.

He proposed in his inimitable way by saying, "Look, if you want to marry me, you better do it today! Don't let this moment get away!" Guess that was his manly self-assurance speaking. On the cusps of forty,

I wasn't too worried about what others would say or think. I wanted to be comfortable with myself and what I felt and decided to go for it and take the risk! And so with an electric kiss we sealed our commitment to take our vows. Nothing could stop us now. We asked his brother to drop us down at the city hall, me wearing a red T-shirt and jean skirt, he the clothes he'd worn all along. There was no wedding song, three-tiered cake, stretch limo, or well-wishers waving us on. But love propelled us, and a shower of raindrops fell to bless us. Our only gift—a red rose in a water globe—foretold of a singular struggle. Since then, we've always had to stand alone, without much support.

I'd always been so nicey-nicey, so obedient to life. But I was no longer afraid of being my own person, to follow a dream and hope it would open up a whole new chapter. Now there was someone in it with me to help with the responsibility. I wouldn't have to be out there playing superwoman, struggling with two dependents. Finally I could be the person I wanted to be and do things for *me*. I'd made so many sacrifices. All my anxiety abated when Howard was near. His bouquets of sweet-smelling roses made me feel pursued and placed on a pedestal. I felt special in his eyes, healthy, and *alive*. It actually unimpaired me in spirit and gave me a legacy of loving memories to hold on to.

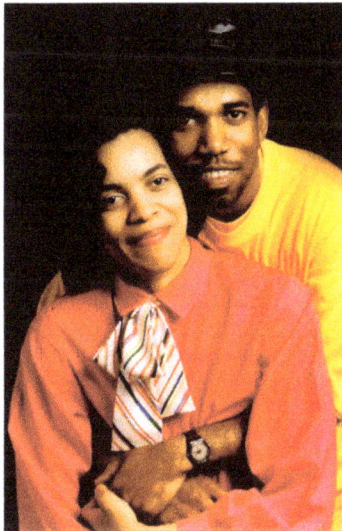

Howard and I when first married.

True love chose the proper time to come and find me. The success of a lot of things depends on *timing*. I had always wanted that "right relationship" and tried several times to make one work, but it never happened. Suddenly when I least expected it, there it was! He has taken on an awful big responsibility, and it certainly tests our wedding vows, but it's been well worth the wait. I don't believe we made a mistake. God took me from being overloaded, overwhelmed, and stressed out, gave me an "M-R-S" and helped me reopen my family practice. Not that it is free of problems, but I can focus more and concentrate on how to solve them. And I find it leads me to many creative thoughts. When frustrated I get to fall into the arms of the one I love, see his tender smile, be caressed, and know I'm not alone. It means so much! Without partnership, we are limited. But with partnership, we can do what we can't do on our own. Love can be a guide and a source of strength. I took hold to the hands of courage and commitment I'd found.

We knew our relationship would be challenged by my sons as well as our disabilities, but we made the choice and listened to our inner voice. God's mercy brought us to each other and these roles. But as with most rejoined families with a stepfather and stepsons, there were many adjustments to make and strong feelings of rejection and apprehension on their part. They had never had a chance to move into a bond of friendship, having only been together a few times. Culture also came into play, black American, Jamaican, and Hispanic. At first everyone panicked!

Because Howard and I quickly bonded, I guess I didn't realize what a struggle it would be for my sons to accept this new person in Mom's life. In hindsight, I realize Malik was asked to make lots of adjustments—to an adopted brother, my illness, and a new stepfather. Hector, having spent years in a group home, had to endure much coming and going in his life too. It's been a lot to go through. Forming a blended family and blending disabilities aren't easy, especially when there are learning and emotional difficulties. We tugged and sometimes bumped each other's lines and took it one day at a time. We went one step forward and two steps back but somehow still remained on track.

One never knows how skills they've learned will come in handy. Techniques I used with squabbling kids in school, I had to apply to my "big guys" at home to work out conflicts and boundary issues. I had to develop new economies to stretch our budget and apply salesmanship to sell myself as a person with disabilities to my in-law family. Industry is always necessary when you don't have a lot because you have to make use of what you've got. Gladly, all of us believed in *family* enough to try to make it work. One thing is for sure, I wasn't just spending my time home squeezing the Charmin, checking to see if it had more sheets. I stayed involved with things constructive and placed accent on the positive. The good part is, I moved from being "instructional" to being more "relational" in personality. Relationships are the basis of good communication in families.

We were in a new era. Howard was not the type of hubby my daddy was. Although I was still chief cook and bottle washer, he did the cleaning of the house and the laundry (a fair division of labor, I would say). He also spent most of his time at home and didn't assert that male right to be "out with the boys," experiencing other joys. How men had grown!

He began working as a house parent with deaf clients, and I remained home as I could no longer get van service to continue school. At social gatherings, people would say, "Well what do you do?" If I said I was a wife, a mother and stayed home, it was like I was nothing, like I just took up space and my mind had gone to waste. I didn't want a paycheck to be the measure of my value. I wanted to feel okay as who I was and what I had to offer. I believed a woman at home could still make a great difference in the lives of those around her.

Being a disabled housewife has its problems. With Howard and I, it's not just a matter of his seeing me without makeup, wearing an old dress. It's seeing me in total ugliness and nakedness, bearing those times when I am down and miserable, commiserating and lampooning him with my anger and frustrations; when I'm physically not well and must be waited on; when I'm emotionally drained and trying to "drink from his cup" as mine is empty; when I can't meet my husband's needs because all the energy has been drained out of me by my day; when I forget that he is walled behind silence and that there is the drone of tinnitus ringing in his ears, driving him to bursts of anger or reducing him to tears. I share his pain of unrealized dreams because of his disability and sit wondering what might have been if I hadn't developed mine. It gets hard sometimes! He is extremely tidy, and I am kind of cluttery. And there are all the "who's worse off" wars and "who deserves sympathy today" battles we've been through. We learn to work around those too. We have our marriage vows put to the test regularly, in sickness and in health, for better or for worse. But this is still better!

LaGuardia College held a special assembly and gave award certificates to various students from our program. I received one, and so did he. It felt like someone knew we came through a rough period and *made it*. That paper trophy meant as much as my college degree for it was just as hard won. I still remember the tears that warmed my cheek when they called our names. Howard went up and accepted for us both, then signed "I love you" from the stage. The deaf students looked around to see, not believing I was now "Mrs. G," sitting there in my wheelchair. How they stared! But I didn't care; I was happy as can be. Happiness in marriage comes when romance is followed by a solid base of commitment. No matter how things worked out, I knew he would not forsake me.

On returning to New York, we saw all the city's problems compounding our own and began dreaming of going back to Atlanta, to buy a home in an area much safer for me. In the face of reports of a chilling new rite of passage for teens—killing a person—I felt I had to get my sons out of the city to try to find a better environment that they also might have a future. I was ready to give up my daily dose of smog, dirt, and overbrewed coffee, which I gulped down with the *Daily News* and escape in search of clean air and open space. It was a beautiful dream, but we weren't sure we could pull it off. Yet we were willing to stand up to the critics and naysayers who didn't think it was a good idea. It would mean heading out with nothing but a dream, having no money or help and no one to lean on, Howard at the lowest salary level, placed in a spot we had to sink or swim. Frederick Douglas believed the South was the best place for black people to achieve great results. We thought we would go and see if he was right. Mama and Daddy had come here because of a dream of a better life. Now we would go in search of the one they left behind, said we wouldn't quit, had to make it.

It would require paying a big price, putting the house up for sale, and using all our savings for moving expenses. The timing didn't seem right, for a little after we got married, Daddy suffered two strokes, one right behind the other. We clung more tenaciously to each other with Dad lingering in that twilight between life and death. Mom had to place him in a nursing home, and she was now home alone. How difficult it would be to leave her, although I knew she'd have my sister and brother. Up against love for my mother, the dream seemed to lose its luster. It would take all the strength I could muster to wave goodbye.

But this *would* give me a chance to start over. And I'd be known for the person I'd become, not who I was before. Moving would broaden my horizons and allow me to experience a new culture. The problem is, the thing I believed God was leading me to do just wasn't comfortable and brought great emotional pain. The things I felt down inside were so hard to contain. I looked for an answer that would have been easier. There was such twanging and plucking of my heartstrings. It would just be one of those *hard* things that life sometimes calls on us to do. Parting always is...We've all gone through that at one time or another.

And we've all dreamed dreams of greener pastures, poppy fields we'd like to pick, slopes we'd like to roll down. But things happen, and those dreams get placed on hold. We keep holding on to them until they're covered with mold. I dreamed of going back to those red clay fields down home, back to where Grandma left off to pick up her dreams again and find a life simple like hers was, close to the land and God. So I decided with much anguish of heart to dust that dream off and go live it.

I know the importance of dreams to a person's life, how they can be a driving force, how without the ability to dream and reasonable expectation of achieving them, life seems not worth living. There's nothing to aspire to. Not aspire in terms of achievement of title or things, but for the self-satisfaction that you derive in doing it. Following my dream meant getting out of my comfort zone into uncharted waters and facing ambiguity and uncertainty. I wondered if I would be able to adapt and deal with the change in culture and the feelings of displacement. Would our self-worth be strong enough for us to survive? Could we evaluate our gifts, put them together, and make use of them? We knew who we were and what we were about would be tested. But we didn't know if we could stand the test.

Like characters in *The Wizard of Oz*, we had finally found our courage, been given new hearts, had our minds renewed, and were ready to follow the yellow brick road to find our dream. We were two disabled people headed off to what seemed like no-man's-land, leaving the comforts of what's familiar, willing to take the risk, believing God was on our side. We thought we were leaving crime and grime behind. We didn't know it, but we were headed for a city that, although very pretty, is just as highly impacted by drugs, robbery, violence, and a pollution problem practically unequaled in the nation. That shows we always think the grass is greener somewhere else, until we get there and find out what we're running from is waiting right there to greet us. I just hoped we wouldn't end up as *failures* and have to come back home.

My experience taught me that partnering and teamwork are very important rather than observing life from a safe position. Best of all, I've learned the value of making connections and forming relationships instead of isolating myself and trying to go at it alone.

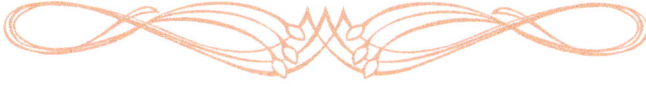

CHAPTER THIRTY-THREE
Getting On with Our Lives

BEFORE leaving New York, there were lots of preparations, first to ready the old house for sale, in and of itself no small undertaking. What we lived with might not be acceptable to somebody else, so we began fixing, repairing, and replacing. You know that feeling of opening yourself up to the prying eyes of the world, hoping no one finds any fault? Had to keep everything perfect, never knowing when an agent or prospective buyer might stop by and we'd be put on display. Day after day being on guard is a lot of pressure. Moving is something no one wants to do often. That's for sure!

Meanwhile, I began eating, sleeping, and drinking Atlanta, kept it foremost in mind, even ordered *The Atlanta Constitution and Journal*. I had it delivered up north to my home each weekend to keep abreast of the happenings there so I'd be aware. How's that for determination? I was so focused I could close my eyes and almost picture myself in the country, waking up to a hearty breakfast of smoked ham and eggs, then Howard running out to stretch his legs, while I sipped the last dregs of fresh coffee. Or going fly fishing by a quiet stream or just the two of us on a porch swing in the cool of evening. Envisioned green pastureland with herds of bovine lowing as they graze and chew. Imagined sleepy little towns with lush mountain settings behind we'd pass through. Could smell country scents of wood burning and Southern pine and jasmine and honeysuckle blooming on the vine. Could practically taste stacks of flapjacks and molasses, and my toes felt like dangling in tall tickly grasses. I thought it would be a ball to have down-home folk with that Southern drawl pass by and say, "Hi, y'all?" Ahhh, such stuff dreams are made of!

We began experimenting to find where we'd fit in. There was a deafness program Howard wanted to attend, so we selected a college in North Georgia about 150 miles outside of Atlanta in a small city called Rome, tucked comfortably in the breasts of the Tennessee Mountains. That's not far from Cave Spring, a rural area with a large deaf institute and many deaf residents in the surrounding farm community. It is an area of immense beauty with rolling hills dotted with irreparable old barns and other rustic evidences of the past. Also near is the lovely campus of Berry College, on which can be found back up in her woods an old grist mill with a giant water wheel whose turning plays music to the restless soul. We could sit there listening until we grew quite old, so we thought. But that's not the real world, is it? Only a nice place to go visit and find tranquility and peace of mind. That winding road leading deep into the silent forest started me dreaming about tomorrow...or was it yesterday I was trying to get back to?

Georgia has a wide assortment of creek ponds and toad frogs and a wealth of wildlife in her lush overgrowth. But her real beauty is in her people, who have a particular love for hearth and home, yard and garden, birds, nature, and family. Honesty and Christianity seemed to abound in her small backwater towns, but just like yelping bloodhounds chasing an elusive prey, the people hadn't always caught up with today. Some spoke proudly of a New South, while others held tenaciously to her old legacy. Yet it was peaceful and quiet as can be in Dixie. Church folk still filled her many houses of worship on Sunday mornings before going out to eat. When done they sat in shady places to keep out of the sun and waved to folks passing through even if they didn't know you. They treated people nicely most days, but then there were those other ways no one liked talking about.

Rome's comfortable look and feel lulled one into a false sense of security. It seemed homey and idyllic (nice little city) but economically depressed and undergoing job stress. Yet a real cracker barrel place to go kick your shoes off and throw back in one of the rockers on everybody's front porch, or warm by a fireplace in a grand room. A place a person felt they could settle down amid the cornfields and kudzu that grew rampantly on the trees. Where kids still picked wind-flowers and chased bumblebees. Where residents put wagon wheels and old pitcher pumps in their yards as icons of yesterday, showing they stubbornly held on to things they could long have let go of, even their biases. Had plenty of hardworking folk there who didn't have much, so they didn't bother with a whole lot of fuss. I liked that. Women had a fresh-scrubbed look, and a lot of them still carried little pocketbooks on their arms, not afraid of anyone snatching it or doing them any harm. Just threw it down anywhere you know. It was that kind of place, slow paced. Everybody smilin' and greetin' each other, even if you were a black sister or brother, they said hi to you too! We thought this was just right for big-city people turned country. Got ready for barbeque, bandannas, and sweet Southern manners. We imagined fitting in and finding acceptance despite our disabilities, yet we were prepared to demonstrate our ability.

Howard went down that August 1989 to register for fall classes. He made his first solo long-distance drive more than a thousand miles just after passing the driver's test on a quest to locate an apart-ment. He used to call while canvassing neighborhoods, telling me everything was going good and things were falling in place as they should. But my growing hopes suddenly dimmed when doctors said Dad's chances for recovery were slim. Every day I spit-polished my dream in order to see its amber glow. It was tough though! I had such feelings I was abandoning ship just when he needed me most. I got all tangled up in mixed emotions, especially guilt. It's hard to prepare to go on living when someone dear may be dying.

Malik had been dating a girl in his training program and didn't want to leave her; he was slated to go into job placement too. Moving to Atlanta would place his employment and the relationship in jeop-ardy. His reaction was sullenness and hostility toward me. Hector finished college and was working as a pastry chef, so the effect on him wasn't so drastically felt. But I had to deal with the issue of trusting his maturity to remain behind and take care of the house until it was sold. Really both their reactions were cold because of what they felt they were losing. Going was as hard as could possibly be! But we went. The plan had been laid in cement.

Our small two-bedroom duplex was in a remote enclave on the north end of the city called Armuchee. It's too bad we didn't realize the north side of town is almost always where mostly whites live. There were still very clear lines of demarcation between the white and black communities. We unknowingly had rented on the wrong side of the line. That's what happens when you're new in an area and don't yet know your place. Georgia's chicken wire fences couldn't hold back the intrusion of hate into our dreams.

A moving company drove our furnishings down while we traveled by train. But I didn't know Malik was in so much pain. I tugged him by the shirttail and practically dragged him in the cab as we left for the trip. He pounded the walls of the house, even knocked a hole in the siding in his anger, feeling he'd never see his girl again. That immediately changed our relationship as he began passively and sometimes actively resisting our attempts to appease him. Now I realize out of guilt, we probably played into the game of control that later created lots of ups and downs in our household. It got to the point he and Howard couldn't pass close to each other in a room without it being read as provocation. I began living in fear it would erupt into a physical confrontation.

We came south looking for peace but brought an internal war with us, making adjustment even more difficult. Daily I tried to hold the hostile fires to a minimum. We had problems making ourselves understood and finding ways of expressing our expectations of one another without explosions. Howard and I communicated in sign language; Malik didn't, leaving him alone. He began grieving deeply the loss of family, friends, and job opportunities. The fact the person he called Dad lay near death made it doubly hard to accept the stepfather he had left. We couldn't tune into where he was coming from, and he couldn't tune into where we had come to—a backwoods place with only a few channels on the TV set. Boy, was he upset!

But he was lucky. At least he could make a call, because for us, there was no relay service at all. I had to phone home if I wanted to talk 'cause Mama had a TTY she'd bought. Poor communication and the change in family dynamics wore away the newness of our romance and soon challenged loyalties between us. They were like kids playing tug-o'-war with me as the rope. That heart game was a lost hope, for it seemed I was being asked to choose who'd lose.

Upon arrival we immediately faced hostility from neighbors who weren't happy to see a black family move in *their* community. We were met by harsh realities of the South that we knew little about. Racial bias was alive and well, waiting right there to greet us. You didn't have to travel too far outside of Atlanta, "the city too busy to hate," to find people for whom hating was a way of life. As my son jumped out of the car and stood in the common area between sides of the bungalow, our white neighbor yelled to her son, "Go out there and tell them niggers to get out of my driveway!" What a welcoming committee for arrivals from New York City! We weren't accustomed to their style. For this had we traveled a thousand miles?

That was just the beginning. When we'd leave the house and return, ugly things were sprayed on our back door, and there would be footprints where they pounded and kicked it some more, all because they wanted us out. If we went into the Laundromat nearby, they treated us like undesirables, rolled their eyes, tried their best to ignore, hoping we'd get the message and walk back out of the door. Poor Malik was followed all around the quick-stop store like a thief. Then late one night we had a really strange visit from the police. Got so nervous we slept with our car parked right up to the front door, not knowing if they'd come back and harass us some more.

These were people who hated us without even knowing us, who thought we were thieves, there to destroy the community simply because we were black, who looked on my husband as less than a man, wouldn't give him a job anywhere up there, didn't care that we needed to eat and get on our feet. Although we were Northerners, we knew how to garden and make things grow, but we didn't know how to nurture relationships with those people and make them grow, for they were sewn from the same old seed. Having folks tolerate you and just barely put up with having you around is not the same as accepting you. Economically, we found it very hard to make ends meet, and support systems were not there to sustain us; neither did the culture. We began to struggle financially, emotionally, and in many other ways. Yet we got out there, flapped our wings, and tried making it. Malik signed up for drivers ed, said the other kids put junk in his head questioning if he was a drug pusher because they saw him ride up in a new automobile. Didn't know it was a rental. Figured the only way we got something was to sell drugs or steal. They lived under certain illusions and drew the wrong conclusion about him because he was young, black, and from the city. It's a pity because Malik was already struggling to leave New York behind and put it out of his mind.

We managed at last to buy our own first car, an old one, but good enough to get where we were going. Got it off a folksy-talking used-car salesman who had that Andy Taylor style that fools Northerners into trust. He sure fooled us. Half the time the car wasn't running; it wouldn't even start. We kept taking it back, and they said it was this or could be that, but a lemon is what it was. We needed a good set of wheels on our odyssey of searching for but not finding jobs, friends, or acceptance. There was much resistance. We had no connection with the black community, and whites certainly weren't opening welcoming arms to us. Malik finally got a little job stacking newspapers. Howard was hired by a rehab center as a house parent but shortly after got a letter stating there was no longer a need for his services. He believes it was because the job entailed supervising young white females alone overnight, and it made them uptight.

At that point our resources both financially and emotionally were running on empty, and Malik kept acting out his need for friends. So we took up the responsibility to take him where young people hang out wherever they gathered. This meant parking outside theaters, game parlors, music stores, and fast-food joints, waiting hours for him to come out just so he could have some livelihood. Didn't do a whole lot of good. Being responsible for a young man's happiness so completely and his being so dependent upon us were a lot of stress. Instead of getting along better, we got along less. His needs controlling our schedule and activities created more friction and antagonism. We got worn down in the process.

Before I knew it, I was beating on the doors of heaven to keep us from beating on each other emotionally. The money shortage we fell into, coupled with isolation, loneliness, and estrangement from family, nearly sank us into turmoil. Things weren't going well at all. We just couldn't connect despite our gallant efforts to help ourselves. Bad economic times, job shortages, and cutbacks were hard on residents of the area and even harder on us. A constant diet of fast foods and disappointments had our stomachs churning with despair. Something told us it was time to leave there, but we weren't going running. We took a stand and actually drew a line in the sand, let 'em know we weren't gonna back down. We stood our ground and left when we were ready. Oddly enough, it was a game of ball that dispelled tension between us. Guess it gave a chance to throw some shots without anyone getting hot.

With every hurdle we face in life, we have to do battle with our fears as well as that which wars against us. The biggest battle is most often in our minds. We had to overcome the psychological hurdle and not let fear stand in the way of our desire to succeed. Something kept saying, "Why did we come to this godforsaken place? It's all a big mistake!" But Howard said, "No, let's go to Atlanta where job possibilities will be brighter!" He said God told him in a dream He'd be waiting. Sure enough He opened a door, provided just what we had been hoping for, an accessible two-bedroom apartment in a quiet complex. We had passed our first survival test.

But that meant packing our belongings and moving *again*. Never forget that day we rented the U-Haul truck, got it loaded up, and headed for the highway. The thing is, Howard had never driven a truck before. I held his arm, and Malik hugged the door as the old clunker jostled along. It turned into a real adventure once we hit I-75 and started rolling, then began to fly, not letting other cars pass us by. In Atlanta, people drive fast, so if you are going to keep up with the pack, you can't hold back. That's one of the lessons I wish Howard never learned because of all the rubber he now burns.

Once we got settled, they were on the go looking for jobs, facing a mob of competition. Howard headed out early seeking work. Malik walked up and down the road, going door to door, fast food stores, anywhere he could pop into. If they said no, he'd dust the dirt off his worn-out sneakers and go. Often hard times bring out the best in us. They cause us to stretch ourselves to our limits, let us see how many megabytes we have upstairs in our computer and develop stamina. Anyway, he finally found something, stripping upholstery. Didn't pay much or last long, but at least he had the gumption to get out there. It showed me things I was unaware, that he could be persistent and was intent on making it.

Howard landed a job at Goodwill and did very well. The whole staff liked him! And the maintenance work he was doing was a cinch because he is neat as a finch. He had the IRS offices spiffed to a shine in no time! Before long he was cleaning the entire building alone. He'd be so tired when he came home he'd just drop right in bed. Hard work is not something he dreads to get what he wants. Once revved up, it's hard for him to stop. Just winds down until he runs out, gives it all he's got. But I felt he could do more. After all, what had he gone to college for? Was that all going to waste? I made haste to encourage him to sign up with DRS and start taking state tests. We did our best together, writing and studying, me helping and going along for the big exam to interpret. Nail biting as it was, we got through it. And he got his foot in the door and landed the kind of job he had been hoping for in rehabilitation. He rose to the occasion as far as adversity was concerned.

And we all learned as we went—neighborhoods, the people, the lay of the city. It really is very pretty! Hadn't forgotten our dream of getting ourselves a nice house, so we began looking about, searching here, there, and everywhere. We wanted an older one, really comfortable and homelike with a big yard space for flowers to grace. Out driving one day in Stone Mountain, we saw one off the main road near a bus line. We thought it would do fine; that way Malik could get around. It seemed the perfect home we had found! But we didn't know how the white residents would react when they saw we were black. All we wanted was a home, not conflict like in Rome. Didn't want a fight or to make people uptight. Yet there were already several For Sale signs up in the area. We should have known then, it was white flight.

The house was owned by a Chinese lady eager to move to Roswell and very motivated to sell, so we bought it. This time around, we were greeted cheerfully enough by white neighbors who came to introduce themselves and I'm sure to look us over. Guess they must have said, "Poor handicapped people, must be some government program, a group home or something." It seldom occurs to folks we can get things and own property on our own. Anyway, it looked like they decided to keep their eyes on us, because I'd see them across the street at the pool, peeking and staring, looking from behind bushes, just gawking and watching. For what? I don't know! In the summer, teenage kids would climb atop the clubhouse, sit, sun, and stare, then throw coal from the barbeque pit, our windows to try and hit. On MLK's birthday, someone sent us an awful gift but left no name slip—just put feces and urine in baggies and bombarded the front door. What for? This time I'm not sure it was so much about race as just the fact that we were out of place—*different*, disabled. You see, residents of neighborhoods have little tolerance for people who aren't quite like *them*. So there we were again. If we stayed, we were going to have to sink or swim.

The house we bought was in good shape, but the yard needed a lot of TLC. That was no problem for an outdoors man like Howard. He looked forward to the job of dolling her up. He traded the car in for a pickup truck and began cutting down trees and hauling debris. Forty exactly! There were plenty of tasks for me too, buying furnishings piece by piece and making my own curtains. Whew! What we didn't do to that place! Cut down, dug up, planted, designed, decorated, and worked wonders before everyone's eyes. Were the neighbors surprised as they watched it evolve from an eyesore to one of the nicest in the area and best taken care of.

To our dismay, we got ripped off by an agent "friend" in whom we placed confidence to have it painted, then we were charged way too high by another guy to have it made accessible. There aren't a lot of companies who do alterations, so the disabled get taken advantage of in these situations. The government needs to fund programs for home modification so we won't get victimized out there by ourselves. Assistance should not be limited to those at abject poverty level receiving Medicaid because many wheelchair users don't qualify for public aid.

Happily, I got busy learning to put up jellies from fruits 'n' vegies and baking cakes without too many mistakes, had my men coming home to hot dinners and the smell of freshly baked bread. I was getting along quite well without use of my legs. But as a disabled housewife, home alone, it was hard for me to get friendships going for support.

Yet the Lord, in His ever wisdom, had planted us right next door to a white lady and her husband who was a Baptist minister. And they did indeed administer grace to us with their loving kindness. On short visits, the wife brought treats and small gifts from their missionary travels. I got to see some of the world through her eyes. Her warmth filled my living room, as did colorful mementos from their trips. Sometimes when they were away, I babysat their little lop-eared rabbit. He was a great companion too. Though we both were mute, he was awfully cute and showed me a trick or two he could do.

On Women's Day she invited me to her all-white church. I was placed at the head of the table, as if to make a statement to the others it was time to erase some of the lines. Reaching out, *including*, is what Christianity is supposed to be about. It's wonderful how even one special friendship across lines can heal the hurt and anger we all feel toward members of certain groups in our communities. True to convictions, they remained behind as the steady march of For Sale signs continued going up and residents moved to escape the influx of black families into the area. The problem was the same north and south; when blacks came, whites went.

But I gained a new understanding of their fears in a painful way. While watching TV, one day, I saw a familiar-looking face. But they were saying the girl was dead—raped, then shot in the head by a guy who took her car and left her body in a garage. The face didn't register at first, but when a news truck appeared next door and a crowd gathered, I knew something was astir. I regret to say, it was my neighbor's daughter who had been killed that day by a *black* assailant! "Oh my god! Not that! Not to them! Why *them*?" I asked Him. But He did not answer. Just somehow used me to go hold her, let her cry upon my shoulder, and give her a little water globe with an angel in it. And just for that moment in time, in her anguish at losing her child, and in me imagining what if it were mine, we became as one.

I experienced deep grief and loss too when Daddy died, and I went back home to say goodbye. I felt like a part of me died with him. I know the good times did, in a lot of ways.

Life is often one pain on top of the other, and our issues get compounded. We never realize the role people play until they're gone and sorrow lingers long. It left Malik reeling too, for once back in Atlanta, a terrible period of anger ensued resulting in his being in a shelter and our lives going totally helter-skelter because of *pain*. We entered family therapy to try to pull together again. The South doesn't have a lot of services for people with disabilities. And when problems are as complex as in our family, there's just nowhere to turn for support, leaving no resort but to draw on our own limited resources and determination to improve communication. We sought vocational help and placement for him due to recurrent difficulties. They kept sending him here and there, and we were getting nowhere. But the Lord helped us begin to heal our hurts and divide. Slowly we began reconciling our differences and letting go of the past. We came out on the other side *better*, stronger, behaving more like family, learning to assist, support, understand, and forgive. Reconciliation didn't come to the larger community, however. The pattern of whites running continued until only those who couldn't escape remained.

Five years passed with us scrimping, sacrificing, and going through hardships often down to the penny, overdrawn and participating in food cooperatives to eat healthily. Like so many families in the '90s, we struggled but held on and tried to self-correct some of our own problems. We didn't have an easy time of, but God gave increased potential to work things through, and we kept going, going, and going like Eveready batteries.

With time, the steady dribble out and trickle in brought changes in the neighborhood for the worse. Before long, the area grew unsafe due to a new negative element. And so we decided to pick up and go after all we'd put into it. This time we hoped to head for the outlying area south of Atlanta away from the urban crush. All of us at times feel the need to escape some of our own. We hunted and pecked at homes, trying to be careful to make the best choice, hoping this would be the *last* time. Our desire was to have one built just right for me and my chair.

Oh, the dreams we had of how it was going to look. Not too fancy, mind you, just flat, open 'n' wide, with a modified kitchen and bath and a beautiful garden accessed by a specially laid path. We spent hours drawing it out, thought of every imaginable kind. We visited so many places and looked at every plan we could find. But none were designed with a disabled person in mind. Builders never think about us when they construct things, although they plan for children, even a family pet. Hasn't hit 'em yet that they need to plan accessibility into their housing communities.

We sold our old house at a loss due to the area turning down, unable to get what it should have cost. Then needing a temporary residence, we located a complex that included accessibility in their advertisements. I called, got an appointment, had an interview, and you wouldn't believe what they put us through! First they said my adult son would not be permitted to live with me despite his disability if he couldn't show proof that he earned an amount equivalent to four times the rent. Second, their model apartments were situated on the top floor, and I couldn't go up and see what I was getting. They *swore* they had one just right for me, so we paid our deposit and security fee. Wouldn't you know when we came to move in, the apartment had no ramp and the mailbox was so far you had to go there by car! The toilet had no grab bars, the cooking nook was only big enough for a little kitchen witch, and there was a host of things that needed to be fixed! We had no choice but to move in anyway. There aren't many accessible apartments around these days. I suppose they thought it was enough to widen the doors. But accessibility can mean many things depending on what an individual needs and is looking for.

That first day, only hours after arrival, a blocked-up toilet ran over and flooded the entire flat, while I sat in water up to my ankles, waiting for my husband to get back. The apartment was located in the rear by itself, so I couldn't get help. The office wouldn't respond to my relay calls at all. Seems the staff resented their "inconvenience." As a consequence, our new furniture got waterlogged and ruined, but the manager said it was not their fault. Were neither the bacteria I ingested drinking water from a broken faucet, nor the termites eating through the closet, not the decrepit patio deck overhead, which could have fallen and knocked me dead, not even the lack of wheelchair parking space in the place. You see *nothing* was their responsibility once you paid your money and accepted the key.

When I went in to see the manager, she tapped me on the head demeaningly with a piece of paper as if to say, "Now you be a good little girl and be *quiet*." I definitely didn't buy it! Found out they were under HUD and decided to file a complaint about inaccessibility, but I didn't even know where to call because that information isn't readily available at all. I was on the phone constantly with no help in sight, trying to fight them. Finally I found a disabled lawyer who took great care in filing a report, sent supporting documents, and told them we would go to court if necessary. They sent an investigator, but after months of calls, copies, and misery, the response we got back said she found "no cause" for further action. Other than in 4 percent of cases, they never do. Not because the problems don't exist, but staffing isn't there to give complaints proper care. So I just prayed for the day to get out of there.

When it came, we were given a blazing sendoff as gunshots thundered like cannon fodder outside my window, and a somber brigade of roaches lined up to say goodbye. A few even tried to come along with us for the ride. But I made sure they remained on the other side! We have to leave some things behind, hard as it may be. Yet we prayed one day to end the wandering and find *stability*.

I didn't let that place really bother me because I felt it was only a matter of time before I'd be in my brand-new home and everything would be *fine*! After all, we laid everything on the line, put down all our savings and more trying to purchase the dream we were chasing—that country house, that simple life, that safe haven to come home to, which would work for me and my disability. We met a fast-talking builder, a fellow New Yorker, who showed us a model and told us building it with modifications would be no problem. He had lots of experience, so he said. Wish I'd realized it was all in his head. Guess the affinity I felt with him turned out to be my undoing. Anyway, we signed a contract and didn't investigate his background like we should have.

We now know what a big mistake that was, 'cuz anything that could go wrong did, while he strung us along with misrepresentations. For six months we cramped up in that squirrel hole, holding on ever so tightly to our dream, not seeing the reality of what he was building and being too inexperienced to pinpoint its failings. When we made our weekly trips out to the site, we viewed our dream home through rose-colored glasses. You know, the filtered lenses we put on sometimes when we allow ourselves to be led blindly by childish emotion and refrain from taking a good look. Maybe because it is fun to *dream* and kid ourselves into believing things that *are not*, for the reason we want them to be so badly. Or that we wrestle so often with issues of being assertive. Or that communication barriers make it hard to get things clear. Or maybe we keep making the same mistake of taking professionals with smiling faces to be "friends," for lack of any, being too trusting, and taking them at their word. I've learned now never to trust people no matter who where large sums of money are concerned. Wish we hadn't because it would have saved our pocketbooks and our innermost feelings a lot of hurt. For we again got taken for jerks. The real estate system found us to be easy victims.

Suffice it to say we went in leading with our hearts instead of our heads. We made the same mistake twice, following bad advice. Being deceived, getting ripped off or taken advantage of is a terrible thing to have happen to one, but when it comes at the hands of people we think are friends whom we *trust*, the experience carries with it so much tonnage.

I must admit that there had been a little voice whispering. I guess I just didn't listen 'cause the builder assured us everything was going well. He said my jitters were perfectly natural. Right up to move-in day, he strung us along singing a sweet little birdsong. But when we screeched up in the heavy-laden truck, carrying all our best hopes and dreams, beaming, and bursting at the seams with glee, we found the place dirty, the house wasn't ready, and (you guessed it) he made a fast exit! His men were still working, and many items on our preinspection list hadn't been done. That was strike one. Then they kept coming back while I tried to unpack. The first four months went like that with me working around handymen trying to get settled. Any woman knows that's a surefire way to get nettled!

As we lived in our "dream home," all sorts of things went wrong, and we saw problems we hadn't noticed before. The ceiling had seams, bulges, and nail pops. A settlement crack appeared running the length of the garage floor. Window screens were warped and rusted. Air whistled in through misaligned doors. They cracked the tub wall when it was installed, and upstairs there was a bowed-out wall. The tiles cracked in the downstairs bath, and an ugly discoloration covered the concrete paths. The drywall was marred by imperfections, and the stucco needed correction, not to mention blobs and paint stains fallen here and there. Evidence of poor workmanship was spattered everywhere. The plumbing was left rough, the wiring was all wrong, and air leaked out where it didn't belong. My handicapped toilet began flushing when not in use, while the builder made up excuse after excuse. Movement of silt our way, when it rained, made it apparent something was wrong with the grading. Our young garden plants stood drowning in standing water. Water also settled in front of the garage door and poured down from the gutters. Before long it was coming in under the walls. Soon it got underneath my wood floors and turned them black, causing further grief. When we saw it settling around the foundation, we knew we had a serious situation. The underlying cause? The house was set too low. As for accessibility, the ramps cracked, kitchen modifications were poor, and the threshold was too high for the chair at the front door. A lowered peephole never got installed, and the flashing doorbell and fire alarm units weren't hooked up at all. I never got my roll under sink, and my special walkway to the backyard began to collapse and sink, as did my elation.

Imagine! We sold a house that when inspected only needed a washer in the sink for something with multiple defects, thinking we would get a problem-free new one and be set for the next ten years. That's enough to bring anyone to tears! We were left open to being victimized by desperation to find someone to meet my accessibility needs, which played right into his greed. Foolishly we turned down a well-known, reputable builder for a novice who made vain promises he couldn't deliver. The guy professed to be a Christian, a man on a mission to make the dream of new home ownership attainable to those of lesser means. He gave us an engraved gold leaf Bible and his blessing at the signing. Guess that was all just a clever ruse to gain our trust. But he grossly underestimated us as folks often do. Never thought we would discover what he was up to, passing himself off as a man of compassion while ripping us off in the name of the almighty buck. However, not finding out soon enough caused us to get stuck.

When one buys a house, they buy a permanent license to worry. Ending up with something like this and can't get it fixed is a nightmare from which we longed to awaken—the mental oppression, the constancy of dreading what will go wrong next. The builder accepted no professional responsibility, which locked us in a legal action that was hard to get through and saddled us with fees we couldn't afford to pay. There we were, up against the struggle of a shattered dream, after taking another one of life's inevitable spills. We slipped into an economic storm, an emotional storm, and a storm of disappointment.

The battle to have our home restored had us mired in uncertainty, and we were left in a quandary. Would they fix it or have to take it back? We didn't know! And then where would we go? Our house had no *warranty*; neither did our future at that point. Any moment things could slip right back out of joint.

We are tempted to say to ourselves when these things happen, "Haven't we suffered enough already?" We wish all that we've come through could exempt us from more of life's problems, but sometimes that's just not God's will. Yet He is with us, and His power is behind us. We shouldn't become discouraged when we can't find that "right place," nor should we give up because of inadequacies we see within ourselves. Happiness never manifests itself in the "things" we keep chasing because it has to come from the inside out. One thing I do know, I've got a perfect house waiting for me in heaven, not built by human hands. God promises things but often requires that we *wait*.

It's hard to accept making a bad choice by listening to the voice of our feelings. I blamed myself because I'm the one who insisted he was *the one*. I sat saying "Dumb me" and berating myself for my stupidity, but I got tired of feeling dumb and stupid. Maybe I didn't have to be to have done this. We decided to "get on with our lives" and just try to live regularly—pay the mortgage, cut the grass each week.

Living in Georgia, I was feeling a world away from New York when hijackers slammed two planes into the World Trade Center while I watched in disbelief by TV. My heart hurried home immediately. Soon the Pentagon in DC was struck too; the whole country was stunned and deeply grieved.

Suddenly it was not me alone confined at home; everyone sat paralyzed by fear. Everyone felt vulnerable and afraid of a hidden enemy who killed indiscriminately. And everyone was feeling worried about their inadequacies. The overwhelming sense of helplessness came because we could not be protected. In the twinkling of an eye, millions of lives were altered and affected. Greater unease followed when bioterrorism hit. Overnight there was a major culture shift. The nation slumped into a quick recess, and American life became so much more complex. Many people were asking, "What's going to happen to us?" Most were just happy to be alive. On every stratum, folks wondered how they would survive. Suddenly no one had any security; no one's future had any warranties. As with me, the country had to deal with pain and loss very unexpectedly.

Concerns about my little house and family all at once seemed trivial, with thousands of innocent victims buried beneath the rubble and the nation headed into war to counter a threat unlike anything we'd ever faced before. Though the president tried to urge everyone back to normalcy, we knew things would not be the same for any of us again.

My life's journey began at World War II's end. Then came war in Korea, Vietnam, and the Persian Gulf. The full span of my lifetime we've spent bickering and fighting among ourselves. In that sense, not much has changed. But something positive resulted from the September 11 tragedy. New attitudes arose. Suddenly Americans of all backgrounds showed solidarity. Images of police and firefighters putting their lives on the line for others prompted folk to look for ways to help their neighbors. Many donated time, money, and blood. Instead of locking themselves away in their private castles, people reached outside of their own households with concern. A sense of responsibility and trend toward service took hold. People behaved a little more civil, kind, and patient. For a period of time, there was a revival of compassion.

Americans talked about coming together in peace. Partnerships formed around the country and across the world. Leaders talked about making a positive difference, feeling compelled by the support and cooperation they were getting. What is it that made us reach out? Perhaps it was the threat of someone taking the American way of life away that made it more precious and meaningful to people regardless of color. Black, white, and brown all stood together, waving flags. Our small differences didn't appear that important anymore. We saw that if we are going to make it, we'll have to do it together. Despite our racial and cultural diversity, we've learned how much we really need each other. Tragedy showed us who we really are—one nation under God. We rediscovered our roots. Crisis awakened us to the fact that we need to stop fighting over small details and focus on what really matters. In mourning, Americans reached out to touch each other and knelt to pray together. Seeing so many lives lost in an instant caused reshaping of priorities and brought new definitions of success and worth. Focus diverted away from the drive to have and achieve in favor of personal time and time to spiritually reflect. More value is being placed on family, friends, and love.

Terror lurking in the shadows is causing many to deeply question. They ask themselves, if they died today or tomorrow, if God would accept them, and they wonder if they've lived good enough lives to make heaven. Many are turning to the Bible for answers to the questions of their lives, realizing the need to have something available down on the inside to get through these difficult times. Everyone is desperate for reassurance and hope.

A lot of people are where I am now, feeling like I feel. Many had towers fall in their lives, even before September 11, and are dealing with loss and grief. Tragedy has sensitized us to the feeling of each other's infirmities. But division has already reared its ugly head with calls for racial profiling and judging people by appearances in the wake of recent events. Hate crimes against Arab Americans have been reported. Now there is a new group of "you people" to be blamed. It's so typical of us to want to put colors on the face of problems. From here on, it will be a challenge for every American to do the ordinary—hop on a plane, get mail, or go see a ball game. No one feels safe maneuvering on urban terrain or in big crowds. And everyone has a problem with tall buildings. We'll all have to learn new coping skills to adapt to the realities of life in the twenty-first century. Nothing remains the same. The one sure thing is *change*. It's going to take time. It takes time to turn life around. The challenge is, once things get better, not to lose the sense of unity and compassion we've found.

I believe we have entered an era of tremendous hope and power! The change in public sentiment provides an open door and a base on which to build. On many levels, people are asking questions. They want to know how members of other communities view them and the cause for all the hatred. They are looking for answers to deal with trouble, particularly spiritual answers. We may be able to look afresh at issues related to social justice, class differences, access, and discriminatory barriers without wallowing in bitterness, with a mind toward seeking peace and finding common ground.

This is an opportunity to triumph over our fear of differences. Now that barriers are coming down, it is a perfect time for communicating across lines to dialogue and share. Communicating doesn't have to mean using a lot of words. It means touching each other by revealing our innermost thoughts and feelings and being accepted for where we're at without having to fear the consequences. As we pull together as Americans to face the future, maybe some of our old hurts will finally heal and lines of demarcation erased. Though our view ahead is overshadowed by fear of impending danger, let's remember that our source of safety and protection is in the Lord. He is our security! We can't lean on our heritage or anything else. We can only lean on *him*.

The new generation has a defining moment to recall when everything changed, just as I can look back on the '60s. The fact that such devastation could happen here has brought the world home. We no longer feel safe and protected. Now they are asking themselves the same profound questions I've tried to answer: Who Am I? What is my purpose? Where is my place? And how can I contribute to ease some of the hurt and ugliness around me?

There is a tremendous need for information, charity, and support so that families in crisis don't feel so all alone. In these times, we must turn away from self-absorption and look for ways to perform acts of service to meet the needs of the poor and hurting. Not everyone in the same way, but each in some way. It's also important to tell others how they are touching our lives and making a positive difference. All we really have in life to prove our worth is the good we leave behind.

What's making the crucial difference in everything going on in our lives right now is that God dwells with us. We are experiencing His presence daily. He has empowered us with new dreams and is taking care of things one at a time. Special provisions have come our way as we continue to progress. My husband has even started a home business to help others with disabilities lead more independent lives. I'm still writing, which is cathartic for me and finding my voice. We haven't overcome every obstacle, and all of our issues haven't been resolved. But faith has centered us and helps us weather storms. We'll stand in faith until our faith changes our circumstances. I have confidence that the goodness of God is going to show up and do what we haven't been able to do on our own!

At least we now live along the beautiful countryside where land space is open and wide. Farms line the dusty road that takes me home. It reminds me of the one that took us out to Grandma's house a long time ago. We're not on the level we want to be yet, but *here* feels right for me!

We found our place; God saw to that. Anyone who puts their hands in His will find theirs too. We're in the process of restructuring, redefining, and refocusing on where we are going and where we've been. In our stumbling, falling down, getting back up, and continuing, we've grown in spirit. It takes faith coupled with patience to accomplish what God intends. People around say I wear an indomitable smile. That's 'cause I plan on being here for a while!

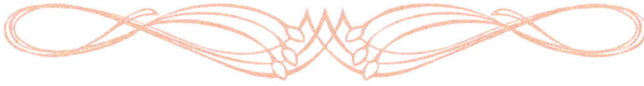

EPILOGUE

EVERY time we think we've gotten to know our *identity*, who we are changes. It happens racially, in relationships with others, and to each of us personally. We have to keep trying to "get to know" and develop intimacy as we enter and exit seasons. This makes making friends hard work, even with ourselves.

Like me, lots of individuals are feeling *excluded* today, isolated and stranded inside the walls of their own existence, being cut off from family, faith, and community. They have attempted to fill their need with things while going online, trying to get in touch with somebody out there who cares to "connect" with. It's amazing how as technology advances, we've gotten less capable of or inclined toward communicating one on one and really struggle to link up and form positive relationships.

Lots of people are yearning for simplicity and sanctity today. There is so much that makes us feel uncomfortable, uneasy, and afraid. In contemporary culture, people seem to worship the vulgar, in-your-face, confrontational style of relating with so much disrespect. Everyone screams and yells or puts each other down viciously. For that reason, maybe it's better I can't talk. Words make such a mess of our lives. I actually have one of the best disabilities because it places me in such demand. People are dying for someone who will listen and not speak to tune into what *they* have to say. We've gotten so far away from standards, values, and character—from basic respect and knowing how to communicate normally and decently. People walk out of the office together but quickly go their way to separate neighborhoods, separate realities and experiences.

There has been lots of talk about reclamation, revisiting, reclaiming what's been lost, about going home physically, spiritually, and emotionally to nesting places, to the old traditions, to where we came from, to celebrate who we are, our cultural identity; to rediscover the roots of our culture, present our issues, and share feelings; to write or tell our own history and not have others tell it for us; to pass on stories to the children to be kept alive from generation to generation. People now tend to have a strong group identity and want to revive a spirit of nationalism and brotherhood with their own, perhaps fearing extermination as we evolve into a multicultural society.

Also many are trying to go back to nature, to a time when our ancestors lived off the land, and there was an abundance of harvest to share, a time when they worked in the soil and relied on the Lord, when despite oppression there was tremendous hope, when we didn't have so many overlapping cultures and feel so mixed up.

Many seekers have gone on a spiritual quest back into the past to find out how their ancestors lived, to revive their old rituals, to experience them personally, not to just read about it in books. We hope, in so doing, to rediscover our soul, to reenergize our life force.

I believe I have good reason to be proud of my upbringing even though society says I am a child of underprivilege, born in the ghetto and reared in the courts of the inner city. There was alcoholism in my family but also virtue, hard work, and real struggles to keep commitment. We suffered as children because of issues my parents couldn't work through, but love was always there for us. We were taught to work, try to have something, take care of what we had, and fight for our self-respect. It imparted a certain validation that gave us a sense of purpose.

Perhaps that is what has impelled me to pen my own history, to leave the legacy of my experience for my sons and grandchildren to know the struggles we faced to get here. Our stories are often told by persons external to our communities with little respect for our ways and values. I struggled for years with an identity crisis, feeling of little worth because of my color and economic status. But I now have a right identity as a child of God, and I've purposed in my mind to have a better life.

African Americans need to remember from whence we have come as a people and as individuals so we can continue the work of healing, restoring dignity, and taking responsibility for our own communities to stop families and communities from disintegrating. We need to focus on ourselves now, to look within and individually heal. We need to share our spiritual pilgrimages and include our failures as well as our successes. It is important to record our spiritual histories and heritage to make young people aware of the battles the Lord has brought us through. When they don't know, they are more vulnerable and can't stand alone. But if they know what we did and why, maybe they can improve upon it.

I remember fondly the old people in my family who've passed on, how their eyes laughed and their good yet simple ways. We could use more of their wisdom these days. The old values displaced in modern society, we ought to bring back. There's still a place for them in this technological world. Our poverty is not only in needing better housing or positions. It is in getting our spiritual house in order, to reconnect and rebuild that dependent relationship on Jesus Christ as the answer to our neediness. In the past, church was the setting where we got training and self-discipline.

A lot of us have gotten away from that old-time religion that was so interwoven into who we were back then. Some don't go to church at all. Others go but concentrate only on what they wear and how they fix their hair instead of concentrating on what's in their hearts. This means biblical principles don't get carried home, to work, or out into the neighborhood where life happens, and they can't influence future generations. A person's life is often measured by what is gained, what is lost, and what is held on to. The same can be said for the life of a group. I hope our group can hold on to that yearning for dignity that was so precious to our forefathers, those values and ideals rooted and grounded in faith and love.

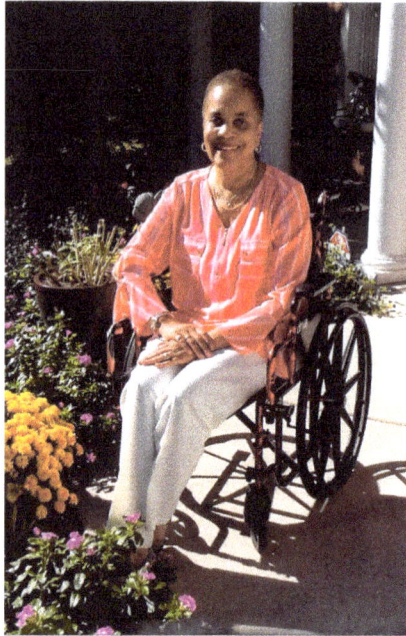

A more recent photo.

I've just entered a new phase—middle age. Years are wonderful things if they give you things to cherish. In my thirties, it was all about ambition. In my forties, I looked for fruition. Now that I am over fifty-five, I see the things I thought meant so much weren't that significant. The school and my job went on without me. I was replaceable! I wasn't that important! The program ran real well after I left. What I did to prepare my sons and other kids for the next generation really is the only thing that has lasted and borne fruit. The Bible says, "Others have labored and we have entered into their labors." In other words, many have planted seeds that have produced fruit in our lives.

Regardless what you find your security in—whether it's job, family, money, health, position, house, car, or whatever—it can be wiped out in a moment, in the twinkling of an eye. The only thing we can do is place our faith in the source of real security, the Lord Jesus Christ, and look forward, not back, to what He wants to do with us. Illness can stir up thinking and bring us to new levels of understanding, forcing us to examine what we believe and apply it to our circumstances, to reshape our priorities and discover what's really meaningful.

I am able to see this old body is fragile and my time on earth is temporal, but I can still have an impact that will live on after I am gone. The challenge is to take the things that have happened to me and learn how to use them to help others rather than being broken by them or made callous. We can choose to be pitiful or powerful by either sitting back and letting others do everything for us or we can find ways to do what we can for ourselves. But we really have to want to and be determined. No one can be determined for us. That has to come from within. Disability is an opportunity to be determined to do what we want with our lives.

My focus has turned with greater interest to adults with disabilities like myself. I feel more in tune with what they go through. One goal in writing this has been to give voice to their struggles so that others will understand and be more sensitive. And I'm trying to find a way to let that special person inside of me out. I'd like to believe my story will have significance to the lives it touches by laying myself open, making myself real, and allowing others to come close and touch me.

I hope to become part of a heritage upon which my sons can stand, by standing for something myself and living it before them. If my life is going to be shortened by illness, I won't have much to leave in a will. I hope this book will give testimony to my faith in Christ and how it operated to strengthen me and change my priorities. If I can leave them my faith, though poor, I believe they'll be rich.

I have reached that age where I'm looking back, doing a review. I want to make sure I've learned the right lessons from what I've been through. And I want to tell all the Lord has done before my time on earth comes to an end. The declining nature of my condition seems to give greater urgency to that need to get it down on paper. When life is over, someone has to put your playing pieces in a box, and all the booty you collected during the game goes to someone else. We have to refocus our eyes to see what's really important and ask what of eternal value we can leave that will help them play their cards right so they don't end up gaining the whole world and losing their souls.

The ending of my story is not yet written. This is actually a beginning with Howard and me heading off, still seeking to improve our lives. God has given us visions beyond our capabilities. Thank God He sent us forth as a twosome. Our marriage reached its third decade, despite the challenges we've faced. We probably put too much store in homes to bring us happiness. But we've moved forward, sold it and continued along the rocky road in our quest to find who we are and where we fit. What's most important is that we endured, in spite of difficulties.

Too often, we find ourselves embroiled in legal battles for our rights or having to defend ourselves from being ripped off and taken advantage of. That's an unwanted reality for people with disabilities that I hope one day will change. I don't know what path God will take us down, but having made it through this, I'm not so afraid to fail, and I won't give up! I've finally found the courage to go on, having learned to accept myself and deal with the lessons of life. I'm still dreaming of a better future.

My life story is not one of greatness. I think I'm pretty ordinary. But the Lord can take the ordinary and do something quite extraordinary when He breaks through with His amazing grace!

A walk down memory lane has awakened me to a lot of pain, yet it's made me realize my ability has not been lost. I am who I am by the design of God. I have to accept myself as right and special for His purposes so that I can evolve into who He wants me to be. I am a work in progress. He is reshaping me, turning my "ugliness" into something beautiful. He is, after all, infinite in answers to life.

Everyone today wants to have that look, walk, talk, style, and savoir-faire that says you are in; you're on top of the game—the image so popularized on TV and in movies. We tend to compare ourselves with them, and if we look as good, we feel good. If we don't, we feel less and unworthy. But I have discovered how you walk, talk, or look really isn't important. It's what's deep inside that makes a person. Not having a voice, having a smile that's twisted, being crippled, has taught me this is all just packaging and you really have to look beneath the wrap to see what you are getting. Sometimes pretty paper masks an ugly gift. Sometimes the paper isn't great, but the gift inside is wonderful, and so it is with people.

So many people today have a struggle with a lack of confidence, with feeling inadequate because of their limitations, with feeling they don't have enough going for them and lack what it takes. But our sufficiency is in God, not in ourselves. It's God's provisions for us we must claim. We can trust Him to put us over when we can't put ourselves over. God has enabling power. He makes us abled. There are times when I physically and emotionally feel I can't do things, but I pull on His power and have faith in His grace. I can be strong in Him.

In man's value system, worth is wrapped up in appearance and performance. But God says we are not valuable because of what we do, have done, or how we look. It has nothing to do with our race but our humanity. Our value is inborn. A person is worth something simply because he is. God showed how much we are worth to Him by sending His son to die on the cross. He invites us to become members of His family so that we won't have to live in anger, disconnection, and vulnerability. Attachment to Him leads to dignity and hope.

In the end, it's not race, sex, or disability that counts most. It's having something inside that says, "I want it, I'm not going to stop until I get it, and nobody's gonna keep me from it!" Through difficult times, God makes us strong and stronger. An old Chinese saying goes, "A diamond can't be polished without pressure; nor a man perfected without trials and tribulations." Victory is not in how much we've suffered, but in the goodness of God as He brings us through. I know I am not perfect and still have a long way to go. I'm not what I ought to be, but not what I used to be. I've come along way, baby, and as Yogi Bera says, "It's not over until it's over!" The keys to success no matter what strikes you have against you—race, poverty, handicap, humble beginnings, or womanhood—are hard work, strength, and faith. You have to have a positive vision for your life, a plan, and willingness to sacrifice to get there. It's important to do the little things you need to do to reach your goals. When you have chronic health problems, progress rarely comes in leaps and bounds. It's those little day-by-day things you *keep* doing that ultimately pay off. Learning to break goals down into manageable chunks is important for a disabled person, and the nondisabled too! That is self-enablement. Love and support of family and friends will help us get through any ordeal.

We all have our challenges and dreams, not only disabled people, and must find the strength and determination deep inside ourselves to pursue them, to find others to coach us and hold on being shored up by faith. And as we achieve, we must never forget who we are and where we've come from.

I set out to teach but ended learning a good deal more. Teaching and learning really are a hand-in-hand process. In the book *To Kill a Mockingbird*, it says you never really understand until you slip into a man's skin and walk around in it for a while. Working with someone who has a disability is not the same as having one, yet we can all grow and learn if we become sensitized to particular issues while at the same time recognizing individual differences. The Lord allowed me to have two kinds of experiences. I was born an outsider in a white society, and I'm now an insider in the disabled community.

What have I learned? I've learned that suffering can be a source of strength if you allow it to refine you. Also, it's not what you see on the surface that determines a person's worth, nor what he has, but what he does with what he has. Many able-bodied people have ability and opportunity and never use it. For many disabled, their abilities lie hidden beneath the surface and opportunities are few. But they can be a wealth of knowledge and resources to others. The normal always presume to teach us when often it is the normal who are taught by us, especially the value of vulnerability. I think that's the Lord's purpose in leaving us as we are.

In today's culture, folks are not so apt to come out and say cruel things anymore, since everyone is so politically correct. It's more what's not said and how we get treated. They're either overly helpful and smothering or completely inattentive to difference and refuse to lend the slightest hand or give any breaks, showing little or no sensitivity to our needs or feelings. There's always that expectation for the disabled person to keep up, measure up, not complain and make do, or be viewed as a whiner or a pain in the neck. Surely, we don't want to be burdens to anybody, so most often we play along, stretching ourselves to the limits of stamina and tolerance to save face.

Bad things happen to good people. But who can say to God, "What doest thou?" We must go on loving ourselves as well as others and be compassionate. And we must take responsibility for ourselves and not let disability, negative environments, or circumstances determine our future. I'm not crazy about the hand I've been dealt, but I try to approach it with a positive spirit and good humor.

Facing the jet age in a wheelchair, I can't say I've gotten very far, especially not physically—around the house, to the mall, a restaurant occasionally. But I can honestly say I've come a long way in who I am by drawing nearer to the Lord. It's all right to go through life at one mile an hour in a wheelchair as long as you keep going. I don't compare my progress with anybody else, and I don't have to live up to what others think. I just have to do my best and know one day I'll reach my ultimate destination. I am not a person with nothing to do and all day to do it in. And I don't sit around being indulged. I am productive and useful and strive for independence. There are lots of advanced technology on the horizon of the twenty-first Century to help Americans with disabilities maximize what we can do. When human compassion and understanding catch up with this technology, new worlds will indeed open for us to explore.

Productivity means making meaningful contributions. Our society defines that generally through work, but each of us has to find ways of using our time and talents to benefit others, for our families, or for important issues in our communities even within our limitations. There is a need for members of the larger community to figure out how to put our talents to use.

Sometimes it takes years to work through these things. They don't all happen instantaneously. We should have goals but realize they won't come overnight. It's a long road with many pitfalls. That's hard to accept in a society where we press buttons and get things we want, voila! But we have to deal with the here and now, and God will give us the tools to move on and grow. If you are facing difficult challenges, these steps will help:

- Avoid things that just give a feel-good effect but have no lasting value.
- Seek real solutions and long-term techniques for working through struggles and accompanying emotions.
- Try to get more comfortable with outward expression to let someone know where you are at, and get feedback from someone you trust.
- Develop intimate relationships.
- Have friends. Don't close the world out!
- If you are a disabled person, find ways to speak up and share your experience so others can know where you are and what you need and respect your boundaries. This will give a much greater sense of self.
- Always develop a sense of responsibility for your problems and take positive steps to find solutions as opposed to manipulating others into doing things you can do for yourself.
- Don't always look for others to come and rescue or bail you out.
- Don't make family members your caretaker for things you can do.
- Avoid temptation to treat yourself like an invalid.
- Maintain healthy relationships with others, and don't hold on to unhealthy ones just to have folks in your life. Believe that you can draw the right kinds of friends and partner with them.
- Don't be overly dependent.
- Set goals and accomplish them. Then set new goals and work toward them. There is nothing more rewarding than reaching a goal you have set for yourself!
- Take things step by step.
- When you know what you want to do, go for it, but be mindful not to be too hard on yourself!

- And don't waddle in self-pity. It rarely helps!
- Remember, there is nothing you are going through that somebody else hasn't already been. Open up and share. You are not the only one!

Having a struggle with disability has helped me realize what a gift each day is to just be able to get up and get started. I can't help but feel gratitude for the grace in which I operate. However, I can't depend on my wheelchair status to exempt me from the cruelness and incivility of these times. If anything, I am often viewed as an easy mark. A person with a disability often gets caught between what is sanctioned or disallowed by law and what according to fairness and compassion would be right. Still, there are wonderful people around. It has allowed me to see there is goodness and spirituality in a lot of places, even in a sprawling urban metropolis like New York. Selflessness and compassion are out there. Maybe we don't experience enough of it, but people do still care about their neighbor. We must focus on and nurture those positive responses.

Life is often not fair and long. The healing process is slow. Look for God's hand at work in difficult times. He sends others to help soften the pain. We must throw ourselves on the altar; let go and let God, make Him our partner, acknowledge our inabilities, and totally depend on Him. While on the road of life, take time to smell the roses, but remember you will sometimes get hurt by thorns. To get through pain and hard times, it is best to stop focusing on yourself and look for someone else to encourage. Bring hope to others, and by doing so, revive your own spirit. Get involved with organizations that dispense what Albert Schweitzer called "light, help and human kindness." Help bring dignity and you'll find it. Change the route of someone else's life for the better and it will redirect yours. Be vulnerable with others, open up, and receive love. Keep a healthy balance in relationships, be accountable to someone, and talk to them about your struggles. Get together and share, develop intimacy, open channels of communication, let others help you through it. Hand in hand, move from can't to *can*. Those who think they *can't* generally can when we learn to identify and reinforce their strengths.

As with racial minorities, society seems to believe the solution to the disabled problem is economic. Find us all jobs and our problems will be solved. And so rehabilitation services have turned into primarily a "find work and close the case" process. They lack a holistic approach to service delivery, and many areas are being cut from the typical agency budget. These are penny-pinching times, and often what gets cut out is what's needed most—more emphasis on education, socialization, independent living, therapy, mobility training, and activities for personal and spiritual enrichment. Meeting the needs of the whole man or woman will give us a better chance. We need to broaden our definition of meaningful contribution beyond gainful employment.

We have a moral obligation to advance opportunities for everybody to get an education and fulfill their potential.

Everyone must have a dream and a genuine opportunity to support their ability to believe in themselves. We should be focusing on building esteem, enhancing a positive self-image, fostering respect, and increasing independence, which brings dignity. This comes by valuing and affirming people for who they are and what they can offer, because we all have something to give.

I remember a toddler at the UCP Center who smiled so beautifully. It was all she was able to do due to paralysis. Yet she did it graciously and better than anyone else I knew. I used to go in each morning, looking forward to seeing her little face. She did something good each day for anyone around who needed cheer. I was so glad to be near and blessed by her presence. Who is to say she wasn't valuable when she gave of her special gift to others every day of her life?

We need to overcome attitudes about inferiority, inequality, and worthlessness. God doesn't make junk. We are all unique, and everyone has a special niche in this world. Disabled adults must strive to open up new frontiers as the marchers did in the '60s to make others more respectful of us, tear down stereotypes, and fight against low or too high expectations. In life we never really learn how to fight until we find something worth fighting for. For the disabled, it is not only a battle for survival from day to day but for respect and dignity as we try to hold on to our independence and self-worth. A great deal could be accomplished on our end through organizing and being proactive to see that our needs are made known. Perseverance and a little tact break down walls of resistance.

From a young age, I've had that gallant sense of wanting to change the world. But God showed me I would have to allow Him to change me. Writing has become a way to let people hear my heart's cry, to give my testimony to His grace and power. Being in a wheelchair is as good an experience as I have had because of what it's taught me, where it's brought me, what it's brought out in me and those around me. It led me to love and marriage and showed me how much I already was loved by my family. And it's given me the strength not to be so namby-pamby. Women, as we get older, do get better!

I suffered a fall in life, but unlike Humpty Dumpty, I've been put back together again and restored. The Lord proved His love for me even when I was in the pit of despair. When I was down, He picked me up. He loved me before I had a career and after I lost my job, speech, and walking ability. He has given me something to do with my reduced abilities and continues to love me because of who He is, not who I am. The experience has caused me to value people more than things and money, to value friends, family, and relationships more than titles and achievements. It's given me a closer daily walk with Him as I face my challenges. And I'm closer to my family and more aware of them than ever before. I know as I grow and change, they are too. We are all in the process of evolution.

I live a very quiet, cloistered life, but so what! The important thing is that I *live*. I haven't crawled up into a corner. I know the warmth of a family's love and a man's love. I feel whole even if I am broken. Now I have the opportunity to ease into the day with a cup of coffee, a warm bath, and a morning show or lie by my window watching the wonders of nature. Whereas I used to watch young drug dealers run into my yard to evade the cops, I now watch grazing deer come in to nibble my plants and hummingbirds sip nectar from my purple hibiscus. I enjoy the beauty of life itself! Soon I am up writing, creating home life, cooking meals, and managing bills. I still can't quote scripture, and I have a long way to go in my spiritual walk. But I've learned enough to know that He is near, that He cares and I can lean on Him.

If you can get quiet long enough, you can ask yourself, Why did God put me here, and what do I have to give? Right now I believe it is the ability to put this experience down on paper. I still wrestle with private fears and aloneness, but I've learned to fill my days in productive ways as I head toward my destiny and calling.

Who am I now? I am ears for my deaf husband, his business partner, and a home manager. I'm a counselor for one son and a coach for the other. I'm also a daughter-in-law, a mother-in-law and a grandmother. My place is along a rural route in Georgia. My purpose is to be a vessel through which God can impact the next generation. Right now I have no 401(k) and lack a retirement plan. I guess to some that makes me a failure.

So how do I measure success? I measure it by how you rise to the challenges life presents you as you struggle to find your place in the sun. I've completed the cycle from the rebellion of the '60s to the consumerism of the '70s and '80s to become a much more spiritually oriented, introspective person, having found all my things have not brought me joy, only whopping credit card bills and no peace of mind. I am back now where Grandma was "clinging to the old rugged cross and hope to exchange it someday for a crown!"

I've concluded the way walls will really have to be broken down, each one has to reach one on a personal level, to touch a life, make a friend, establish a link. If there is to be peace on earth it has to begin with each of us! When we are seeking a way to have an impact, we often overlook the fact that whatever God has assigned you to do, that is what is right for you, so do it with all your heart! There are so many ways we can touch those around us in those little things we do that often seem to have no value because no one tells us. But one day something small is done to let you know you meant something special to someone, and really, that's what matters most when lives are shattered. In compassion, there is power to make a difference.

I have found new purpose in sharing my disability experience with others to promote better understanding and break down barriers. My wheelchair has to be factored into everything I do. But I'm convinced God is in control and watches over me. There have been moments I felt abandoned, like when I came face-to-face with the reality my speech was gone and I laid my head on the table, wincing in heartfelt pain. We go through life trying to juggle a lot of balls, attempting to hold it all together, then when the pieces fall apart, we try to hold everything in and say we are okay. We deny the pain and shame, but it takes up residence inside and eats at us regularly. We carry the weight of it in our broken spirits. Either we can continue in bitter trials and defeat, or we can get ready for freedom by giving ourselves over and letting Him do things with us. I can better understand now what the Bible means when it says, "Though outwardly we are wasting away, inwardly we are being renewed day by day."

I don't have the worse malady in the world. Many have had worse, requiring long hospital stays, surgeries, and painful treatments. But what is important is how things have come together for me to make me who I am, how I view it, and what I chose to do with it.

There is a recreative process that can restore defective bodies as our spirits grow. I've found there is great strength in love, sacrifice, and going through things together, facing the fears and the uncertainty. Only by struggle can strength be gained. When we have been rocking, reeling, and feeling our lives upended, God is teaching us to trust. We have had to stand when there's been no one to stand with us. He allowed trials that helped us develop and made us uncomfortable, so we'd have to take leaps of faith. God has placed us in conflict to teach us to use our spiritual wings and soar. But I am confident that after we have suffered for a while, God will establish us and settle us.

I realize my perspective is limited to my own backyard and narrow sphere of relations. One desire I have is to travel and experience another side of life, to see this country through the eyes of people who have a different view. Perhaps if I begin to reach out to the really less fortunate, I will come to realize my needs have indeed been well met and will learn how to share.

By year 2000 my disability had taken on a devastating new dimension for me because it prevented my helping out my aging mother. And it placed me in a position to have to let others do things for her what I wanted to do myself and hampered my ability to "give back." As never before, I began praying to get out of this chair so I could go there and pitch in. Seeing her becoming weak and needy and knowing I could only do but so much was a very frightening feeling. I was more paralyzed by my sense of helplessness. The desire I had to rescue Mama since childhood came back so powerfully. I asked myself, "Is it right to ask others to take responsibility for *my* mother? How do I find caregivers so many miles away? How do I cope with the fear of losing her, my only friend? How do I bridge the communication gap as age brings changes in her alertness and ability to comprehend? Although she didn't always understand she was *there*. I dreaded the day when she would not be there for me.

I've learned something about dreams and what they cost. Mine cost me Mama and 228 Street. When I think about what I gave up to "break out" of the city, to get the cars and a country home, I ask myself, was it all worth it? I wonder if I really needed all these *things*. Back then we had each other. I long to follow that highway north that takes me to my childhood *home*. Everything I ever really *needed* was right in my own backyard.

Mom died in 2013 after living on 228 Street for more than fifty years. With anguish of heart, I sold Mom's home despite its sentimental value because crime, drugs, and violence had infected the neighborhood. Her block was the corridor that cars from Westchester passed through to buy drugs. Whites had long since packed up and left, fearing loss of property value. Middle-class black neighbors also moved away. A new breed of residents had taken over. Mom was one of the last diehards who remained. Right up until she died, she showed such pride of ownership. Since she passed, I don't go back. It's too painful to see how the new owner let our home seat fall into disrepair.

I fear the same cycle of decline will follow us and destroy the nice community where I live now if black owners won't step up, the government doesn't help out, and whites jump up and run. But if they do, I won't follow. I'll stand resilient even though I sit, and I'll try to make things better like Mama.

I came from an impoverished area of the inner city, began life in Harlem playing in a vacant lot amid shards of broken glass. I've come a long way from the inner city to the exurbs of Atlanta. I've had some successes in getting an education and teaching, and I've been broken by some things that I've had to overcome. Not only have I developed new wings and begun to fly more confidently by finding enablement through self-advocacy, but I've developed wings in spiritual things in having my heart softened toward God. The Lord is carving inroads that go ever deeper. I feel happier and more satisfied being close to Him. I'm going to keep rolling toward my destiny, trusting I can still do what I was born to do. Anything is possible with the right help. I fully believe in my infinite potential now that I have a more informed sense of who I am and can be.

* * * * *

How far have we come? Because of our new self-indulgent lifestyles, we overspend and overburden ourselves with debt then have to work and work to shovel out of it. Then we can't spend time at home because of long job schedules. We are enslaved to credit card companies and cannot save. So intent on getting more and having more, we've become avid consumers. Plastic keeps us stressed out financially, leading to greater family pressure. We teach our kids to "must have now" rather than sacrifice and wait. We focus so much on putting pretty, flashy things around us to outshine the low esteem in us. We still haven't changed the tape playing over and over inside that says we are not worthy.

Some of us constantly complain about a white man holding us down yet have become so rejecting and hostile toward one another for fear someone is going to steal what little we have, or that we might have to give up a little to help someone else. We would rather lock ourselves up in our houses with our possessions than open our doors and hands, not realizing if we pulled together we could protect and help each other. Alone we are more vulnerable and miserable.

Today I am sure most would agree the stabilizers of our society have crumbled. We want to change that but don't know how because we are so fractionalized and fragmented. Through Christ the walls can be broken down. We can rally in His name with all people of goodwill working to achieve one common goal. We need to allow faith to focus us on a higher purpose, to stabilize and rebuild our country and communities that have gone bad. We don't need to be the same but must be able to work together toward one aim. Only God can change the hearts and minds of men and women, not schools, government, politics, or the president.

To make things better, we should ask others to forgive our insensitivity, expand our circle to include persons who are different culturally or ethnically, repent of old behaviors and practices, then begin reaching out in love across lines. Everyone can improve the quality of life by just doing *something*. We have to set all the barriers aside and look at where we are spiritually. Then get out of all our boxes and into the flow of God's grace. The feeling of getting involved, giving time, giving to the future is very rewarding.

Compassion is the power that can change the world.

The civil rights movement was against a system that was unjust in jobs, housing and education. Now we have homes and cars, can move to certain communities, become doctors and lawyers, and even sit on boards in corporate America, so the perception is that the system is "fixed." But the problems with inequity are systemic. It's not easy to see how to fit into the new fight. There aren't clear confrontations anymore with a villain like Bull Connor in Selma. And there aren't clear leaders anymore like Malcolm and Martin, whose voices called us to action. Yet the disparity grows ever wider. It is hard to keep young blacks who have skills involved. The struggles are not easily defined and harder to grasp. Now civil rights issues are often played out in sophisticated court battles, and these efforts at "self-help" go unheralded by the media.

The proponents of the civil rights movement didn't teach hate. They talked of everyone working together hand in hand. Martin L. King had a philosophy of excellence, and he lived it daily, as we should. He was not just a dreamer, but also a fighter. What is most important, he connected himself to a higher source that kept him on course. As African Americans, let us not be so busy looking back that we neglect to see the opportunities that are here and prepare ourselves to meet them.

Let us not fail to teach our children of our hard-won struggles and the cost in lives paid for the privileges today. Let us not fail to honor and revere our grandmothers, moms and dads, and all who have not been exalted by the world's standards (i.e., money, position, and power) but for their lives of service to us in the little ways they made a difference, which made all the difference in the world. We need to have submissive spirits, stay low and humble like the older people, to allow a greater manifestation of God's power. Although we live in a throwaway society, let's not cast off the best of what we had in exchange for the new, because remembering what we've come through will give us the inner resources to get us where we are going! The problem is loss of love and respect for ourselves as a people. We seriously need to turn our eyes inward and look at how we treat our own sisters and brothers.

I feel both proud and ashamed sometimes because of our good and bad. We now have more economic growth and know more about technology but less about God. It has not been an even tradeoff. We're the losers in this equation. In Grandma's time, folks were poor but didn't have barred-up windows and doors. In the past, urban ghettoes like Harlem were pockets of culture and family life where people of like backgrounds huddled together for safety and a sense of identity. Today urban ghettoes are montages of mismatched characters tied together more by deprivation and desperation than oneness, and many are being preyed upon by their own. We must work on loving and helping ourselves before we can expect others to love or respect us.

One way to heal is not to keep bringing up the past. After all, we can't go back and change it. Once the wrong is acknowledged and apologized for, go from there, but don't continue in the same old practices of racism and discrimination. It takes work on all sides and starts with an honest self-assessment of where we all are. Each individual has to answer the question "Do I have biased attitudes?" and make an effort to reach out cross-culturally to build bridges and make friends. Before we can make a difference, we should ask ourselves if we are any different. Face truthfully the fact that we are not. We have the same struggles to do what is right and the same conflicts.

When we realize we aren't but can be with guidance and empowerment, then we can become vessels to pour out light into the world.

Often conflicts are worked out in play. It's necessary to cultivate relationships through activities outside the workplace and in our churches to get to know one another. It will require putting aside our racial and cultural conflicts and allegiances for the cause of Christ and the good of the nation. Forgiveness and a recommitment to go forward can heal wounds of the past. There won't be separate neighborhoods in heaven. There will be people of all nations, and we can't wait for God to work it out. We'll have to get it together down here! Spiritual unity overcomes old attitudes about inequality.

I wanted to get my sons away from the city so they'd have a better chance to succeed. I don't know now if I ran from trouble or to it. Seems moral decay and violence are everywhere, and there are so many broken people out there. Though I don't have any big answers, I have decided to say what I believe, and take part with others who believe likewise. Too many have just simply dropped out, refuse to get involved while hard-won gains are slipping from our grasp. It's time to stop looking the other way as things in our schools and communities crumble around us. We must pull together to reclaim the streets and our kids. Being strong, godly men and women as adults will give the kids someone to emulate and look up to. Rather than sitting back, saying, "What's wrong with them?" it's better to exam ourselves and ask, "What's wrong with us?" because they aren't buying our stuff!

I regret that strong family units don't exist today for so many black youth as it did for me, for it gave us rootedness and identity despite growing up in poverty. My parents drummed in right from wrong and respect for our elders, told us never do things that shame our family so we could hold our heads high. They guided us to be accountable and seize opportunities through hard work and education. They taught us principles and carriage. I hope to pass on a message that kids today need what my folks gave me: good morals and habits founded in Christianity.

Not everything that has been around a long time should be cast out like an old shoe to go along with the new wave and the new age.

Tried-and-true ethics and family values endured because they served us well, giving many lads and lasses who could easily have gone in the wrong direction a story to tell. There is work yet to be done. The new generation desperately needs saving. It *can* be accomplished if all of us work together to overcome differences, share resources, give knowledge, and teach respect!

A word like *housewife* is no longer an offense. It doesn't bother me when people ask my name and then what I do. I feel being "Mrs. G." and "Mom" are worthy occupations. Writing is my side job. I've made the transition to home life. Now I am getting into downsizing, throwing out a lot of my old collection of stuff acquired over the years, cutting back, and trying to get out of the habit of constant consumerism, realizing you can't use material things to fill a spiritual need.

Today the world is more connected and more information is available. I've lived to see email, fax machines, and digital TV, and I'm now surfing the World Wide Web. We have iPhones, social media, and a global economy. I've been trying to add new words to my vocabulary like *tweet* and *twitter*. This is my season to restructure, redefine, and refocus on where I am going and where I have been. In my stumbling, falling down, getting back up, and continuing, I've grown in spirit. We must have faith coupled with patience to accomplish what God intends.

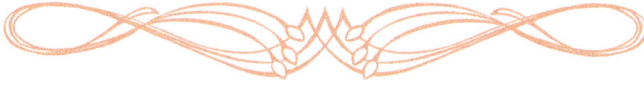

ABOUT THE AUTHOR

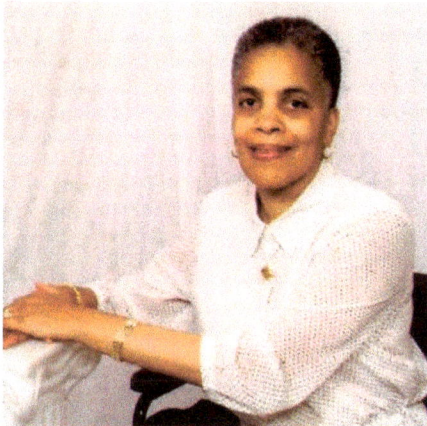

SHE was born in poverty at Harlem Hospital in New York City in 1949. She graduated cum laude, with a BA in education from Herbert H. Lehman College in 1974. And then she earned an MA in education of physically handicapped from Teacher's College, Columbia University in 1977. Her background includes teaching common branch subjects to special education and regular students in elementary school and nontraditional settings. Rolling around in her wheelchair, she feels like a warrior of sorts, fighting her own private battle for dignity on the home front. In 1989, she married and reverse migrated to the Deep South where she has family ties. Jean and her deaf husband, Howard, worked to help others with disabilities learn how to live and work independently in their communities. She has discovered that just because she can't talk doesn't mean she can't speak. And just because she doesn't walk doesn't mean there aren't still peaks to climb in her mind.

Her goal in writing is to reach out to readers and provide a look inward so they can see the world through her eyes. She's hoping to give insight to someone walking where she's been. Or desiring greater social awareness and sensitivity. By unveiling her experience as an African American woman with dual disabilities in a deeply personal way, she attempts to put others in touch with what it feels like to be her, thus the title *Touch Me! I'm for Real*. Retracing her family's journey, she shares what she's been through and what she gained. She traces her spiritual pilgrimage also and recounts the blessings God bestowed on her beginning with the legacy of faith left by her elders. She believes old-time religion can still help people to overcome in these changing times.

CPSIA information can be obtained
at www.ICGtesting.com
Printed in the USA
LVHW010025090623
749128LV00010B/79

9 781644 629376